500
Treatments
for 100 Ailments

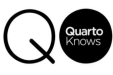

Inspiring | Educating | Creating | Entertaining

Brimming with creative inspiration, how-to projects, and useful information to enrich your everyday life, Quarto Knows is a favorite destination for those pursuing their interests and passions. Visit our site and dig deeper with our books into your area of interest: Quarto Creates, Quarto Cooks, Quarto Homes, Quarto Lives, Quarto Drives, Quarto Explores, Quarto Gifts, or Quarto Kids.

This edition published in 2017 by Chartwell Books
an imprint of The Quarto Group,
142 West 36th Street, 4th Floor,
New York, NY 10018, USA
T (212) 779-4972 **F** (212) 779-6058
www.QuartoKnows.com

Conceived, designed and produced by
Quarto Publishing plc
an imprint of The Quarto Group
The Old Brewery
6 Blundell Street
London N7 9BH

Chartwell titles are also available at discount for retail, wholesale, promotional, and bulk purchase. For details, contact the Special Sales Manager by email at specialsales@quarto.com or by mail at The Quarto Group, Attn: Special Sales Manager, 401 Second Avenue North, Suite 310, Minneapolis, MN 55401, USA.

10 9 8 7 6 5 4 3 2 1

ISBN: 978-0-7858-3564-6

Printed in China

The information in this book is not a substitute for professional medical or health care. The advice in this book is based on the training, experience, and information available to the authors. Each personal situation is unique. The authors and publisher urge the readers to consult a qualified health professional when there is any question regarding the presence or treatment of a health condition.

Because there is always a risk involved, the editors and publisher are not responsible for any adverse effects or consequences resulting from the use of any of the preparations or procedures described in the book. Please do not use this book if you are unwilling to assume the risk. For personalized advice, please consult a physician or other qualified health professional. Even your own opinion of your condition and treatment should be confirmed with second and third opinions of medical professionals.

Research studies and institutions cited in this book should in no way be construed as an endorsement of anything in this book. The authors and publisher expressly disclaim responsibility for any adverse affects arising from the use or application of the information contained herein.

If you have existing allergies you must discuss these with your practitioner so that they may safely prescribe a treatment. If you have any medical conditions or are taking any type of medicine it is imperative that you inform your practitioner, who will be able to advise you on safe use of conventional and complementary treatments.

500 Treatments for 100 Ailments

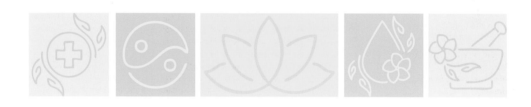

Dr. Christine Gustafson, MD

Dr. Zhuoling Ren, TCMD

Dr. Geovanni Espinosa, ND, LAc, CNS, RH(AHG)

Beth MacEoin, MNCHM, RSHom

Stephanie Caley, BSc (Hons) MNIMH

CHARTWELL
BOOKS

About the Authors

Traditional Chinese Medicine

Dr. Zhuoling Ren, TCMD, is a doctor of TCM with over 20 years' experience, and is also a fellow of AAIM. Dr. Ren is the president and founder of the American Foundation of Integrated Medicine. She is also the president and founder of the China Institute of Traditional Chinese Medicine, with clinics in Minneapolis and St. Paul, Minnesota. Before establishing the China Institute she was doctor-in-charge and head of the acupuncture department at Xiyuan Hospital in Beijing.

Homeopathy

Beth MacEoin, MNCHM, RSHom, trained at the Northern College of Homeopathic Medicine before setting up her own practice and becoming a registered member of the Society of Homeopaths. She is the author of several books. Beth has also taught a course on complementary therapies to medical students in Newcastle, England.

Conventional Medicine

Dr. Christine Gustafson, MD, had a private integrative medical practice in Alpharetta, Georgia that combined traditional and complementary medical therapies. She was board-certified in holistic medicine, and graduated from the Program in Integrative Medicine at the University of Arizona. Unfortunately, she passed away in August of 2012. She was a member of the American Holistic Medical Association and the American Association of Integrative Medicine.

Naturopathy

Dr. Geovanni Espinosa, ND, LAc, CNS, RH(AHG), is a renowned naturopathic doctor recognized as an authority in integrative and functional urology. Dr. Geo is Clinical Assistant Professor at New York University Langone Medical Center (NYULMC), Department of Urology. He is the author of the popular prostate cancer book: *Thrive, Don't Only Survive* and co-authored numerous books on natural medicine in urology and men's health. Dr. Geo is the Chief Medical Officer of XY Wellness, LLC and blogger on living long and strong at DrGeo.com.

Herbalism

Stephanie Caley, BSc (Hons) MNIMH, is a London-based medical herbalist. She trained at the University of Westminster, after a lifelong interest in natural medicines. Stephanie is a member of the National Institute of Medical Herbalists, and runs a busy herbal medicine practice and Caley's Apothecary. She is often interviewed on the benefits of herbal medicine for magazines, newspapers, and TV.

Contents

1
Skin

2
Eyes and Mouth

3
Ears, Nose, and Throat

4

Digestive System and Urinary Tract

5

Respiratory System and Circulation

6

Aches and Pains

7
Personal Complaints

8
Mind and Spirit

9
First Aid

Introduction

This book is an invaluable integrated medical resource that provides real choices in an easy-to-use, at-a-glance format. The 100 ailments are grouped according to type (for example, conditions that affect the mouth and throat, or those that require first aid). For each condition, a diagnosis, the most common symptoms, and the goal of treatment are clearly set out. Remedies are then provided from five different fields of healing—conventional medicine, traditional Chinese medicine, naturopathy, homeopathy, and herbalism—allowing you to compare approaches to the same condition, and consult with a qualified practitioner who can provide more detailed recommendations.

Conventional Medicine

The practice of medicine involves using science as an evidence base in the application of medical knowledge and clinical judgment to determine a treatment plan for an ailment. Medical doctors undergo extensive training at university and within the hospital system to enable them to diagnose illnesses accurately.

A patient–doctor relationship involves first gathering data, by taking a case history, performing a physical examination, and carrying out any necessary tests, including X-ray, blood, or urine tests. This data is then analyzed and assessed to develop a treatment plan. A doctor follows the patient's progress and alters the plan as necessary. The type of treatment offered often includes pharmaceutical drugs, which require a prescription.

Traditional Chinese Medicine

According to traditional Chinese medicine (TCM) theory, illness occurs when a person's inner balance is disturbed. This balance includes the body's Qi (the internal energy), blood, and body fluid. Good health also involves being in harmony with nature—for example, the four seasons and the elements of heat, cold, dampness, dryness, and wind. As such, a red and inflamed rash is "hot" and is treated by using cooling remedies, while a phlegmy cough is "damp" and requires herbs that dispel dampness.

TCM treatment usually involves combining herbal remedies with acupuncture and/or acupressure. The treatment principle is to promote the circulation of Qi, blood, and body fluids, to relieve the pathogenic factors (cold, heat, dampness, etc.), and to rebuild the balance between internal and external organs.

Naturopathy

Naturopathy was founded on the principle of "nature cure," which asserts that the body is essentially self-healing if provided with the right diet, environment, and habits, such as meditation. Naturopathic medicine concentrates on healing the whole person by identifying and resolving the underlying cause of a condition, rather than only treating symptoms. Practitioners will determine the most natural, non-toxic, and least invasive therapies necessary for achieving an effective treatment.

The doses and treatments outlined in the naturopathic sections of this book are primarily intended for adults. However, if an ailment predominantly affects children (for example, chickenpox) the recommended doses are appropriate for children. If an ailment affects adults and children equally, the doses suggested are for adults unless otherwise indicated. The remedies outlined for each ailment (both herbs and supplements) can generally be taken at the same time, and any contraindications are specified in each section.

Homeopathy

At the heart of homeopathy lies the principle of "the law of similars." Much like the process of immunization, homeopathy involves administering a highly dilute amount of a substance to stimulate the body to heal. Because effective homeopathic treatment has the potential for giving broad-spectrum support, it can not only relieve pain and discomfort, but can also reduce the symptoms of emotional distress and mental stress that are often triggered by dealing with nagging pain. To determine the most appropriate homeopathic treatment, make a note of your symptoms and assess the speed with which they have come on, whether there have been any obvious triggers, the location and severity of pain, the time of day that pain is most intense, and any emotional reactions to feeling ill. Then match your symptoms to those described in the homeopathic sections of this book. If a close match does not exist, the remedy will not improve your symptoms.

Homeopathic remedies are available in "first aid" potencies of 6c, 30c, 6x, or 30x. Mild symptoms that have recently developed should respond well to an appropriately selected remedy in a 6c. Established problems that have developed slowly and insidiously over a few days rather than a few hours will respond better to a stronger 30c potency. Work along the same lines with 6x and 30x potencies, if these are the only ones available to you. Unlike conventional medicine, which advocates completing a course of treatment, homeopathy involves taking the appropriate remedy for strictly short-term use.

Herbalism

Herbalism is a traditional medical practice based on the use of plants and plant extracts. Much of modern-day pharmacology owes a debt to herbal medicine, as many of the drugs available to Western physicians are derived from plants that have a long history of use as herbal remedies. Dosage and usage depends on a patient's specific symptom and its severity, personal taste, and/or the form of the plant available (for example, fresh or dried plant material). Consult a herbal medicine practitioner regarding the specific amount to be used to treat a particular ailment.

There are also different philosophies regarding the use of herbs, or any medication for that matter, during pregnancy or lactation, in children, and in combination with conventional medications. But years of experience with herbs has illustrated that some plants can be helpful and safe to take in these situations to ease a variety of complaints. Always consult a herbal expert who will be able to advise and make recommendations specific to your situation.

1

Skin

Dermatitis

Diagnosis

Dermatitis is an umbrella term for a variety of inflammatory skin conditions, the most common being contact dermatitis and eczema. Dermatitis is widespread, affects people of all ages, and is often a temporary problem that resolves on its own. The condition manifests itself as an inflammation of the skin due to an over-reaction from contact with an external substance. The result is red and itchy skin, and a strong impulse to scratch that can lead to infection. Specifically, contact dermatitis is an irritant reaction, caused by the direct effect of prolonged exposure to a substance on the skin, one that would cause a reaction in most individuals if applied in sufficient concentration. It usually flares up on the hands, as they are most often exposed to the problem substance. Common irritants include soaps, detergents, and other household chemicals, metals (especially nickel), drugs, and food.

Symptoms

- Red, itchy, inflamed skin
- A burning sensation
- Blistering and peeling skin
- Occasionally, skin cracks
- Reaction can spread to affect other areas of the body
- A strong urge to scratch
- Skin crusts over

Treatment Goal

The best way to treat dermatitis is to remove the cause by identifying and avoiding the allergen. While there isn't a cure for dermatitis, treatment aims to control and relieve symptoms.

Conventional Medicine

Prevention: Dermatitis lends itself to treatment using mind-body therapies, such as meditation, for stress reduction. Elimination diets are very helpful for the condition, with dairy and gluten being predominant offenders.

Emollients: Topical emollients and soap substitutes (such as Cetaphil®) should be used to treat dry skin on a daily basis. These emulsifying products keep oil in the skin to relieve itchiness and inflammation caused by dryness.

Topical steroids: Many people worry about the effect of topical steroid creams, used to treat dermatitis, on children and are concerned about skin thinning. This complication is prevented by slightly lowering the amount of topical steroid cream used every day over the period of one week. Hydrocortisone (at 0.5% and 1%) and triamcinolone acetonide (0.025%) are mild creams that are suitable for children. A moderate strength cream is triamcinolone acetonide (0.5% and 0.1%). Potent creams are betamethasone dipropionate (0.05%) and fluocinonide (0.05%). These higher potency creams should not be used for more than two weeks continuously, but they can be used intermittently as prescribed. A fingertip unit, the distance from an adult finger tip to the first crease in the palm, is a general dose. This amount usually covers a space twice the size of the adult flat hand.

Oral steroids: These are occasionally used for severe flare-ups. They work well but must be used only rarely because of major adverse effects on the endocrine and immune system.

Newer medications: Steroids such as tacrolimus ointment and ascomycin ointment are being used with some success. Cyclosporine is very effective but very potent, with renal toxicity (kidney damage) as a side effect and rapid relapse with discontinuation.

Anihistamines: Sedating antihistamines can be used at night to decrease itchiness.

Traditional Chinese Medicine

Herbs:
• Internal herbal decoction: Mix 10 g of Ye Ju Hua (wild chrysanthemum flower), 30 g of Huang Jing (Siberian Solomon seal rhizome), 15 g of Huang Bai (phellodendron), and 20 g of Fang Fen (ledebouriella root) in a ceramic pot. Boil the mixture in 3 cups of water for 15 minutes to make about 2 cups of decoction. Take ½ cup three times a day for 10 days to complete one course of treatment. Three courses of treatment may be needed for chronic conditions.

• **External herbal formula:** Combine 30 g each of She Chuang Zi (cnidium seed), Di Fu Zi (broom cypress), Ma Zhi Xian (dried purslane), Tu Fu Ling (glabrous greenbrier rhizome), and Xin Ren (apricot kernel) in a ceramic pot with 6–7 cups of cold water. Bring to the boil, simmer for 30 minutes, and strain the liquid. Add 6 more cups of water to the pot and repeat the process. Wash the affected area with the liquid or add it to warm bath water. Soak the skin in the herbal solution for 20–30 minutes twice a week.

Acupressure: Press the Feng Chi point, located 2 inches from the center point of the base of the skull at the back of the head with your thumbs, using gentle pressure, for one minute. Close your eyes and press the temple points with your thumbs for one minute. Press the Hegu point (in between the index finger and thumb) for two minutes with your thumb once or twice a day. For chronic dermatitis, those pressure points can be used with gentle pressure as long as the condition exists.

Diet: Eat fresh food instead of convenience food and drink plenty of fluids. Avoid shrimp, beef, lamb, and chili pepper since they may interfere with your herbal treatment and increase heat in your body.

Naturopathy

Diet: Omit wheat, rye, oats, and barley from your diet. After six weeks add one food at a time and note any changes with the dermatitis. Avoid dairy products, sugar, white flour, trans-fats, omega-6, saturated fats, fried foods, and processed foods as they tend to cause skin inflammation.

Supplements: Take vitamin E at 400 IU a day to relieve itchiness and dryness. Vitamin A is essential for smooth skin and helps dryness. Take vitamin A at 100,000 IU for one month, bring it down to 50,000 IU for two weeks, and then take 25,000 IU for maintenance. It is advised that vitamin A be taken under the supervision of a doctor because of its toxic potential. Pregnant women should not

Tip: AVOID TRIGGERS

Avoid contact with items known to trigger a reaction. Consider the toiletries you use—scented soaps, bath products, body creams, and lotions may be triggers. Always avoid highly perfumed products.

take more than 10,000 IU of vitamin A a day. Take 30 mg of zinc three times a day to raise immunity and aid skin healing. Evening primrose oil contains gamma linoleic oil (GLA), which is an essential anti-inflammatory for the skin.

Burdock root: Take 4 ml of tincture or a 500 g capsule three times a day to detoxify the skin.

Hydrotherapy: Boil 100 g of chopped oat straw, which benefits skin, in 3 quarts of water for 20 minutes. Add this to warm bath water and soak in the bathtub for 30 minutes.

Homeopathy

Because of its complex nature, dermatitis should be treated by an experienced homeopathic practitioner. The remedies listed below provide an idea of the most common solutions that a practitioner may consider for this condition.

Petroleum: If there is a history of rough, dry skin that festers easily and heals very slowly, Petroleum is helpful. Affected areas itch and burn, and skin eruptions tend to settle in folds of skin. The skin may be broken and bleed as a result of compulsive scratching. This leads to hard, thick crusts developing over sore areas.

Sulphur: This is the most common remedy for skin problems, especially when they are accompanied with localized itchiness that is worse at night or after bathing. It is used to treat intensely itchy, inflamed skin that is aggravated by heat. Symptoms include skin that is dry, rough, scaly, and readily infected. Burning sensations after scratching are especially troublesome when getting too warm in bed.

Graphites: Useful when there is a tendency to develop a thick, honey-colored crust when weeping patches dry out. After scratching, the itchy areas weep a thick, sticky yellow fluid, while the skin feels raw and sore. Affected areas are most likely to include folds of skin, with a strong tendency for the skin to crack around mouth, nose, ears, or nipples.

Arsenicum album: This is indicated if the skin is dry with associated sore, burning sensations in the eruptions that are unusually soothed by contact with warmth (for instance, in the form of warm compresses or warm bathing). The overall texture of the skin may be dry and rough, while patches of eczema develop blistery eruptions that feel intensely itchy. This sets up an itch-scratch-itch cycle that leads to burning in the affected areas.you may feel weepy and tearful when in discomfort.

Herbalism

Treatment will depend on the type of dermatitis, the cause of the inflammation, and the specific symptoms involved. However, some general suggestions for using herbal medicines are mentioned below.

Calendula: Use a cream or lotion that includes extracts of calendula, which helps calm the redness and irritation associated with this condition. Alternatively, pour 1 cup of boiling water over 2 tsp of calendula flowers. Let the water sit for 10 minutes, strain it, and soak an absorbent cloth in the mixture. Apply the cloth to the inflamed skin. The resins in calendula are particularly useful in helping the skin to heal, but are most readily available in a 90% tincture. Many practitioners use this extract as part of a cream for dermatitis.

Demulcents: This category of plant contains mucilaginous compounds that form a protective, soothing layer over the skin, which can improve dermatitis. These plants, which include aloe vera, slippery elm bark, marshmallow root, fenugreek, chickweed, and comfrey leaves or roots, are commonly used as poultices, or in creams and lotions.

Chickweed: Most commonly used topically for the relief of irritation and itching, it can be applied fresh as a poultice. The dried herb can also be steeped in boiling water for 10 minutes to make an infusion, which can be applied as a compress. Macerated, or infused, oils can also be used as part of a cream to relieve the itching of dermatitis.

Witch hazel: Functioning as an astringent, witch hazel is used on the skin as either an aqueous distillate, an ointment, or a gel, and can be applied up to three times daily. It should not be ingested, and it occasionally can worsen the dermatitis. Keep a close watch on your symptoms to see if the dermatitis is improving.

Oak: Another approach to dermatitis is to think of it in terms of a wet or dry condition. Some herbal experts feel that the reason treatment fails is that this principle is applied inaccurately. The herb oak is effective for the beginning stages of contact dermatitis, when it is in the wet form. The bark of the oak tree is astringent in nature because of its high tannin content. To make a decoction, boil 25–50 g of small pieces of oak bark, available from herb stores, in about 1 quart of water for 15–20 minutes. Apply the liquid as a compress three times daily. Each treatment should be made from fresh water.

Eczema

Diagnosis

Eczema is an inflammation of the skin that causes itching and discomfort. It can be triggered by stress, house dust, animal fur, pollen, food allergies, and environmental conditions. It is closely associated with asthma and hay fever. It is an unpredictable disease and there is often no apparent reason for its onset. It can be very upsetting, particularly for children. There are many different types of eczema, with the main ones being contact eczema, caused when an allergen comes into contact with the skin, and atopic eczema, which is passed on genetically.

Symptoms

- Patches of rough, flaky red skin, mainly on face, armpits, elbows, hands, and knees
- Inflamed, itchy skin
- Tiny red pimples
- Patches of dry, scaly skin
- Scratch marks where skin is irritated
- Blisters or cracks, and sometimes bleeding
- Weeping sores, with a thin, watery, or crusty yellow discharge
- Disturbed sleep patterns

Treatment Goal

By identifying specific allergens that cause outbreaks and alleviating the discomfort of irritated skin, the itch-scratch-itch cycle can be prevented and potential infection avoided.

Conventional Medicine

Identify the triggers: Avoid any known triggers. Common triggers of eczema include foods (particularly dairy products and gluten), and environmental allergens such as dust mites and pet dander. Food allergy testing can be important in the process of identifying potential food triggers.

Diet: Essential fatty acids (EPA/DHA or fish oil) decrease inflammatory mediators in the body. Serve oily fish two to three times a week, or give 4 g of omega-3 fish oil supplements daily to significantly improve symptoms and reduce outbreaks.

Topical steroids: If inflammation continues, topical steroids such as hydrocortisone and triamcinolone acetonide, which are moderate-strength ointments, are prescribed.

Tip: USE AN EMOLLIENT

For general flare-ups, emollients should be applied liberally and frequently to keep skin from drying and cracking. Emollients can also be used in between steroid cream treatments during the day.

Betamethasone dipropionate and fluocinonide are more potent steroid creams that can be used if moderate-potency steroids are ineffective. The least potent should be chosen, as even topical steroids have side effects.

Prescription drugs: Oral prednisone or intramuscular triamcinolone can be used. These have side effects, including immune alteration, emotional changes, weight gain, and glucose intolerance. In the most recalcitrant cases, cyclosporine, a potent chemotherapeutic agent (a drug that can alter the DNA of a cell) can be prescribed. This is for extreme cases only and should be prescribed by a specialist only after alternatives have been explored.

Antibiotics: Medical care must be sought in cases of secondary infections occurring from a rash. In this case, doctors do not usually obtain a skin swab for a culture, because 90% of patients have skin that is colonized with staph aureus whether it is infected or not. Staph is the most common infecting organism; Streptococcus pyogenes is another common organism that causes infections in an eczema rash. An antibiotic that treats both should be used, such as erythromycin, cephalexin, or dicloxacillin.

Traditional Chinese Medicine

To treat eczema, an internal and external herbal treatment is commonly used to dispel dampness and cleanse blood heat. Consult your doctor before the long-term use of any treatment.

Herbs:
• Jin Yin Hua tea: Combine 10 g each of the herbs Jin Yin Hua (honeysuckle flower) and Jin Lian Hua (gold lotus flower) in a teapot. Add 3–4 cups of hot water and let the herbs steep for five minutes. Let the tea cool, then strain it and give ½ cup three times a day.
• Long Dan Xie Gan Wan pills: These pills treat chronic eczema. Herbal medicine can be used for several weeks to several months.

• Herbal paste: Mix together the following herb powders: 10 g of Huang Bai (phellodendron), 8 g of Da Huang (rhubarb root and rhizome), 10 g of Huang Lian (coptis root), 10 g of Huang Qin (scutellaria root), and 15 g of Di Yu (burnet-bloodwort root). Add olive oil to make a paste. Apply to the affected skin once a day for seven days as one course of treatment.

Diet: Fruits such as pears, cranberries, blueberries, and bananas are recommended. Avoid foods that are rich and fatty.

Naturopathy

Diet: Food allergies appear to be a major cause of eczema, particularly an allergy to milk in infants. In others, an allergy to gluten is a prime culprit. Foods that contain gluten include wheat, oats, rye, and barley. Eliminate these foods, and any others to which you may be allergic, from your diet for six weeks.

Reintroduce one type of food each week and take note of any changes in your skin. It is also important to increase the intake of cold-water fish such as herring, salmon, and mackerel. For children, add 1 tsp of fish oil to food twice a day. The types of fats found in fish oil decrease inflammation and moisten the skin. Drink

Tip: TAKE PREVENTATIVE MEASURES

Keep damaged skin moist using an oil-based cream.
Avoiding mental stress is also helpful in reducing the occurrence of eczema.

10 glasses of water every day to keep skin hydrated. Eat plenty of different colored vegetables. They contain high amounts of beta-carotene, which is particularly beneficial to skin.

Herbs: Burdock root has a nourishing, cleansing effect on the skin. Adults should take 500 mg in capsule form or 3 ml of tincture a day. Children should take 150 mg or 0.5 ml a day.

Topical: Calendula has antiseptic properties and heals broken, damaged skin. Apply calendula cream, available from health food stores, around the affected area twice a day. Neem oil can also be helpful in healing inflamed, red, and itchy skin. Apply it to the affected area twice a day.

Supplements: Children should take 1 tsp of fish oil, added to food, twice a day. Adults can take a 3 g total of EPA/DHA combination. Vitamin C with bioflavonoids promotes skin healing and raises immunity; take 1,000 mg three times a day. Adults can take 3,000 mg of evening primrose oil, and children should take 1,000 mg. Gamma-linoleic acid (GLA) is an essential anti-inflammatory for the skin. Vitamin E is useful for the prevention of oxidation of essential oils and for its skin-healing properties; adults should take 400 IU and children should take 100 IU a day.

Homeopathy

Due to its complex nature, eczema should be treated by an experienced homeopathic practitioner. The remedies listed below demonstrate some of the treatments your practitioner will consider.

Petroleum: To treat rough, dry skin that festers easily and heals very slowly, Petroleum is often selected. Symptoms include affected areas that itch and burn, with skin eruptions showing a strong tendency to occur in folds of skin, and itchiness that is so maddening that the skin may be broken and bleed as a result of compulsive scratching.

Sulphur: To treat intensely itchy, inflamed skin that reacts badly to bathing or showering, and is aggravated by heat, Sulphur is a classic remedy. Use Sulphur for skin that is dry, rough, scaly, and readily infected, and when burning sensations after scratching are especially troublesome when too warm in bed.

Graphites: If, after scratching, the itchy areas weep a thick yellow fluid and the skin looks raw and sore, and if a honey-colored crust develops when the weeping patches dry out, Graphites is appropriate. Affected areas are most likely to include folds of skin, with a strong tendency for the skin to crack around the mouth, nose, ears, or nipples.

Herbalism

Evening primrose oil: This oil is an effective anti-inflammatory when ingested, helping to improve skin condition. It is thought to exert many of its effects because it contains the skin-boosting omega-6 fatty acid, gamma-linolenic acid (GLA). Evening primrose oil is a common treatment for atopic dermatitis in children. Your child's recommended dose will be ascertained by your herbal medicine practitioner. Topical creams made of 12.5% evening primrose oil have also been shown to improve symptoms of eczema.

Calendula: Calendula may be used to soothe the skin and help calm redness and irritation. The resin content is particularly useful in aiding healing. The resins are best extracted in a high percentage tincture, and are often added to creams. Poultices of the flowers can also be applied topically.

Demulcents: Soothing poultices, creams, and lotions can be made from aloe vera, slippery elm bark, marshmallow root, fenugreek, chickweed, and comfrey leaves or roots. The moist properties of the plants will coat the skin, holding in the natural oils and relieving the symptoms of eczema.

Chickweeds: This herb helps to relieve itching and irritation caused by eczema. It can be applied as a poultice, using the fresh herb. The dried herb can also be used, by steeping in boiling water for 10 minutes and applying as a compress. The infused oil of chickweed can also be used as part of a cream, to aid relief from itching.

Oats or oatmeal: Use oats to soothe the inflammation associated with eczema and dermatitis, and to calm itchiness, redness, and scaling. Mix about 1 cup of oats with enough cool water to create a mash, which should be left to macerate for 5–10 minutes. Dab the liquid from the mash onto affected skin with a clean washcloth several times a day. A film will form on the skin, which is calming, but the treatment can also stick to clothing. The mash itself can also be placed directly on the skin for 10–15 minutes, rather like a poultice. Alternatively, a cup of oats can be added to bathwater to achieve a similar skin-soothing effect. This is best done by tying a cup of oats into muslin cloth and allowing the bath water to run through it. The muslin bag can then be added to the bath water to steep longer, and will be easy to remove.

To treat wet eczema: Another approach to eczema is to think of it in terms of whether it is wet or dry. Some herbal experts feel that the reason treatment fails is due to the inaccurate application of this principle. One treatment that applies this principle is the use of plants like oak, which is effective for wet eczema. The bark of the oak tree is astringent in nature, because of its high tannin content. A decoction made from the boiled bark can be used to make a compress and applied as instructed by your herbal medicine practitioner. For best results, the decoction should be made daily and used the same day. A decoction of mallow bark can be used in the same way to treat wet eczema. Also, there is a close link between the digestive tract and eczema, so if someone is constipated an internal treatment may be required.

Psoriasis

Diagnosis

Psoriasis is a chronic, recurring skin disease. It can vary from mild outbreaks, where the person may not even be aware that he or she has psoriasis, to severe cases, which can be very distressing. The condition tends to run in families, although it is by no means certain that it will ever develop in those with a genetic predisposition. The condition can also be triggered by stress, emotional upsets, and exposure to certain stimuli such as medicines. Psoriasis is not contagious. The main type of psoriasis is discoid psoriasis, which manifests as plaques of affected skin on the elbows and knees. Pustular psoriasis generally affects the hands and soles of feet.

Symptoms

- Red- or pink-colored spots or patches
- Patches grow bigger and become covered with silver-colored scales
- Shedding of silvery scales to expose red patches beneath
- Small spots of blood can be seen underneath
- Psoriasis of the nail often manifests itself as small pits in the nails. The outbreak can be so severe that the nail thickens and crumbles away
- Flexural psoriasis occurs in skin folds (flexures). Red, itchy plaques appear in the armpits, under the breasts, on the stomach, in the groin, or on the buttocks. The plaques are often infected by the yeastlike fungus Candida albicans
- The scalp is usually affected, with loss of scales and matting of hair

Treatment Goal

There is no absolute cure for this condition, but treatments aim to control and manage it.

Conventional Medicine

Drugs are generally prescribed to treat initial outbreaks of psoriasis and to treat any exacerbations of the condition. Non-pharmaceutical treatment is often effective to keep the condition in remission.

Eliminate triggers: Stress can trigger psoriasis. Daily meditation as well as other stress reduction techniques, in conjunction with other therapy, can improve the condition. Certain medications are known to make psoriasis worse and should be avoided. These are commonly beta blockers used for hypertension, lithium used for bipolar disease, and antimalarials. Eliminate dairy and gluten from your diet as a trial to see if this is effective. Use probiotics and prebiotics to optimize intestinal health and relieve symptoms. Check vitamin D3 levels (25 hydroxy D), as vitamin D3 therapy leads to improvement in some patients; recent studies correlate psoriasis with a low vitamin D3 level. Amounts of 1,000 IU daily are often used initially.

Sun exposure: Sunbathing generally leads to an improvement in psoriasis but sun protection must be used. UVB exposure three times weekly along with oral PUVA (psoralen plus ultraviolet A) given two to three times weekly is effective.

Topical treatments: Bathing daily in tepid water with non-detergent soap, and applying lotion such as Cetaphil® immediately after bathing leads to improvement. Topical steroids can provide a brief remission, but they decrease in effect with continued use. They do not help the arthritis that can accompany psoriasis. Salicyclic acid at a strength of 2–10% can decrease scaling. Do not use salicyclic acid at the same time as Dovonex®.

For severe conditions: Systemic methotrexate taken at 25 mg a week can be used, as can cyclosporine, to treat severe psoriasis. Side effects of these drugs are extensive. Consult a specialist if the extent of the disease requires this type of medication.

Traditional Chinese Medicine

Herbs:
• **To treat highly inflamed psoriasis:** If the skin is red, itchy, warm, and damp, make a decoction from 15 g of Huang Qin (baical skullcap root), 12 g of Jin Yin Hua (honeysuckle flower), 18 g of Bai Xian Pi (dictamnus root bark), 15 g of Cang Zhu (atractylodes rhizome), and 5 g of Gan Cao (licorice root). Boil these

herbs in 3 cups of water and drink 1 cup of the liquid twice a day for one to four weeks.
• **To treat patches of psoriasis:** If the skin is dry and the psoriasis patches are thick and dull-colored with white flakes, make a decoction from 18 g of Xuan Shen (ningpo figwort root), 15 g of Dan Shen (salvia root), 18 g of Huang Jing (Siberian Solomon seal

rhizome), and 5 g of Gan Cao (licorice root). Boil the herbs in 3 cups of water and drink 1 cup of the liquid twice a day for one to four weeks. Consult a practitioner for treatment if the condition persists.

• **Herbal bath:** Add 18 g of Ma Zhi Xian (dried purslane), 15 g of Jing Jie (schizonepeta stem and bud), 20 g of Tao Ren (peach kernel), 15 g of Huang Bai (phellodendron), and 15 g of Ku Shen (sophora root) to 5–6 cups of water. Boil for 20 minutes, strain and add it to warm bath water. Soak your body for 20–30 minutes once a day. If the skin becomes irritated, stop the treatment and consult a TCM practitioner.

• **Poultice:** Pound 50 g of garlic and 50 g of chives together and warm them over heat. Rub the poultice into inflamed skin one to two times a day for several days.

Acupressure: Press the Feng Chi point, at the base of the skull, with your thumb. Press and release about 20 times. Press the Hegu points (between thumb and first finger). Also press the Tai Chong points, found on the instep of the foot between the first and second toe. While sitting, press these points for one minute, repeating the treatment two to three times a day.

Diet: Eat foods that dispel dampness and heat, such as mung beans, watermelon peel, lotus root, purslane, wax gourd, red beans, banana, and grapefruit. Avoid foods that promote heat and dampness in the body, such as pepper, dried garlic, cloves, dried ginger, green peppers, leeks, green onion, and liver.

Naturopathy

Diet: Cut alcohol out of your diet as it worsens the condition by impairing function of the liver and gut tissues, increasing the amount of toxins that are absorbed by the body. Also eliminate gluten, found in wheat, barley, and rye; psoriasis patients have been clinically proven to benefit from abstaining from gluten products. Stay away from corn, dairy and dairy products, and any other foods to which you may be allergic. Fresh fruits, vegetables, whole grains, and beans are high in fiber and will eliminate many gut-derived toxins, which is beneficial to those suffering from psoriasis.

Topical herbs: Cayenne contains a resinous and pungent substance known as capsaicin.

This chemical relieves pain and itchiness by depleting certain neurotransmitters from sensory nerves. Creams containing 0.025–0.075% capsaicin are generally helpful. The first application may give a slight burning sensation, but this should subside with each application. Ointments containing a 10% concentration of Oregon grape have been shown to be mildly effective against mild psoriasis in clinical trials. Apply the ointments three times a day.

Herbs: Polyamines, metabolites of proteins, have been found in high amounts in patients with psoriasis. Berberine, the active ingredient in goldenseal, has been shown to inhibit the formation of polyamines. Take 250–500 mg of a standardized berberine extract 250–500 mg three times a day, or 2–4 ml of a fluid extract three times a day. Smilax sarsaparilla has been used traditionally as a skin tonic and reduces the effects of the bacterial toxins that aggravate psoriasis; take 500 mg in capsule form or 4 ml of tincture three times a day. Milk thistle has an active ingredient, silymarin, that is reportedly useful in relieving psoriasis. Milk thistle seed contains at least eight anti-inflammatory compounds that may act on the skin. Take 70–210 mg of an 80–85% silymarin extract three times a day. Fumitory contains fumaric acid, a compound that has been shown in studies to be useful for treating psoriasis. Topical and oral forms can be taken, but studies have shown some side effects such as flushing, pain, and mild liver and kidney disturbances. Use this substance only under the supervision of a doctor. However, you can brew a strong fumitory tea and apply it directly to the affected area with a cotton ball or clean cloth two to three times a day. The herbs listed here are all available from health food stores.

Supplements: Fish oils, which are anti-inflammatory and nourishing for the skin, have been found to improve skin lesions associated with psoriasis. Take 10–12 g a day. This dosage is safe as long as other anticoagulants, such as Coumadin®, are not taken in conjunction. Some studies have shown that some patients with skin conditions have both low amounts of stomach acid and the pancreatic enzyme lipase. Take 2–4 pills containing this digestive enzyme with each meal. Betaine hydrochloride improves stomach acidity and digestion, especially of proteins. Take 1–3 capsules with each meal, but reduce the dose if you experience a warming or burning sensation. Vitamin B12 injections have been shown to improve psoriasis after six weeks of treatment. Ask your doctor to inject 1cc of B12 daily for 10 days. Sublingual B12 may also be used at 400–800 mcg a day. Folic acid is helpful, especially if you are taking methotextrate for psoriasis. Take 400 mcg a day.

Tip: COMBINE TREATMENTS

For more severe and complicated cases of psoriasis, a combination of treatments that includes Chinese herbal medicine, acupuncture, and dietary therapy is recommended. Getting enough sleep is also important.

Homeopathy

This condition should be treated by a homeopathic practitioner. The suggestions below give an idea of the remedies that a practitioner might consider when treating a patient with this condition.

Prevention: Soaking in an oatmeal bath can help sooth skin. Suspend a small muslin bag that has been filled (but not stuffed) with oats under the hot tap as the water is running.

Arsenicum album: This remedy can ease the soreness of rough, scaly skin that is so dry it looks like paper. Signature features include burning sensations and soreness as a result of scratching, and symptoms that are eased by contact with warmth. Stress and anxiety noticeably aggravate skin problems, and skin eruptions may alternate with asthma.

Lycopodium: Use if dry, raw skin is combined with urinary or gastric problems when feeling rundown. Anticipatory anxiety aggravates skin symptoms. Skin tends to feel sore and raw in areas of folds, while the skin on the hands and the soles of the feet can be especially dry.

Calc carb: Consider if skin is rough and scaly and becomes readily cracked and chapped, especially in cold weather. The skin has a generally unhealthy look to it with a tendency to become sweaty and clammy, and is also slow to heal.

Graphites: Useful for when areas of skin affected by psoriasis become very easily cracked, weepy, and bleed after scratching. Thickened, scaly skin weeps a yellowish-colored discharge that dries to a crust.

Herbalism

Aloe vera: Take the gel from a fresh cut aloe leaf and apply directly to the affected area. If fresh leaves are unavailable, you will find a variety of gels and lotions containing aloe vera at your local health store.

Burdock root: Burdock can be taken internally as a tea or tincture, or it can be applied directly to the affected area as an essential oil, an ointment, or a poultice. Although there are few reported adverse reactions to burdock, there is the potential for burdock, as with herbs used topically, to aggravate symptoms. If this happens, discontinue use immediately.

Cleavers: Cleavers is thought to have many healing properties and is a wonderful adjunct in the treatment of psoriasis. It can be utilized as a tea or tincture, and can also be prepared

for use as an ointment or in a poultice. It is recommended that cleavers be combined with burdock for the most effective treatment. Do not take for an extended period of time.

Barberry: Barberry is a specific herb for psoriasis. It contains a compound called berberine, which is responsible for many of its medicinal properties. Topical application is the best way to administer barberry. Apply it as a poultice, or use the tincture mixed into a cream base with other herb extracts useful in treating psoriasis. Barberry has been known to cause skin irritation and allergic reactions when applied topically, so be aware of any adverse reactions.

Calendula: Calendula can be applied topically as an ointment or tincture.

Scabies

Diagnosis

Scabies is a contagious disease caused by a parasitic mite that feeds off dead skin cells. It appears as an itchy rash, usually starting off on the hands. It spreads from person to person via close skin-to-skin contact, such as occurs when sharing a bed. When there is an outbreak of scabies, it is important that everyone in the family is treated at the same time even if they do not have symptoms. If this is not done, the mites may return after a couple of weeks because they have survived on the skin of some members of the family, who have re-infected others.

Scabies is transferred when fertilized female mites tunnel their way through the top layer of skin and lay their eggs. This tunneling produces tiny lines on the skin that are sometimes visible. Approximately three weeks later the eggs hatch and a new generation of mites are ready to reproduce and lay more eggs. After a few weeks the body develops an allergic response to the insects' excrement, which manifests itself as an itchy rash. Scratching can cause the skin to form a crust, which looks like psoriasis.

Symptoms

- Intense itchiness, especially at night
- The mites prefer certain areas of the body, such as the web spaces of the fingers and toes, palms of the hands and soles of the feet, wrists, armpits, skin around the navel, nipples, and scrotum
- The tunneling shows up as a telltale dark red line
- Itchy red spots and blotches appear
- Intense scratching, particularly at night if you are overheated
- Sore, bleeding areas of skin
- Clear blisters

Treatment Goal

Treatment aims to relieve itchiness and other symptoms, and rid the body of the parasites and their eggs.

Conventional Medicine

The mite that causes scabies is Sarcoptes scabiei. Treatment depends on an accurate diagnosis, which is made by the pattern of the rash that scabies causes. The mites, eggs, and mite feces can be microscopically observed after obtaining a sample from the skin using mineral oil on top of a lesion.

Prevention: If scabies is suspected, remove all bed linen, clothes, and towels used by the infected person within the past two days and launder them in hot water with detergent. Good hygiene—especially in crowded institutional settings—is a must in prevention.

Lindane (Kwell®) lotion: Apply lindane lotion to the entire body, below the neck, after bathing. If scabies is on the face, lindane can be carefully applied there, taking care to avoid the eyes. Leave the lotion on for about 12 hours before washing it off in the shower with soap. Repeat this treatment one week later. Generally, treatment is recommended for the whole family, as well as for those in close contact, such as care givers. Lindane should not be used on infants or pregnant women as it is potentially neurotoxic. Permethrin cream is a better choice for these patients, massaged into the skin from head to toe and left on for 12 hours. Only one treatment is needed.

Traditional Chinese Medicine

Herbs: Combine 30 g of She Chuang Zi (cnidium seed), 30 g of Di Fu Zi (broom cypress), 20 g of Tu Fu Ling (glabrous greenbrier rhizome), and 20 g of Ku Shen (sophora root). Boil the herbs in 4 cups of water for 30 minutes. Strain the liquid and wait until it has cooled to a tolerable temperature. Soak the affected skin in the liquid for about 20 minutes. Discard the liquid after use. The herbs can be reboiled one more time to repeat the process twice a day (mornings and evenings), for five to seven days. Itchiness should lessen immediately after soaking, but to prevent it from returning continued treatment is needed.

Diet: Food that helps clear heat in the blood, remove damp, and moisten dryness are recommended. This includes mustard greens, water spinach, towel gourd (found in Chinese groceries), mung beans, and honey. Avoid food that tends to dry the blood and agitate wind, increase damp, and cause infection, such as chilies, pepper, fish, and shrimp.

Naturopathy

Diet: Eat foods that are high in zinc to boost immunity. Such foods include eggs, turkey, fish, milk, wheat germ, and black strap molasses. Eliminate any foods to which you are allergic.

> *Tip:* HOT LINEN WASH
>
> Wash all bed linen, towels, and clothes in water that is as hot as possible.

Herbs: Tea tree oil is a powerful herbal disinfectant. Apply undiluted tea tree oil to the affected area twice a day. Comfrey also makes an excellent topical salve and can be applied twice a day. Calendula ointment is healing and soothing to the skin. Add some goldenseal tincture, or purchase the calendula ointment mixed with goldenseal, for its antimicrobial properties.

Hydrotherapy: A cool oatmeal bath may help relieve itchiness. Put 1 cup of oatmeal into a cheese cloth and tie it with a string. Hang it under the faucet or float it in the tub. Soak in warm water, immersing in the tub for 20–30 minutes.

Homeopathy

The following homeopathic advice can be used in a complementary way alongside any conventional medical steps that may need to be taken (such as using an insecticide lotion to destroy the mites that cause the intense itching on the areas of skin affected).

Sulphur: This remedy has a strong reputation for treating scabies. However, it needs to be taken with caution by anyone who has suffered from a preexisting skin condition (such as eczema or psoriasis) before developing scabies. In this case, it would be most helpful to consult a homeopathic practitioner in order

to manage the progress of the condition most smoothly. Common symptoms that call for this remedy include maddening itchiness of the skin that is at its most intense at night in bed, after washing, and after scratching. The skin burns when scratched and feels intensely sensitive to contact with fresh air. Skin becomes infected easily while also healing very slowly.

Herbalism

It is important to exterminate the parasitic mite that causes scabies as opposed to simply treating the symptoms. If proper measures are taken to treat the scabies infestation, herbal remedies can be employed to help deal with the unpleasant symptoms.

Chrysanthemum: Along with other plants in the daisy family, chrysanthemum produces natural insecticides called pyrethrins. While it is known that pyrethrins are effective in treating head lice, there is limited evidence that pyrethrin extracts are useful in treating scabies. Be cautious when dealing with pyrethrins: these compounds can be toxic when ingested or inhaled. Do not use chrysanthemum if you have asthma or if you are allergic to plants in the daisy family. If you choose to use this course of treatment, consult a herbal medicine practioner. Although there is the potential for serious side effects, these can be avoided with proper administration.

Anise: Oil of anise can be used topically to treat scabies. Apply it directly to the affected area two to three times a day in an ointment base. The most common side effects are irritation and dermatitis. Combining a small amount of the anise essential oil with a high-quality oil used in skin care (for example, olive oil or almond oil) may help lessen these effects. Side effects may occur if anise is taken internally.

Black pepper: This has been used externally to treat scabies. Apply an ointment that incorporates black pepper topically. Such products are available at health food stores.

Neem: A decoction can be used topically on the skin for scabies. Add a handful of neem to a saucepan with 2 cups of water. Bring to a boil and simmer for 15-20 minutes while covered. Neem has insect repellent properties.

Quassia: Quassia bark is also very useful for aiding getting rid of scabies, fleas, and lice. Use a decoction or make a cold infusion by steeping overnight. Use topically.

Boils

Diagnosis

A boil is a skin infection that results in an inflamed lump under the surface of the skin. It starts as a painful red lump that then swells and fills with pus, which hardens to form a yellow head. It is very tender and can be very distressing, particularly if it is noticeable. Boils usually appear on the face, neck, buttocks, back, armpits, or groin but can also appear on other areas of the body. They are caused by bacteria entering the skin, and can also result from conditions such as eczema and scabies. Some people are prone to recurrent infection, and boils can spread if you are in close contact with someone who is infected. Boils can often be left alone until they discharge of their own accord. If it is large and particularly painful, a boil can be lanced. Antibiotics may be prescribed, particularly if there is recurrent infection. As soon as the pus is released and the core of the boil is gone, the skin should start to heal.

Symptoms

- A hard, sore lump under the surface of the skin
- Soreness around the affected area
- Swollen glands
- Fever
- Enlarged lymph glands
- Infected hair follicle
- Infected sebaceous gland
- Impaired resistance to infection
- Feeling rundown/general poor health
- Constipation
- Diabetes

Treatment Goal

Boils usually run their natural course and are best left alone. But there are ways you can help relieve the symptoms and prevent the infection from spreading.

Conventional Medicine

Prevention: Boils can be caused by a virus, bacteria, fungus, chemical irritation, or a physical impact to the skin. However, they are usually bacterial, caused by staphylococcus and streptococcus, both of which live naturally on the skin. They are more common in diabetics and those with weakened immune systems, and in those who are obese, have poor hygiene, perspire a great deal, or wear overly tight clothing. Losing weight, improving hygiene, and wearing looser clothing is a straightforward way to prevent or reduce the occurrence of boils. You should also eliminate any possible mechanical or chemical skin irritants.

Topical ointments: Use mupirocin or benzoyl peroxide in conjunction with an oral antibiotic. Usually, cephalexin (Keflex®) is a first choice for common boils. A herpectic boil (caused by the Herpes simplex virus) is treated with acyclovir. If the source of the infection comes from a fungus rather than bacteria, the boil is treated with a topical antifungal such as econazole. Zeasorb™, which comes as a powder as well as an ointment, is topical and available over the counter. It can be useful in decreasing moisture in prone areas.

Traditional Chinese Medicine

Internal herbal formulas:
• Wu Wei Xiao Tu Yin: To treat boils that look red and may have a current infection, take Wu Wei Xiao Tu Yin for one month.
• Tuo Li Xiao Tu Shan: Take this formula for one to three months to treat recurring chronic boils at different stages.

External herbal formulas:
• Jin Huang Gao and Si Huang Gao: Apply either of these herbs in cream form once or twice a day on boils that are broken or infected.
• Herbal wash: Combine 30 g of Zi Hua Di Ding (Yedeon's violet), 18 g of Pu Gong Ying (dandelion), 30 g of Huang Bai (phellodendron), 30 g of Bai Jiang Cao (patrinia), and 30 g of Jin

Yin Hua (honeysuckle flower) in a ceramic pot. Add 6 cups of water and let the mixture boil for five minutes, then simmer for a further 10 minutes. Strain the decoction, add 6 cups of water to the herbs and reboil. Repeat the same procedure as above and use the decoction to wash boils once or twice a day.

Diet: Light, fresh foods such as oyster, crab, mussels, water chestnuts, celery, spinach, bamboo shoots, pears, and watermelon are beneficial. Avoid garlic, onion, chilies, and mustard greens, as well as fatty foods.

Naturopathy

Diet: Eat plenty of multicolored vegetables to provide your body with all the nutrients and photochemicals needed to strengthen the immune system. Avoid all foods that depress the immune system, such as junk food, food containing hydrogenated oils and trans-fatty acids, simple carbohydrates, and sugars. Also eliminate foods to which you may be allergic or intolerant, such as dairy, wheat, and corn.

Herbs and spices: Add herbs and spices to your cooking that enhance the immune system and have antiseptic properties, such as garlic and ginger. Take 4 ml of burdock root as a tincture or 500 mg in capsule form a day to detoxify the skin. Take 4 ml of goldenseal as a tincture or 500 mg in capsule form a day to benefit from its antibacterial, anti-inflammatory, and immunity enhancing properties.

Detox: A three-day juice fast will help eliminate impurities, reduce inflammation, and provide you with the nutrients you need to boost your immune system. The juices should be primarily green vegetables and carrots. Celery and cucumbers are great for juicing because their high water content yields plenty of juice.

Topical treatments: Tea tree oil is an effective antibacterial agent. Apply the oil as a cream or 10–15 drops diluted in ½ oz of water two to three times a day. Oregano oil can also be used topically for its strong antibacterial effects. Use the oil directly once or twice a day.

Supplements: Take 3,000 mg of vitamin C with bioflavanoids a day—1,500 mg in the morning and 1,500 mg in the evening. These two nutrients work synergistically to support the immune system and reduce skin inflammation. Take 30 mg of zinc twice a day to support skin function and the immune system. Zinc can deplete the body's stores of copper, so 3 mg of copper should be taken with this supplement.

Hydrotherapy: Alternate applying hot and cold water (three minutes hot, followed by 30 seconds cold) to drain pus. Be careful not to burn yourself by using extreme temperatures. Do not use this treatment in areas where you have numbness due to nerve damage.

Homeopathy

Remedies listed below can help speed up recovery from a mild to moderate boil, but recurrent or severe episodes will need treatment from a practitioner to eliminate the underlying problem.

Belladonna: Taken early, this remedy can stop the boil developing further, or will move it to the next stage where pus is formed. Belladonna is effective when taken at the first sign of boil formation where throbbing, heat, and redness of the affected area are noticeable.

Hepar sulph: This is the most common remedy for this problem, especially when the patient is irritable and chilly. It is useful if the boil has reached the next stage, where there are lots of drawing pains and where suppuration needs to be supported before the boil will resolve itself. The affected area will be hypersensitive to cold air, which aggravates the splintering, sharp pains, and pus when it forms will be yellow in color and thick in texture. This remedy is useful where there is a history of skin being easily infected and slow to heal.

Silica: For festering boils that produce a thin, clear discharge, use Silica. It is also useful for treating boil formation in skin that is stubborn to heal, and tends to scar. Scars are also likely to remain sensitive and painful for a lengthy period of time.

Mercurius: Use if boils emerge around the time of menstruation. Pains in the affected area are characteristically stinging and burning, and very sensitive to the slightest variation of temperature from warmth to cold. Pus formation looks thin with a greenish tinge, or may be blood-tinged.

Herbalism

Echinacea: Take as a tincture 3–4 ml three times daily. Echinacea is an immune-modulating herb and helps to fight off infection.

Goldenseal: Take goldenseal in capsule form (500 mg) or as a tincture (3 ml) three times a day for its antibacterial, anti-inflammatory, and immunity enhancing properties. It can also be used topically as a tincture, or poultice. It should be purchased from manufacturers who use cultivated goldenseal as its populations are threatened or endangered in some areas.

Calendula: The plant contains flavonoids, carotenes, carotenoid pigments, and volatile oil, which are anti-inflammatory, astringent, and antifungal. Steep the flowers in hot water, let the liquid cool slightly, and then soak a clean cloth or piece of gauze in the liquid and apply it to the affected area. Alternatively, apply warm masses of plant material or a cold cream containing calendula to the affected area. Your practitioner may also be able to provide 90% calendula tincture, to use topically.

Tea tree essential oil: Gently massage a few drops of the essential oil or linament into the boil for its antibacterial and antiseptic effects. May also be diluted in a little base oil, or added to liquid castile soap to use as a wash.

Slippery elm and myrrh poultice: Mix 2 tsp of slippery elm with a little hot water to make a paste. Add a few drops of myrrh tincture to enhance its antiseptic action. Calendula tincture, goldenseal tincture, or tea tree essential oil could also be added. Apply the paste topically and cover with a dressing to hold in place. Reapply every 3 hours.

Cradle Cap

Diagnosis

Cradle cap is a harmless skin irritation that can affect the scalp of babies and young children. It is caused by the overproduction of sebum, the oily substance produced by the skin's sebaceous glands. This causes a build-up of a greasylike crust on the scalp. Occasionally, cradle cap can spread beyond the scalp, and it can also be a precursor to eczema. Never try to pick off the crusts or rub the scalp vigorously, as this could cause soreness, bleeding, or even infection. Any loose, flaky areas can be removed with a soft brush. Cradle cap is best left alone to allow the condition to settle. Avoid overwashing your child's hair, as this can aggravate the condition.

Symptoms

- Dry, scaly, or crusty patches on the scalp. These are yellow, orange, or dark brown, and can eventually become quite hard and thick
- In babies, it usually covers the fontanelles—soft areas of the head
- A build-up of dead skin that looks like dandruff, but is visible to the eye
- Affected areas may be red and sore
- Flaky skin spreads to the forehead, behind the ears, and occasionally even around the eyebrows
- The scales may smell and have a build-up of pus underneath

Treatment Goal

While unsightly to look at, cradle cap is a harmless condition. Treatment aims to relieve any discomfort caused by the condition and protect against infection.

Conventional Medicine

The medical term for cradle cap is seborrheic dermatitis. The exact cause of cradle cap is unknown, but it is a common condition. An overgrowth of a yeast organism that usually grows on the skin, pityrosporum ovale, is often present in cradle cap. It also parallels an increase in sebaceous gland activity and tends to run in families. It is more prevalent in cold, dry weather. Although it usually occurs by itself, cradle cap can accompany other medical conditions, such as zinc deficiency, vitamin B deficiency, or any illness that lowers the number or function of the cells that fight infection.

Non-medicated shampoo: Cradle cap usually resolves itself within one to eight months. The first choice for treatment is a mild, non-medicated shampoo for scale removal. Tar-based or anti-seborrheic shampoos should not be used on infants, as they are too harsh.

Using GENTLE friction on the skin to remove the oily scales is essential. Cradle cap often occurs over the soft spot of babies' heads, because parents are often reluctant to touch this area.

Medicated shampoo or cream: If the condition does not clear up, the second choice for treatment is 1% ketoconazole shampoo or cream. This shampoo kills and stops the fungus from growing. The cream contains sulfites, which can cause allergic-type reactions, some of which are serious. Contact with the eyes should also be avoided. With this treatment, the cradle cap should clear up in several days. This treatment can be used for children, but other milder treatments are preferred.

Traditional Chinese Medicine

Herbs: Combine 30 g of Xin Ren (apricot kernel) with 30 g of Tao Ren (peach kernel). Boil in 4 cups of water for 30 minutes, then strain the liquid to remove the cooked herbs. Let the liquid cool until it is a little warmer than body temperature. Soak a clean, dry washcloth in the liquid and place it on the cradle cap, letting it moisten the area for 5–10 minutes. Gently remove the washcloth and dry the area with a clean cotton wool ball. Apply a thin layer of olive oil to the problem area.

Repeat this procedure once a day for three days, letting the scales flake off naturally.

Acupressure: Press the Feng Chi point, located 2 inches from the center point of the base of the skull at the back of the head. It is level with the hairline, and in the depression lateral to the big muscle on the nape of the neck. Apply gentle pressure with your thumbs, slightly turning them in a small circle to massage the points, for one minute twice a day.

Naturopathy

Diet: A nursing mother should eliminate any food allergens and saturated fats from her diet. Eat plenty of cold-water fish such as salmon, mackerel, and herring. A non-nursing child should also eliminate allergenic foods such as cow's milk.

Topical: Massage the head with calendula lotion and vitamin E oil alternatively. Allow the oil to remain on the scalp for 15 minutes then shampoo and gently comb away the loosened scales. This treatment works well for adults as well.

Tip: PLANTAIN WITH VIOLET AND LAVENDER

Try a gentle wash made from the infusion of plantain leaf combined with the leaves and flowers of violet, and lavender flowers. Add equal parts of each plant, approximately 25–30 g of each, to 5 cups of boiling water. Let the leaves steep for five minutes. Strain the water and, when cool, squeeze out the extra liquid from the plant material. Using a soft washcloth, gently wash your baby's head.

Homeopathy

Homeopathic remedies can be administered as appropriately and safely to newborns.

Natrum mur: For cradle cap that affects the margins of the hairline, use Natrum mur. Skin texture may generally show a tendency to be sensitive and dry, with cracks breaking out around the corners of the mouth or in the center of the bottom lip.

Graphites: For moist cradle cap that inclines toward weepiness, Graphites may be useful. The scales of cradle cap are characteristically thick, with the head becoming easily sweaty. There may also be a tendency to cracked, dry eruptions in skin folds.

Lycopodium: Use this remedy if the cradle cap is typically more irritating and itchy when covered. Eruptions on the head will look typically brownish and scaly, like heavy dandruff. Irritation and itching is eased temporarily be exposing the affected area to fresh air.

Rhus tox: If the cradle cap is intensely itchy at night, leading to restlessness, Rhus tox can

help. Itchiness is more intense when the child is too hot, but cold, damp conditions also cause distress. The child compulsively rubs and scratches at the scalp, leading to a tendency for crusts to become moist and weepy.

 # Herbalism

The herbal medicine approach to this disorder of the scalp is based on the fact that there are abnormalities in the sebaceous glands involving inflammation of the skin, perhaps also with a fungal infection. There are several herbs that can be useful. Your herbal medicine practitioner should make sure that there is not a particular fungal infection from Tinea capitis present, which can appear like cradle cap in some infants and children, and for which there are other more appropriate treatments.

Tip FRESH AIR

Keep the child's head uncovered and exposed to fresh air whenever possible.

Calendula and chamomile: These topical anti-inflammatory plants can calm the inflammation associated with this disorder. Calendula and chamomile flowers are often made into creams that can be easily applied to an inflamed scalp. Infusions may be also made and applied by steeping 1–2 tbsp of the flowers in a cup of boiling water for 10 minutes while covered. Strain and apply using cotton wool. These plants are gentle enough in their action that they are safe for use on infants.

Olive oil: A small amount of olive oil massaged into the affected scalp can be enough to provide some anti-inflammatory and soothing qualities for cradle cap. Oils can help to loosen scales, but can be warming and cause irritation from the heat. For this reason, it can be best to use a combination of oils and infusions as treatments. Avocado oil is also very effective.

Acne

Diagnosis

Acne is a common skin disorder affecting young people during puberty, with boys tending to be more prone to it than girls. It is caused by the inflammation of the oil-producing sebaceous glands, which become overactive, flooding the pores with grease. Acne is also linked with an increased number of bacteria on the skin that become trapped inside hair follicles and oil ducts.

Triggers include stress, squeezing or picking at the pimples, and a reaction to some medicines and chemicals. There is no clear evidence that cutting out fatty foods prevents acne breakouts, but a healthy balanced diet should help. If pimples are squeezed and the skin is damaged, there is a danger of infection, which can cause permanent scarring.

Symptoms

- Small, tender, red spots
- Blackheads and whiteheads
- Pus-filled pimples
- Spots on the face, back of the neck, upper back and chest, and occasionally in the armpits and on the buttocks
- Inflammation lasting a few days or weeks, depending on the severity
- Psychological stress

Treatment Goal

To bring relief from symptoms, help with the stress of dealing with this condition, and minimize the risk of any long-term scarring.

Conventional Medicine

To treat non-inflammatory acne (blackheads): A topical retinoid is usually prescribed to prevent and resolve the condition. Tretinoin, adapalene, and tazorotene are common retinoids. Azelaic acid, with its antimicrobial properties, is a more natural option. Salicyclic acid used topically is also effective. Antibiotics are not necessary for this type of acne.

To treat pustular, mildly inflamed acne (whiteheads): Antibiotics (oral or topical) may be used to inhibit the growth of bacteria, thus decreasing the concentration of free fatty acids and the resulting lesions. Topical antibiotics such as erythromycin or clindamycin are usually the first choice. They may be combined with benzoyl peroxide. Topical metronidazole or flagyl is useful for other types of bacteria. Dapsone topical gel 5% was approved by the FDA in August 2005 for the treatment of mild-to-moderate acne. Oral antibiotics are used if topical agents are not working. Doxycycline, minocycline, and tetracycline, which have anti-inflammatory properties, are the most effective.

To treat severely inflamed acne: A topical antibiotic such as benzoyl peroxide is prescribed with an oral antibiotic. These contain tetracyclines (or erythromycin for pregnant women, young children, or others unable to tolerate tetracyclines). Occasionally an injection of corticosteroids is effective for treating individual painful and unsightly lesions.

If acne does not respond to the above treatments: Oral isotretinoin is highly effective in treating all types of acne and leads to a prolonged remission. It may not be used by women of reproductive years without contraception as it harms developing babies.

Oral contraceptives: These can be prescribed for women when not contraindicated and when acceptable to the patient (especially when using isotretinoin). It is effective in treating moderate inflammatory acne caused by excessive androgen (male hormone) secretion.

Natural alternatives: As a rich source of chromium, brewer's yeast may be a natural alternative for treating acne. Zinc has also been shown to treat acne.

To treat excessive scarring: Cryotherapy, dermabrasion, laser resurfacing, chemical peels, punch grafting, and collagen injections can reduce the appearance of scars.

Traditional Chinese Medicine

Herbs: Chrysanthemum dispels heat and relieves body toxicity. Add 6–8 g of dried flowers to 2–3 cups of boiled water. Let them steep for a few minutes, strain the liquid, and refill once or twice more. Drink the tea throughout the day. It usually takes six to eight weeks for acne to clear.

Acupressure: To improve local circulation, self-massage the Yang Bai point, located on the forehead directly above the pupil, 1 inch above the eyebrow. The Yang Bai point is especially useful for treating acne on the forehead. If there is more acne on the cheeks, press the Quan Liao point, located in the depression directly below the cheekbone, about 3 inches from the nostril, in the depression directly below the cheekbone.

Diet: Drink sufficient water daily. Eat plenty of fresh fruit and vegetables, and avoid food that has heating or warming properties, such as hot chili peppers, beef, and lamb. Also steer clear of deep-fried, fatty, and greasy food.

Naturopathy

Diet: Eat plenty of dark green and orange vegetables for their high beta carotene content. They are best eaten steamed or lightly cooked so that they retain nutrients and fiber. Eat meat products once a day only, or make sure they are organic and free range, and are hormone- and antibiotic-free. Eat plenty of high-yielding proteins—especially those that are high in omega-3 fatty acids, such as cold-water fish. Raw almonds, walnuts, and pumpkin seeds are a good source of skin-healthy vitamin E and essential fatty acids. If you are taking antibiotics, eat plenty of unsweetened cultured foods such as kefir, yogurt, and raw cabbage. Antibiotics destroy the healthy bacteria in your digestive tract that are important for good health. Ground flaxseeds provide an adequate amount of fiber for regulation and essential fatty acids. Mix 2 tbsp with food or take it with a glass of water. Avoid junk foods, which have high amounts of toxins that contribute to acne formation. Simple carbohydrates and sugars encourage oil production and feed bacteria and yeast. Also, the sugar-regulating hormone insulin increases skin inflammation. Avoid food allergens such as wheat, milk, and corn and any foods to which you may be intolerant.

Supplements: Take 50 mg of zinc picolinate three times a day for one to three months to enhance the immune system, nourish the skin, and reduce build-up of dihydrotestosterone (DHT). Take 10,000 IU of vitamin A twice a day to reduce sebum production. A high dosage (up to 50,000 IU a day) is needed to be effective against acne, which is best taken under the supervision of a doctor because of its potential toxicity. Pregnant women should not take more than 10,000 IU of vitamin A a day—a dosage that may be too low to treat acne. Vitamin E (taken at 400 IU daily) increases the benefits of vitamin A and selenium. Selenium (taken at 200 mcg daily) works with vitamin E to reduce inflammation.

Topical treatment: Tea tree oil is a natural antiseptic. Apply 5 drops of a 5–15% solution in diluted water to a cotton ball and dab on the affected area.

Tip: TREAT SKIN GENTLY

Avoid using harsh cleansing and exfoliating products that can aggravate the problem by encouraging the skin to produce more oil to redress the balance.

Homeopathy

The following remedies can speed up recovery from a fairly mild, recently occurring episode of acne. Recurring breakouts suggest a more deep-seated problem, which can benefit from treatment by a homeopathic practitioner.

Belladonna: Taken at the first sign of inflammation, Belladonna can stop large, red spots from occurring, or bring them to a head. Use if there is a rapid onset of symptoms with heat, redness, and throbbing tender spots.

Pulsatilla: This remedy is ideal for spots that have emerged in response to a rich and fatty diet. Spots may be noticeably worse at times of major hormonal shifts, such as during puberty, around the time of a period, after pregnancy, and approaching the menopause.

Natrum mur: This can help resolve spots that emerge as a result of excess oil and sebum production. Spots are usually preceded by blocked pores and blackheads. Although greasy in patches, the skin is generally dry and cracked, especially around the lips and mouth.

Nux vomica: Use this detoxing remedy to treat itchy, burning spots that result from getting too little sleep, and consuming too much junk food, alcohol, caffeine, and cigarettes.

Hepar sulph: This is useful for slow-healing skin, where scars of large, yellow, pus-filled sensitive spots remain for a long time. This remedy can also encourage "blind" spots to come to a head and resolve themselves.

Herbalism

Hormone balance often needs to be addressed in acne cases. Hormones are not the simplest area to self-treat, and it is advisable to consult a practitioner of herbal medicine. In some cases the immune system may also need support.

Burdock root: This can be boiled and the tea drunk to act as a blood purifier to improve acne. One method is to boil 2 g of the root and take this tea three or four times daily. Often, skin conditions can worsen before improving; especially when eliminating toxins. Seek advice from your herbal practitioner if you are uncertain.

Tea tree essential oil: Use tea tree essential oil for its antibacterial and antiseptic properties. Apply a couple of drops to a piece of cotton wool and quickly run water over it to dilute it slightly. Dab on the site of acne, avoiding the eyes. This oil can be drying. Discontinue use if any irritation occurs.

Calendula: Also called marigold, calendula is valued for its anti-inflammatory, astringent, antifungal, and wound-healing properties. Use a cream base containing calendula. An infusion of the flowers may also be taken by drinking 1 cup three times daily. Used this way, it has a useful lymphatic effect. Cleavers is also a useful lymphatic herb.

Echinacea: Secondary infections may occur in acne cases, and echinacea is useful to support the immune system, as an immune-modulator. A tincture can be taken at 3–4 ml in a little water three times daily.

Eliminating toxins: Persistent acne may require herbal treatments to assist the body in eliminating toxins by using blood-purifying and gastrointestinal tract stimulants. Try drinking a cup of tea containing nettles, dandelion root and herb, and rosehip twice daily to assist the body in blood purification. Mix equal ratios of the dry plants and fill a tea ball with the mixture. Let the plants steep in hot water for five minutes before drinking.

Impetigo

Diagnosis

Impetigo is a common skin disease caused by a bacterial infection. Bacteria infect broken skin by entering through cuts, grazes, and cold sores. Impetigo usually first occurs around the nose and mouth, appearing as an area of reddened skin that then develops into a crop of blisters. It sometimes spreads to the rest of the body. Mostly affecting children, impetigo is highly contagious and easily spread through contact. Impetigo can be a complication that develops from constantly scratching the skin, so children with eczema are more at risk. It is important to avoid touching the affected area, and children with the condition should be isolated until it clears up. Keeping the skin clean is also important in treating and preventing impetigo, and in stopping the condition from spreading.

Symptoms

- First appears as a small scratch or an itchy patch of reddened skin
- A small red, itchy spot develops into a blister containing a clear liquid
- The blister spreads into a small crop of blisters, which become crusty and weep, in the same place or on other parts of the body
- Usually occurs first on the face, especially around the corners of the mouth, the nose, and the back of the ears
- A scabby, itchy yellow crust that forms over the affected area
- In severe cases, feelings of being unwell
- Raised temperature
- Swollen lymph glands

Treatment Goal

To eliminate the rash, thereby eradicating the infecting organism, and preventing the spread of infection.

Conventional Medicine

Impetigo is an infection of the skin. There are two types, bullous (with blisters) and non-bullous. They are both caused by the bacterium Staphylococcus aureus. Many physicians choose to treat impetigo with ointment, but in more severe cases oral antibiotics are necessary. However, there are also other simple treatments to control this condition.

Antibiotics: Topical antibiotics in the form of a cream or oral antibiotics are prescribed for this condition. The type of antibiotic used depends on how extensive the rash is and what environment the patient is in. Oral antibiotics will prevent the rash from spreading more effectively than topical antibiotics. The most common topical antibiotic used is mupirocin ointment. Success rates are more than 90% with this particular antibiotic if it is used twice a day for a period of two weeks. If the rash is extensive, erythromycin is the antibiotic most frequently used, usually for a period of about seven days. Sometimes the bacteria can become resistant to erythromycin and a cephalosporin is used. Penicillin and amoxicillin are not generally used because impetigo is often resistant to these antibiotics. Symptoms should completely resolve in around 7–10 days.

Antibacterial soap: Washing with antibacterial soaps and soaking the affected area with wet compresses to remove the crusts should be practiced in addition to using antibiotics. Good hygiene is also an important part of preventing a recurrence of the condition.

Traditional Chinese Medicine

Herbs:
• Xia Ku Cao: Take 1 tbsp of the syrup three times a day, or drink 1 cup of tea made from 12 g of the dried herb three times a day.
• Shan Huang Shan: This patent powder form is available online. Take 1–3 g of the powder and apply it to the surface of impetigo. Cover the area with a sterilized cloth pad and tape it down to keep in place. Change the pad twice a day. If the condition does not seem to be improving after three days, or it is getting worse, make an appointment to see a dermatologist to discuss treatment.

Diet: Include plenty of mung beans, red adzuki beans, bean sprouts, wax gourd, pears, watermelon, purslane, and duck meat in your diet. These foods have cooling properties and dispel heat and damp. Avoid rich, fatty foods and deep-fried and roast cooking methods. Also avoid foods such as shrimp, onion, and chili pepper.

Allergies and Medication

If you have existing allergies you must discuss these with your practitioner so that they may safely prescribe a treatment. If you have any medical conditions, or are taking any type of medicine, it is imperative that you inform your practitioner, who will be able to advise you on safe use of complementary treatments.

Naturopathy

Diet: Eat a gluten-free diet for six weeks, omitting wheat, rye, oats, and barley. After six weeks introduce one food at a time and note any changes with the impetigo. Avoid dairy products, sugar, white flour, hydrogenated and saturated fats, fried foods, and processed foods, as they are common food allergens.

Supplements: Vitamin E taken at 400 IU a day relieves itchiness and dryness. Take vitamin A at 100,000 IU for one month, then bring the dosage down to 50,000 IU for two weeks, then to 25,000 IU for long-term maintenance. Pregnant women should not take more than 10,000 IU of vitamin A a day. Vitamin A is essential for smooth skin and aids in relieving dryness. It is advised that vitamin A be taken with the supervision of knowledgable doctor as it is potentially toxic in large doses. Take 30 mg of zinc three times a day to raise immunity and aid the skin in healing. Eveing primrose oil contains gamma linoleic oil (GLA), which is an essential anti-inflammatory for the skin.

Herbs: Burdock root is a great skin detoxifier. Adults should take 4 ml of tincture or 500 mg in capsule form three times a day; children should take 0.5 ml or 150 mg twice a day. Calendula gel or cream is a mild antiseptic and helps to soothe the skin.

Homeopathy

Any of the following homeopathic remedies can be used to speed up recovery from infection. They can be used as a first resort or in combination with conventional treatment in a complementary, supportive role.

Calendula: In addition to taking an appropriate homeopathic remedy orally, it can be helpful to apply a diluted tincture of Calendula to the infected areas. Dilute one part tincture in 10 parts boiled, cooled water and swab the affected areas as often as feels soothing during the day. Calendula can play an important antiseptic role while also speeding up the healing of tissue.

Arsenicum album: This remedy should be considered for children who are pale, chilly, and anxious, and prostrated as a result of being rundown. Blisters especially affect the area around the mouth and lips and burn violently. Discomfort from burning may be soothed temporarily by warm compresses.

Antimonium crudum: This remedy is especially well indicated where yellow, crusted eruptions affect the cheeks and the chin. The latter may be covered by small, sore, honey-colored granules that are worse for cold bathing or for becoming overheated. Children feel unusually cross, peevish, and weepy when it is time to be washed.

Herbalism

Poultices: A variety of poultices and compresses have been traditionally used help to draw out infections and soothe the redness and inflammation associated with impetigo. Chop up a whole marshmallow plant and let 25–30 g stand in 4 cups of cold water for a few hours. Either apply this thick mixture to the skin directly (as a poultice) or soak a clean cloth or piece of gauze in this mixture and apply it to the area (as a compress) several times a day. To make a violet compress, add 25–30 g of the flowers to 5 cups of hot water. Let them steep for five minutes, strain the liquid and let it cool until it is hot to the touch, but not hot enough to burn the skin. Soak a clean cloth or piece of gauze in the liquid and apply it to the infected area.

Cold Sores

Diagnosis

Small blisters that come up around the mouth and nostrils, cold sores usually appear toward the end of a cold and are often passed on by kissing. The first sign is a tingling sensation, followed by a blister. After a couple of days the blister will crust over, eventually healing. Cold sores are not a serious problem. However, once caught, the cold sore virus will lie dormant in the system and can be a recurring problem. Cold sores are caused by the Herpes simplex virus, to which most of us have a natural immunity. In susceptible people, a trigger such as a cold or sore throat will cause it to flare up. Extreme weather conditions can also cause a reaction. It is thought that there is a tendency for certain families to be susceptible to cold sores.

Symptoms

- An itchy, tingling sensation
- Small blisters around or on the lips, inside the mouth, around the nostrils, and sometimes elsewhere on the face
- Blisters filled with yellow liquid that feel hot and itchy, and eventually burst
- Tenderness and pain in the affected area
- Feeling rundown

Treatment Goal

There is no way of removing the virus from your system and once the blisters have formed there is no treatment available to stop them. However, there are steps you can take to help relieve symptoms and stop the cold sore from becoming infected, thus reducing the need for antibiotics.

Conventional Medicine

Prevention: A cold sore can take up to 26 days to erupt, with four to six days being the average. It takes between one to six weeks for a cold sore to heal. After the first infection, the virus can migrate up a sensory nerve and lie dormant until it is reactivated. A large part of treatment lies in learning the triggers for your cold sores and implementing strategies to prevent outbreaks.

Nutritional supplements: Studies have shown that high amounts of vitamin C (500 mg taken daily for seven days), and zinc (at a dose of 25 mg daily) are effective. Zinc can also be obtained over the counter in a lip balm or ointment. This should be applied at the first sign of occurrence, or when in UV light and windy conditions, to cut down the risk of an outbreak. Supplements or a diet rich in lysine (found in vegetables, beans, fish, turkey, and chicken) and low in arginine (found in chocolate, peanuts, almonds, cashews, and sunflower seeds) also suppress outbreaks.

Pharmaceuticals: Acyclovir, famcyclovir, and valacyclovir treat severe cold sore outbreaks by stopping the virus from spreading. Because of this, the medicine must be prescribed at the first sign of outbreak. For recurrences the same medications are used in less frequent doses. For people who have more than six outbreaks a year or very severe symptoms, a prophylactic approach is required. The same medications are used but at about half the dose. However, if outbreaks are occurring this frequently, it is wise to look for an underlying problem with nutrition, stress, or immune function and act accordingly.

Traditional Chinese Medicine

Herbs:
• **Watermelon frost:** To help stop the pain and heal the sores, apply watermelon frost. Do not worry about swallowing the powder as it is harmless.
• **Niu Huang Jie Du Pian:** If the cold sores are infected, take three Niu Huang Jie Du Pian pills three times a day, or as instructed.
• **Herbal tea:** Combine 3 g of peppermint, 5 g of Da Qing Ye (woad leaf), 5 g of Zi Cao (groomwell root), and 2 g of raw licorice in a teapot. Add 2–3 cups of boiling water, let the mixture steep for five minutes, and strain. Drink a cup of this three to four times a day. The herbal tea can be refilled two to three times. When there is a cold sore outbreak, take the tea daily. Only to be used at the acute stage.

Acupressure: Press the Jia Che points, located at the attachment of the masseter muscles to the jawbone. When the teeth are clenched, you can feel these muscles tense. When the mouth is open, there are diagonal depressions on each side of the head above the jawbone. Place your index fingers on each of the depressions.

Apply gentle to medium pressure, on and off, ten times. Press the Hegu points, located between your index fingers and thumbs, with your thumb ten times on and off. Press these points once or twice a day to treat both acute and chronic conditions.

Tip: DAIKON JUICE

Drinking the juice from daikons, a large, juicy Chinese radish, will help heal cold sores. Wash the radish and cut it into small chunks and juice them in a juicer.

Naturopathy

Diet: Eat plenty of legumes, fish, chicken, eggs, meat (preferably grass fed and organic), and potatoes, and take brewer's yeast (1 tbsp twice a day) for their high levels of the amino acid L-lysine, which inhibits herpes replication. Foods that help with tissue repair, such as cold-water fish, are also suggested. Avoid foods that are high in the amino acid L-arginine, such as chocolate, seeds, almonds, peanuts, gelatin, carob, and raisins, as they may stimulate the replication of the herpes virus.

Supplements: Take 2,000 mg of L-lysine three times a day between meals to inhibit the spread of cold sores. To prevent cold sores from forming, take 500 mg two times a day. Vitamin C with bioflavonoids will boost the immune system and decrease the duration of the infection. Take 1,000 mg and 500 mg respectively. Take 30 mg of zinc picolinate a day to inhibit viral replication.

Herbs: The herb Lomatium root is helpful for its immune-enhancing and antiviral properties. Take 500 mg three times a day.

Homeopathy

The treatments below are indicated for cold sores that have appeared as a result of overexposure to sunshine or are associated with a cold. Cold sores that emerge persistently and severely should be treated by an experienced practitioner.

Calendula: If cold sores affect the lips or the sides of the mouth, use a dab of Calendula cream to soothe any soreness or itchiness.

Natrum mur: Helps relieve eruptions that tingle and numbness of the affected area. This is an especially strong remedy to consider where cold sores have developed after exposure to sunshine, or as a result of a heavy head cold. Areas especially vulnerable to develop cold sores include the mouth and lips. There may be an associated tendency for the lips to be dry, sensitive, and to crack easily.

Sepia: An appropriate remedy for cold sores that affect the lips and corners of the mouth. The lower lip may become swollen as well as cracked and dry. Signature symptoms include an overwhelming feeling of being drained mentally, emotionally, and physically.

Rhus tox: Consider if you have dry lips that have a tendency to split at the corners. Cold sores often develop around the mouth and lips, starting as a blister. Symptoms characteristically affect only the left side of the face, or move from the left-hand side to the right. Localized crawling sensations in the affected area are aggravated by contact with cold air and jarring movements, and are soothed by warm conditions. Rhus tox is usually used to treat cold sores that develop after exposure to cold, or from being exhausted.

Arsenicum album: This is a common remedy to treat cold sores that burn. Sufferers tend to feel chilly and anxious.

Herbalism

Echinacea: Also known as purple coneflower, Echinacea purpurea has immuno-modulating effects, changing the counts of any of a number of cells that comprise the immune system. Take 3–4 ml of an echinacea tincture in a little water three times daily at the first sign of tingling to help prevent an outbreak.

Lemon balm: Lemon balm is a specific herb used for cold sores due to its antiviral properties. Tinctures are used, as are lotions containing lemon balm. A lemon balm tincture, lotion, or cream should be applied to the cold sore three times a day or more during an outbreak. It can also be taken orally as an infusion, 3 cups daily. This is beneficial as it is has antiviral and nervine properties.

St. John's wort: One of the main active constituents in St. John's wort is hypericin. This has antiviral properties that work against the herpes simplex virus and is also anti-inflammatory and aids wound healing. An ointment or oil of St. John's wort can be used on the sores.

Garlic: The antimicrobial effects of garlic may help in the prevention and treatment of cold sores. Take garlic capsules or tinctures, although eating more fresh garlic may be just as effective in preventing outbreaks. Fresh garlic may also be rubbed onto the cold sore to speed up healing. The allicin content is very active in its antiviral an antimicrobial effects.

Licorice: The antiviral properties of licorice may be helpful internally as well as externally for cold sores. Take a licorice lozenge several times a day, or prepare a root decoction. Licorice root should not be used at high doses or long term in those with high blood pressure, so consult a practitioner if needed for advice.

Abscess

Diagnosis

Formed when a follicle, pore, or gland becomes infected, abscesses are puss-filled lumps that can occur anywhere on the body and occasionally affect internal organs. They include smaller superficial abscesses such as styes, boils, and pimples, and more serious internal abscesses of the liver or brain, which require surgical treatment.

Abscesses usually either burst, are drained by a doctor, or clear up of their own accord. Depending on the severity of the abscess, you may need to seek medical help. Antibiotics may be needed to stop the infection spreading. There is a danger that an abscess may release pus and bacteria into the bloodstream causing blood poisoning (septicemia). This is what happens when an abscess in the appendix bursts, causing the condition of peritonitis (inflammation of the abdominal lining).

Symptoms

- Red painful swelling that fills with pus
- Skin feels hot to the touch
- Sense of discomfort
- Build-up of pressure in the affected area
- Fever and sweating
- Feeling generally unwell
- Swollen, tender glands

Treatment Goal

To work on the infection that has caused the abscess and bring rapid relief from the symptoms.

Conventional Medicine

Antiseptic wash: External abscesses usually give obvious warning through pain and inflammation prior to formation. They are generally formed from a boil or furuncle (the inflammation of a hair follicle and the skin around it) and then a carbuncle (a group of furuncles coming together). When they present like this, prior to complete abscess, they can be treated and abscess formation can be prevented. At the first sign of skin inflammation or irritated hair follicles, clean the area with an antiseptic wash. Try an over-the-counter product such as Betadine® solution, which is like iodide, or an antiseptic scrub solution.

Antibiotic ointment: After you have cleaned the infected area, apply Neosporin®, a topical, over-the-counter antibiotic ointment, or tea tree oil three times a day.

Epsom salt compress: Soak a gauze pad or clean washcloth in 1 cup of hot water and 2 tbsp of salt. Apply the gauze to the infected area as a compress three times a day for 15 minutes to help relieve the infection.

When should I see my doctor? If your symptoms do not improve within seven days, see your doctor. If redness around the area progresses, or if the pus under the skin accumulates, the abscess probably needs to be lanced and drained. This is a procedure that, depending on the location of the abscess, can usually be performed in the doctor's office.

Antibiotics: If there are any systematic signs of infection—if you have a fever and are generally feeling under the weather—you may need a course of antibiotics. Cephalosporin is the kind of antibiotic most commonly used to prevent or treat early infection. If you are put on antibiotics, be sure to use a good strong probiotic to replace the beneficial flora in the gut that antibiotics can kill. Florastore™, a product that contains the probiotic Saccharomyces boullardii, is available through health care practitioners. Probiotics known as mixed Bifidus and Lactobacillus species can be found in many health food store products.

Traditional Chinese Medicine

Herbs:
• Watermelon frost: This dry powder will help to reduce the infection and eliminate pain. Gather some watermelon frost on the tip of a cotton wool bud and dab it on the surface of the abscess. Repeat every couple of hours to bring relief.
• Chuan Xin Lian: This Chinese medicine has heat and fire toxicity cleaning actions. Take 9 g of the powder three times a day for three to five days. The herb has a very bitter taste, and you may prefer to take it in capsule form.
• Niu Huang Shang Qin Wan: Take this patent Chinese herbal pill according to instructions for one week. If your condition does not improve, see a doctor.

Acupressure: Use the tip of your thumb to apply strong pressure to the Hegu points—located on your hands in the depression between the thumb and the index finger—for one to two minutes. Repeat on the other hand. It will relieve the pain temporarily.

Diet: Eat light, fresh food. Include plenty of turnips, celery, spinach, eggplant, and mung beans in your diet. Foods to be avoided include ginger, chilies, mustard greens, and mutton. These foods increase your body heat, which may make the abscess worse.

Naturopathy

Diet: Eat plenty of multicolored vegetables to obtain the nutrients and phytochemicals needed to strengthen the immune system. Avoid all foods that decrease your immunity, such as junk food, anything containing hydrogenated oils and trans-fatty acids, simple carbohydrates, and sugars. Eliminate foods to which you may be allergic or intolerant, such as dairy products, wheat, and corn, which can cause inflammation and decrease your immunity.

Herbs and spices: Add herbs and spices to your cooking that enhance the immune system and have antiseptic properties, such as garlic and ginger. Burdock root is a great skin detoxifier; take 500 mg of the capsule or 4 ml of tincture three times a day. Take 500 mg in capsule form or 4 ml of tincture of goldenseal three times a day for its antibacterial, anti-inflammatory, and immune-enhancing properties.

Detox: A three-day juice fast will help eliminate impurities, reduce inflammation, and provide you with the nutrients you need to boost your immune system. Drink juices primarily from green vegetables or carrots. Celery and cucumbers are great for juicing because their high water content yields plenty of juice.

Topical: Tea tree oil is an effective antibacterial agent. Apply it as a cream, or 10–15 drops of the oil diluted in a ½ oz of water, two to three times a day. Oregano oil can also be used topically for its antibacterial effects. Use the oil directly on the abscess once or twice a day.

Supplements: Take 1,000 mg of vitamin C with bioflavonoids three times a day. These nutrients work synergistically to support the immune system and reduce skin inflammation. Zinc also supports skin function and the immune system. Zinc can deplete the body's stores of copper, so 3 mg of copper should be taken with this supplement.

Hydrotherapy: Apply hot and cold water (three minutes hot, followed by 30 seconds cold) to the affected area to drain pus. Do not use extreme temperatures, and do not use this treatment in areas where there is any numbness due to nerve damage.

Homeopathy

For a treatment to work effectively, choose a remedy based on the stage of the abscess. If no relief occurs after a period of 24–48 hours, seek conventional care.

Belladonna: Useful in the early stages of inflammation where heat, redness, and throbbing pains are characteristic, but where there is little or no swelling. The affected area will be tender to the touch and sensitive to contact with cold air.

Hepar sulph: This is the most common remedy for abscesses, especially when the patient is irritable and chilly. When there are drawing, sticking, or splintering pains in the affected area, Hepar sulph helps to speed up pus formation to resolve the abscess.

Silica: Can be helpful where an abscess has been developing slowly and insidiously, often in deep tissue. Use this remedy if the lymph glands in the area near the abscess are swollen and tender, and if there is a tendency for the abscess to be disinclined to resolve itself. This remedy can be especially useful where an abscess has been incised, but isn't healing very well, or if the abscess has resulted from a foreign body embedded in the skin.

Mercurius: This is used if there is tenderness and inflammation of the glands near the abscess, plus a noticeable increase in the amount of saliva produced, and a nasty metallic taste in the mouth. If pains associated with the abscess are pulsating, and if contact with heat or cold makes the pain more intense, use Mercurius.

Herbalism

Tea tree oil: Apply this antibacterial oil to the abscess. Tea tree oils can be diluted with any number of base oils. Oil that is 15% tea tree oil would likely provide the best results. If the skin becomes irritated, dilute the oil with vegetable oil to reduce its strength.

Calendula: Calendula is valued for its anti-inflammatory and wound-healing properties. Steep calendula flowers in freshly boiled water, let cool, and then soak a clean cloth or piece of gauze in the liquid and apply it to the affected area as a compress. Calendula cream may also be used. A tincture of 90% of calendula is also very beneficial, as a high alcohol percentage extracts the healing resins effectively.

Comfrey: Also known as knitbone, comfrey contains allantoin, which helps heal the skin. To make a decoction, add 50 g of fresh, peeled root to 4 cups of water; bring it to a boil and simmer for 10 minutes. Let cool, then strain the warm decoction and soak a clean cloth or piece of gauze in the liquid. Hold the cloth against the abscess for 10–15 minutes at a time three times daily. Do not use on broken skin.

Echinacea: Echinacea stimulates the immune system. Take 3–4 ml of tincture three times daily in a little water. A premade tincture of echinacea can be also be added to a compress or poultice of the plants mentioned above, or a cream applied to the abscess to speed up the healing process.

Burdock root: This plant is a great skin detoxifier. Infuse the roots to make a tea or a tincture and take 4 ml, or take 500 mg in capsule form, three times a day. Also, a salve of burdock can be applied to the skin. Macerate the burdock root and mix it with a small amount of water to make a thick paste. Apply the mixture two to three times a day until there is less swelling or redness.

Marshmallow: Chop up a fresh marshmallow root and let 25 g stand in 4 cups of cold water overnight. Apply this thick mixture to the abscess as a poultice, or soak a clean cloth or piece of gauze in the mixture and apply it as a compress several times a day. Slippery Elm powder could be used in conjuction with the marshmallow root cold infusion as a poultice, or used instead of the marshmallow root.

Goldenseal: Take goldenseal in capsule form (500 mg) or as a tincture (3–4 ml) three times a day. This herb has antibacterial, anti-inflammatory, and immune-enhancing properties. This herb can also be used topically on the abscess.

Garlic: Crush some garlic to make a poultice and apply it to the abscess for its antibacterial properties. 🌿

Ringworm

Diagnosis

Ringworm is a fairly common skin disease caused by the infectious fungus tinea. It looks rather like a bull's eye—a ring-shaped mark with a paler area in the center. The condition has nothing to do with worms; it is caught by coming into contact with the fungus, either by touching infected skin directly or by coming into contact with items used by those infected—for example, washcloths and towels, hats, or brushes.

Ringworm particularly affects children, and can spread quickly around schools and nurseries. It is most common in children between the ages of two and 10. Warm, moist environments such as bathrooms and swimming pools are an ideal breeding ground for the fungus.

Symptoms

- Round or oval-shaped patches of reddish-pink skin, starting with a small irritation and then spreading
- Marks are paler in the center, growing redder and slightly raised towards the outside
- Sometimes patches are dry and scaly
- Most commonly found on the face, although they can appear elsewhere on the body, particularly the groin, arms, legs, and scalp
- Sores can be itchy and become inflamed if scratched
- Sores can also appear on the scalp, causing hair to break off, leaving bald patches

Treatment Goal

Ringworm is not a serious condition but is very contagious and an infected person should avoid contact with others. Treatment aims to clear up the rash, and prevent the fungus from spreading.

Conventional Medicine

Treating ringworm requires an accurate diagnosis. The rash can be confused with psoriasis, seborrheic dermatitis, and candidiasis. Fungal skin conditions such as ringworm can be diagnosed by sending a scraping of skin cells to a hospital laboratory for examination under a microscope. Cultures are usually not needed.

Prevention: Identify the source of the fungus to avoid it spreading. Keep the area clean and dry. Many people mistakenly think the ringworm is a dry spot and apply ointments and emollients, which can make the lesion grow. Applying tea tree oil three times daily in the initial stages of the rash can help; continue to apply the oil for a two-week period. Tight clothing or bandages should be avoided, as should hydrocortisone cream.

Antifungal agents: Topical antifungal agents such as lotrimin, lamisil, and lotrisone can be applied twice a day for two to three weeks. If these don't work, oral antifungal agents—for example, 100 mg of itraconazole or 200 mg of diflucan a day—can be used. These drugs can be harsh on the liver and liver enzyme testing is sometimes done. Taking milk thistle together with these drugs can protect the liver and does not reduce their effect nor cause significant interactions. Using undiluted tea tree oil topically in conjunction with these medications is also appropriate. If there is no resolution within two to three weeks, or if infection recurs, see your doctor.

Traditional Chinese Medicine

Herbs: External herbal medicines are the primary methods for treating ringworm in traditional Chinese medicine.
• **Herbal formula:** Soak 9 g of Din Xiang (clove flower bud), and 15 g of Da Huang (rhubarb root and rhizome) in 90 ml of rice vinegar for seven days. Apply an adequate amount of this formula to affected skin twice a day.
• **Herbal paste:** Combine 30 g of garlic and 30 g of fresh Chinese chives. Pound the garlic and chives together to make a paste and apply it to the inflamed skin, repeating once or twice a day for several days.

Diet: Encourage eating foods that help clear heat in the blood, remove damp, and moisten dryness such as mustard greens, water spinach, mung beans, and honey.

Naturopathy

Ringworm is a fungal infection and is often associated with other infections. Once a person has multiple fungal infections they may develop systemic candidiasis. A naturopathic treatment for ringworm should include a plan to rid systemic candidiasis, if this is suspected.

Diet: The following dietary measures are part of the standard diet to control candida. Eat chicken, eggs, fish, yogurt, vegetables, nuts, seeds, oils, and lots of raw garlic. Eliminate refined and simple sugars, including white or brown sugar, raw sugar, honey, molasses, or sweeteners. Stevia is a sugar substitute that is allowed. Avoid alcohol, milk, fruit or dried fruit, and mushrooms. Avoid foods that contain yeast or mold, including all breads, muffins, cakes, baked goods, cheese, dried fruits, melons, and peanuts. Increase your fiber intake; take 1 tsp to 1 tbsp of soluble fiber containing guar gum, psyllium husks, flaxseeds, or pectin mixed in 8 oz of water twice a day on an empty stomach.

Environmental considerations: Ringworm spores can live in the environment for over a year. Because of this, it is prudent to clean the house as well as possible to rid it of the fungus. Vacuum rugs and carpets frequently and clean all smooth surfaces (floors, counters, windowsills, and so on) with a 5% bleach solution for several weeks. Ringworm fungi collect in tubs, on bathroom floors, and in hampers and dresser drawers. Regularly clean these breeding grounds with a mixture of tree tea oil, thyme, and rosemary oil. Use 10–20 drops of each in a bucket of water. Wash all exposed textiles (clothing, bedding, pillows, and so on) in a 5% bleach solution and hot water.

Dry everything in a hot dryer, as high temperatures kill the fungus. Combs and hats should also be thoroughly cleaned and disinfected. Keep your pets free of fungi. If you suspect the ringworm is coming from a pet, take the animal to the vet for a thorough examination and professional treatment. Thoroughly wash any pet bedding.

Herbs: Oregano oil has strong antifungal effects. Take 5 drops of liquid under the tongue or mixed with a glass of water. You can also take 500 mg a day in capsule form. Garlic fights fungus and boosts the immune system; take 500 mg twice a day. Take 200 mg of grapefruit seed extract twice a day for its antifungal properties. Undecylenic acid, a derivative from the castor bean oil, has been shown to have strong antifungal activity. Take 200 mg three times a day. Pau d'Arco has strong antifungal properties. Take 2 cups of the tea a day. Take 200–500 mg of barberry a day for its antimicrobial and antifungal properties.

Supplements: Caprylic acid is a fatty acid shown to have antifungal properties. Take 1,000 mg three times a day. Taking 1,000 mg of vitamin C a day helps enhance immune function. Take a high-potency multivitamin for the many nutrients it provides to support immune function. Take probiotics with about four billion micro-organisms twice daily 30 minutes before each meal. These micro-organisms provide acidophilus and bifidus, which are friendly bacteria that prevent yeast overgrowth and fights candida.

General considerations: You can't wash away ringworm, but a daily bath or shower may hinder its spread and provide some relief from itchiness. No astringent, gritty, or germ-fighting soaps are needed, just use a plain, gentle soap to keep the area clean. Avoid harsh scrubbing; it will only aggravate the lesions. Ringworm fungi thrive in moisture. After bathing, thoroughly pat the affected area dry and then sprinkle on some absorbent powder. (Do not use cornstarch; fungi will use it as food.) You'll also see improvement if you air out problem areas with an electric hair dryer set on cool.

Homeopathy

Either of the following homeopathic remedies can be used in a complementary way with conventional treatment in order to speed up recovery from a ringworm infection.

Sepia: This remedy may be helpful where the classic circular patches particularly affect the skin of the scalp on the crown and/or back of the head, potentially affecting the growth, fullness, and quality of the hair.

Sulphur: If symptoms of ringworm set in within the context of a history of poor-quality skin and hair, with a tendency to spots, boils, and easily infected skin, use Sulphur. Symptoms include skin that feels very uncomfortable for washing, showering, and getting overheated (especially in bed).

Herbalism

Goldenseal: This herb has been shown to be of use in treating conditions of bacterial, fungal, and protozoal origin. Ringworm, being of fungal origin, responds well to topical treatment with goldenseal. Berberine and hydrastine are well researched phytochemicals of this herb. The dilute tincture may be applied topically as a compress. A poultice may also be made by making a paste of the powder, applying it to the affected area, and covering. A poultice may be changed twice daily. When sourcing goldenseal, check that the source is sustainable, as it is endangered in its natural environment.

Garlic: When used topically, garlic has antiseptic and antifungal properties. Crushed raw garlic can be applied directly to the affected area two to three times a day for one to two weeks. A more effective and tolerable method of delivery is a garlic oil, which can be purchased from your local health food store. Ajoene, an organosulfur compound in garlic, is known to have powerful antifungal properties and has been shown to work just as well as over-the-counter antifungal medications. Look for a gel containing 1% ajoene, if possible, and apply twice daily for 7–10 days. Garlic has virtually no side effects when used topically, although minor irritation of the application site can sometimes occur.

Tea tree oil: Tea tree oil can be used topically as an antifungal and antibacterial agent. Apply it to the infected area either as a 70–100% tea tree oil solution (or neat); although be cautious of applying to sensitive skin. The oil is known to cause dermatitis in prolonged, or frequently repeated use. For those with more sensitive skin, a 20% tea tree oil solution, or a 5–15% tea tree oil cream, may be used, but stronger doses have been shown to be more effective for fungal infections. Dermatitis is the only significant side effect associated with the prolonged, repeated topical use of tea tree oil.

Calendula: Calendula can be applied topically as an ointment or tincture to treat fungal infections. Dosing recommendations are highly varied, depending on the product and formulation. A 90% tincture is most often recommended. Calendula has very few contraindications or adverse reactions when used topically, although there is potential for an allergic reaction.

Cloves: When applied topically, cloves have known antifungal properties. Use them as an oil or salve several times daily. Potential adverse reactions with topical application include dermatitis and mucous membrane irritation. Not to be taken internally for fungal infection.

Myrrh: Topically, myrrh is very useful as an antifungal. The undiluted tincture may be applied frequently to the affected area. The myrrh tincture should be 90%, to ensure the constituents are extracted well. The oil may also be used. Contact dermatitis may occur with repeated use, so stop use if affected in this way.

Tip MANAGE THE INFECTION

After washing make sure that affected areas are dried gently, but thoroughly, since warm, damp conditions are an ideal environment for fungal infections to thrive in. Since ringworm is highly contagious, destroy any items that may have been in contact with the infection, such as combs, brushes, and/or hairbands. Also check pets for symptoms, since they may need separate treatment.

Warts

Diagnosis

Warts are benign tumors caused by the human papilloma virus (HPV). They are very common, occurring mostly in children and teenagers, and are often spread by close physical contact.

Plantar warts are generally found on the soles of the feet. Genital warts are sexually transmitted but are still caused by HPV, and can affect both men and women. The virus can stay in the body for life, periodically flaring up. Some types of genital wart virus (particularly HPV types 16 and 18) are linked with an increased risk of developing cervical cancer. These high-risk wart viruses do not cause visible warts, however. Wart viruses that do cause visible genital warts do not appear to increase the risk of cervical cancer.

Symptoms

- Warts on the hands are found most frequently around the nails and on the fingers
- Usually light brown in color
- They appear singly or in cauliflower-shaped clusters
- They may itch and bleed

Treatment Goal

To clear up any warts, ease painful symptoms, and prevent a recurrence.

Conventional Medicine

Genital warts should always be treated by a health care professional.

Duct tape occlusion: Warts that are not painful do not need to be treated, but can be removed through duct tape occlusion. The area surrounding the wart is completely covered with duct tape and left for about a week. The tape is removed and the area is soaked and debrided with a pumice stone. After a day, the duct tape is reapplied. This treatment is continued until the wart is gone.

Topical treatments: A 17% salicylic acid, obtained over the counter, can be applied to a wart twice a day for 12 weeks. The area should be clean and dry before application and bandaged after treatment. Liquid nitrogen is sometimes used successfully if other treatments fail, as is electrocautery. If the wart is very large or does not respond to any of the above, the wart may be cut off in a doctor's office. If all of these treatments fail, bleomycin, a chemotherapeutic agent, can be injected into the wart to remove it.

Laser therapy: For warts that are painful, laser therapy can be used. This results in a wound that takes four to six weeks to heal.

Traditional Chinese Medicine

Herbs: In general, internal herbal medicines are not used to treat warts. However, if the condition is severe, or warts grow quickly in a short period of time, use the internal formula suggested for plantar warts (see p. 80).

Moxibustion: Performed by a trained practitioner, this treatment can successfully remove warts. The practitioner will burn a small cone of Moxa (a herb) to force the wart to become loose and be detached from skin immediately.

Acupressure: Press and push the wart from its root to remove it. This treatment should always be performed by a trained practitioner.

Naturopathy

Diet: Eat a diet based on whole foods to support your immune system. Avoid processed foods that are high in simple carbohydrates, which can weaken your immune system and reduce the ability to fight viruses that cause warts.

Supplements: The following nutritional supplements will support immune function and healing, which will help combat the viral infections that cause warts. Take 500 mg of vitamin C two times a day; 100,000 IU of beta carotene a day; 400 IU of vitamin E a day; 200 mcg of selenium a day; and 15–20 g of zinc a day. Taking 50–100 mg a day of B-complex helps to reduce the effects of stress, which can weaken your immune system.

Herbs: Thuja has a caustic effect on the wart and also has antiviral properties. Apply 1 drop two to four times a day. Take 500 mg of olive leaf extract twice a day for its antiviral properties. Garlic also has antiviral properties. Apply 1 drop of tincture two to four times a day. You can also use a raw garlic patch. Cover the wart and surrounding skin with a thin layer of castor oil or olive oil. Apply a thin slice of fresh garlic and tape it in place, leaving it on overnight. To maximize the benefit, place 2–4 drops of greater celandine on the wart before covering with garlic. This application may need to be repeated nightly for up to three weeks. The wart will turn black as it begins to die.

Tip: BOOST YOUR IMMUNE SYSTEM

The appearance of warts is thought to be associated with the presence of a virus in the system, so it can be helpful to take practical steps to boost immune function. Simple helpful steps include avoiding alcohol, tea and coffee, and convenience foods that are packed with chemical additives. Eat immunity-boosting foods that are a rich source of antioxidant nutrients, such as tomatoes, strawberries, peppers, citrus fruit, blueberries, and broccoli.

Homeopathy

Any established tendency to develop warts should be treated by an experienced homeopathic practitioner, who will aim to eradicate the tendency from inside. A minor, recently developed wart can benefit from the following treatments. Also refer to the advice given to treat plantar warts (see p. 81).

Nitric ac: This is a suitable remedy for warts that are cauliflower-shaped and have a dry texture. Warts may produce sharp, sticking pains, be very sensitive to the touch, and bleed readily after touching or washing.

Dulcamara: Consider this remedy if warts are fleshy in texture and appear on the hands and fingers. Warts look smooth and flat and may be combined with a tendency for the palms of the hands to become moist and sweaty.

Natrum mur: If warts have a tendency to develop on the palms of the hands, this remedy may be a possible choice. Additional symptoms include a tendency to develop very dry, sensitive skin that cracks easily in cold weather. Alternatively, greasy patches of skin and blackheads can also be present, with breakouts of acne or cold sores being a common occurrence, especially when emotionally stressed or rundown.

Thuja: This is one of the leading remedies used for warts, especially if they appear after vaccinations. The condition feels worse when exposed to cold and dampness, and is soothed by exposure to warmth.

Herbalism

The herbal approach for the treatment of warts is often very similar to that for plantar warts (see p. 82).

Thuja: This tincture may be applied topically, directly onto the warts three times daily. Warts can be very persistent, so it is important to persevere with applications. Thuja is high in thujone, and has antimicrobial and antimitotic properties.

Greater celandine: A herb restricted to practitioner use, the tincture can be applied topically to the warts. Fresh juice from plants can also be used topically.

Echinacea: It is important to support the immune system, and echinacea can be used as an immuno-modulatory herb. Take 4 ml of tincture three times daily. Alternatively, make a decoction by boiling 2–3 g of dried root in 1¼ cups of water for 10 minutes.

Diaper Rash

Diagnosis

Diaper rash is a form of irritant dermatitis that is caused by exposure to urine and heat, and further aggravated by the friction and chafing that result from wearing a diaper. The most common symptom is a red and sore diaper area. Triggers include wearing wet or soiled diapers for long periods of time, skin getting overheated, and overuse of baby wipes or cleansing agents. Some babies develop diaper rash when they begin eating solid food. It can be triggered by a reaction to the new foods, particularly citrus fruit, peas, and raisins, which are not digested easily. In some cases, diaper rash can become severe and be very distressing for the baby. Occasionally, the rash can become infected with bacteria or fungus. Diaper rash should always be treated, and can usually be done so from the home.

Symptoms

- Red spots or patches of inflamed skin in the diaper area
- Skin has a tight, shiny appearance
- Scaly skin
- A bright red rash around the anus
- Red, irritated patches in the skin creases of the leg and groin area
- A strong fishy odor
- Pus-filled blisters and spots can develop if the rash becomes infected with bacteria

Treatment Goal

To identify and eliminate the cause of the rash and bring rapid relief from the symptoms.

Conventional Medicine

The four common causes of diaper rash are candida (yeast), irritant dermatitis, bacterial infection, and seborrheic dermatitis. Treatment depends on the cause.

Prevention: Change diapers as soon as possible after they are soiled and avoid using plastic pants. Cleanse the skin carefully to remove any urine or feces and dry the skin thoroughly when changing diapers. Check for a bad reaction to a particular brand of diaper. Often a food allergy can aggravate the condition. Eliminating casein (milk protein) from the diet can help. Opt for a soy- or rice-based alternative.

Topical creams: To treat irritant or contact dermatitis, zinc oxide can be applied to protect the skin, as can Desitin® or A and D ointment. Sometimes a low-potency hydrocortisone cream can be used if the above combination does not work.

Antibiotics: If a bacterial infection is diagnosed by the doctor, topical antibiotics such as mupirocin is applied as an ointment. Cases resistant to topical antibiotics are treated with oral erythromycin or penicillin.

Nystatin cream: Diaper rashes caused by candida (yeast) are treated with topical nystatin cream, which can be used in conjunction with hydrocortisone cream.

Traditional Chinese Medicine

Herbs: Both internal and external herbal formulas can help reduce itchiness and treat the rash. The herbs needed are suitable for babies.
• **Internal herbal formula:** Add 8 g of Jin Yin Hua (honeysuckle flower), 3 g of Shen Gan Cao (raw licorice), and 3 g of Bo He (field mint) to 3 cups of boiled water in a teapot. Allow the herbs to steep for 5–10 minutes, then strain. Feed your baby 2–3 tbsp of the tea, diluted in a bottle, three to four times a day for three to five days in a row. If the rash gets worse, stop treatment immediately and see your doctor.

• **External formula:** Combine 15 g of She Chuang Zi (cnidium seed), 15 g of Di Fu Zi (broom cypress), 12 g of Jing Jie (schizonepeta stem and bud), 15 g of Fang Fen (ledebouriella root), and 15 g of Xin Ren (apricot kernel) in a ceramic or glass cooking pot. Add 4–5 cups of water and bring to a boil. Turn down the heat and let the herbs simmer for 15–20 minutes. Strain the decoction and mix it in warm bath water. Gently lower your baby into the water and keep him or her in the bath for as long as is comfortable. Do not rinse the herbal solution off. Thoroughly dry your baby with a soft cotton towel. Repeat on a daily basis. If you notice any signs of discomfort, rinse your baby's body with clear water and stop the treatment.

Acupressure: Press the Nei Guan point, which is located in the center of the wrist on the palm side, about 2 inches below the crease. The San Yin Jiao point is located about 3 inches above the anklebone on the center of the inside leg. Press for about one minute.

Tip: TAKE PREVENTATIVE STEPS

Gently but thoroughly dry the affected area after bathing your baby, and make sure that as much air as possible comes into contact with the affected skin. With this in mind, leave diapers off as often as possible. Change diapers frequently to avoid your baby coming into contact with feces and/or urine for long periods, which can increase the sensitivity of already sore skin.

Naturopathy

Diet: Make sure your baby is getting plenty of fluids, especially water. This dilutes the irritating acids present in the urine and stool. Observe your child carefully when introducing new foods. A breastfeeding mother should reduce or eliminate any food allergens from her diet—especially, dairy, wheat, citrus fruits and juices, sugar, and caffeine.

Supplements: Probiotics are essential for infants and for a child's general health. Take 1 tsp of the powder a day mixed with juice or water. A bottle-fed infant can be given ½ tsp in his or her formula. A breastfeeding mother should take ½ tsp twice a day. Vitamin E should be applied topically as a cream or oil.

Herbs: Calendula has soothing and healing properties. Apply a lotion, gel, or cream to the rash when you change the diaper. Evening primose oil or lotion serves as a gentle anti-inflammatory treatment. Apply it each time you change your baby's diaper.

General recommendations: Avoid using diapers as much as possible to allow the baby's bottom to be exposed to the air. Change your baby's diaper as soon as he or she urinates or has a bowel movement. Use diaper wipes that are unscented, or that have witch hazel or calendula. Other diaper wipes contain chemicals that can be irritating to your baby's skin. When washing your baby, avoid using harsh soaps and scrubbing vigorously. Instead, use a mild soap with gentle friction, cleaning well between the skin folds, and pat dry.

Homeopathy

Either of these homeopathic remedies can help clear up a recent, fairly mild flare-up of diaper rash. Inflammation, irritation, soreness, and general discomfort should decrease within a day or so. If the diaper rash has approached a more chronic phase where severe, established symptoms have emerged, it should be treated by an experienced homeopathic practitioner.

Tip DIET

Breastfeeding mothers should eat cooling foods, such as purslane, mung beans, lotus, lettuce, mango, cucumber, eggplant, spinach, strawberries, and pears.

Belladonna: Consider this remedy to treat the first signs of diaper rash, especially if symptoms have developed abruptly and dramatically. Symptoms include spots that look bright red and angry and feel noticeably hot to the touch. Normally calm, placid babies become fractious and irritable.

Cantharis: As a result of poor sleep, the baby becomes drowsy and out of sorts during the day. If diaper rash causes particular distress at night, and results in spots that are noticeably sore and burning after urinating, use Cantharis.

Herbalism

Salves: Herbal medicines, in a salve form, can treat diaper rash by serving as a protective barrier between the skin and the diaper, as well as helping to alleviate redness, irritation, and inflammation. Salves that include plantain leaf, calendula flowers, and chamomile flowers have a combination of antimicrobial, anti-inflammatory, and skin-soothing and healing effects that help to relieve the symptoms of diaper rash. Calendula flower extracts added to a lotion or ointment, have many skin-healing properties that can be beneficial.

Aloe vera: The gel of this plant is very cooling and soothing to the skin, and helps to form a protective layer over the affected area. The gel can be used fresh from the stripped leaves, or is readily available in health food stores.

Calendula: This can be used topically in a salve, as mentioned above, but can also be used as a diluted tincture or infused oil. Water infusions are also of great use to wash the nappy area in between nappy changes, to help heal the skin, and calm inflammation and irritation.

Athlete's Foot

Diagnosis

Athlete's foot is a very common fungal infection. We all have one or more of the fungi that can cause athlete's foot to be present on our bodies. They feed on dead skin cells and are usually harmless. Athlete's foot is primarily a problem for people who suffer from sweaty feet, wear sneakers for long periods of time, or do not dry their feet properly. The contagious condition is usually picked up through communal changing rooms and other damp environments. It can spread quickly by direct skin-to-skin contact and indirectly through towels. The fungus thrives in the damp conditions between the toes, where it multiplies, eating the dead skin that is shed by the body every day.

Symptoms

- Irritation and itchiness between the toes and around the base of the foot
- A red, itchy rash in the spaces between the toes
- Small pustules (sometimes, but not always)
- Peeling skin and blisters
- Unpleasant odor
- Often a small degree of scaling
- Painful cracks between the toes
- Toenails can become infected too, sometimes separating from the nail bed
- The infection can spread to the rest of the foot and other parts of the body

Treatment Goal

To clear up the condition without recourse to a dermatologist.

Conventional Medicine

Prevention: Athlete's foot is a superficial fungal infection known as tinea pedis. There are about five fungal organisms that produce athlete's foot, all of which thrive in moist, warm places. For this reason keeping the feet dry and cool is important in prevention and treatment. Over-the-counter powders such as Tinactin® are effective in prevention and in early treatment, as is tea tree oil. Avoiding communal changing areas and showers is advisable. Changing socks daily or whenever they are damp and keeping up a diet rich in antioxidants also helps.

Fungicidal agents: Treatment consists of applying an over-the-counter fungicidal agent such as terbinafine, naftifine, or butenafine for four weeks. These agents are associated with higher cure rates and quicker response times than some of the older topical treatments. Sometimes a once-weekly internal antifungal medicine called Diflucan (fluconazole) is used, especially in severe cases.

Traditional Chinese Medicine

Herbs:
• **Herbal footbath:** Add 30 g of Ku Shen (sophora root), 30 g of Huang Bai (phellodendron), 18 g of Ma Zhi Xian (dried purslane), 20 g of Cang Zhu (atractylodes rhizome), and 30 g of Bai Xian Pi (dictamnus root bark) to 6 cups of fresh water in a ceramic cooking pot. Boil the herbs for five minutes. Turn down the heat and simmer for 30 minutes, then strain. You will get approximately 4 cups of liquid. Pour 2 cups into a pan, add hot water, and soak your feet in the herbal footbath for 20 minutes once a day before going to bed.
• **Herbal powder formula:** Ask a Chinese herbalist to mix the following powders well: 10 g of Huang Lian (coptis root), 10 g of Huang Bai (phellodendron), and 6 g of Da Huang (rhubarb root and rhizome). Store the herbs in a sealed container. Wash your feet with warm water and dry them thoroughly. Apply the powder—about 1 tsp—to the affected area with a cotton wool bud. Leave the powder on for up to 12 hours. Apply twice a day for three days. Stop for one day, then use again for three days. Repeat this procedure for one month. If your skin feels irritated, stop using the powder and consult your doctor.

Diet: Those with athlete's foot should avoid hot, fatty, greasy foods, which can aggravate this condition. Sweet foods should also be avoided.

Naturopathy

Diet: Eat plenty of fresh vegetables, lean protein, and whole grains. These foods will support your immune system. Add unsweetened cultured foods to your diet such as kefir, yogurt, miso, and raw sauerkraut, which contain friendly bacteria that fight off systemic fungus. Avoid sugar and processed carbohydrates, which fuel yeast and help athlete's foot to reproduce. Avoid or reduce fruits and avoid fruit juice altogether. Most fruits and all fruits juices are too high in sugar and fuel yeast. Drink 10 glasses of water a day to assist in flushing out yeast toxins. Drink two glasses a day of a green drink made from spirulina, wheat grass, and barley grass powder. These substances will help raise your immunity levels and feed healthy bacteria.

> ### *Tip:* USE COTTON SOCKS
> Clean and thoroughly dry your feet daily, and expose them to the open air as often as possible. Use cotton socks so that your feet can breathe, and change your socks every day

Topical: Tea tree oil has antifungal properties and can be applied directly to the infected area. If the toenail is infected, cut the nail back as much as possible and apply pure tea tree oil to the infected area.

Herbs: Use oregano oil for its strong antifungal effects. Take 5 drops of liquid under the tongue or mixed with a glass of water. Undiluted drops may be too strong for some people and you may belch the oregano. You can also take oregano oil in capsule form at 500 mg a day. Garlic fights fungus and boosts the immune system; take 500 mg twice a day. Grapefruit seed extract has antifungal properties. Take 200 mg twice a day. Caprylic acid is a fatty acid shown to have antifungal properties; take 1,000 mg three times a day. Undecylenic acid is a derivative of castor bean oil and has been shown to have strong antifungal properties. Take 200 mg three times a day. Pau d'Arco tea, available in bulk or as tea bags at health food stores, has strong antifungal properties. Take 2 cups of the tea a day.

Supplements: Take 1,000 mg of vitamin C twice a day for its immune-enhancing functions. Take a high-potency multivitamin. It will provide many nutrients that will support immune function.

Homeopathy

If symptoms are severe or have a tendency to recur, the best results will be obtained by consulting a homeopathic practitioner.

Causticum: Use if there is severe itchiness between the toes, with a tendency for recently healed-over cracks to reopen easily. It is helpful in relieving soreness that develop in folds of skin.

Rhus tox: If the rash looks blistery and crusty, and feels very itchy at night, use Rhus tox. It is especially helpful for moist athlete's foot that is made more noticeably irritating if it gets cold, damp, or wet.

Sepia: For athlete's foot that has a tendency to flare up periodically, use Sepia. Symptoms will include intense blistery eruptions between the toes. There may also be a noticeable tendency to develop dry, cracked skin, and you may feel rundown and drained.

Calc carb: Use Calc carb if your feet have a tendency to be cold and clammy; if the skin is generally cold and damp to the touch, while also tending to chap and crack; if the least physical effort sets off a bout of sweating, with irritation being made worse by bathing, socks, and contact with cold air; or if it improves in dry, warm weather, and becomes more comfortable for being carefully rubbed.

Herbalism

Athlete's foot can be treated fairly easily with herbal medicine in addition to proper foot hygiene. Almost all herbal remedies used for athlete's foot are applied topically, directly to the infected area. This method increases effectiveness and limits unwanted side-effects. However, if symptoms do not resolve, it is advisable to seek medical attention as a more aggressive mode of therapy may be indicated.

Garlic: Garlic is antiseptic and antifungal. It contains the compound ajoene, known to have powerful antifungal properties, and has been shown to work just as well as over-the-counter antifungal medications. Garlic has virtually no side-effects when used topically, although minor irritation is sometimes reported. When taken internally at high, therapeutic doses, garlic may interfere with certain antithrombotic drugs. Crushed raw garlic can be applied directly to the affected area two to three times a day for one to two weeks, although the odor can act as a deterrent. Apply twice daily for 7–10 days.

Tea tree oil: There are many competing recommendations regarding the dosage and effectiveness of tea tree oil for use in treating athlete's foot. It can be used topically as an antifungal and antibacterial agent and has been shown to work well to relieve symptoms. Apply a 5–15% tea tree oil solution or a 5–15% tea tree oil cream topically to the infected area. A much stronger dose of either the solution or cream is needed to produce a cure. Recommendations range from applying a 25–100% strength oil or cream two to three times daily. Dermatitis may be a side-effect associated with the prolonged and repeated topical use of tea tree oil.

Calendula: Also referred to as marigold, calendula is easily accessible and can be applied topically as an ointment or tincture. Dosing recommendations are highly varied, and consultation with a local herbal therapist may be warranted. A practitioner would often use a 90% tincture topically, as this method of extraction is best for extracting the resin content which is particularly beneficial. Calendula has very few contraindications or adverse reactions when used topically.

Cloves: When applied topically, cloves have known antifungal properties. Use this herb as a dilute essential oil, available over the counter, several times a day. There are several potential adverse reactions to the topical application of cloves, including dermatitis and mucous membrane irritation. Do not take this herb internally to treat fungal infections.

Myrrh: Myrrh has known antifungal properties, and can be used topically for athlete's foot. This can be purchased as an essential oil, and applied diluted in a base oil three to four times daily. Practitioners also use the tincture topically.

Professional Medical Advice

The information in this book is a not a substitute for professional medical advice or health care. Consult a qualified health professional when there is any question regarding the presence or treatment of any health condition.

Corns and Calluses

Diagnosis

Both corns and calluses are a build-up of hard skin that forms in response to pressure or rubbing in a particular area. The skin thickens as a form of protection. Corns are usually found on the feet. Wearing badly fitting shoes or high heels is a contributory factor. Calluses are found on the feet but may also appear on the hands or knees. They usually develop over a bony prominence. Corns can be pared, or filed down—the skin is dead, so you do not feel anything if the top layers are shaved off. Care is needed, however, and anyone with circulatory problems in their feet or diabetes should get expert advice before attempting to remove corns themselves. Both conditions occur most often in people who have a high foot arch, as this increases downward pressure on the toes.

Symptoms

Corns
- Dead skin cells build up causing pain and discomfort
- A small raised bump appears with a hard center
- The affected area looks yellow
- Aching sensation
- Usually appear on the feet

Calluses
- A rough patch of skin develops, usually over a bone
- Skin becomes hard, thick, and raised
- Usually appear on the feet, hands, or knees

Treatment Goal

While uncomfortable and painful, corns and calluses are harmless. Treatment aims to identify and remove the source of pressure or friction and relieve any immediate discomfort.

Conventional Medicine

Use a pumice stone: Usually, a callus or corn can be taken care of at home. Try using a file or a pumice stone to soften and rub away excess skin. Continue to do so until the callus or corn disappears.

Salicylic acid: After filing away the callus or corn, apply a plaster of 40% salicylic acid, which is available over the counter, to an area slightly larger than the callus or corn and put a corn ring on top to relieve the pressure. You can also apply a skin softening cream to help skin stay soft.

For persistent calluses and corns: Seek advice from a doctor if the callus or corn does not go away within four weeks of removing the cause, or if it tends to crack open as this could cause infection. Medical treatment usually involves surgical paring of the thickened skin by a doctor or surgeon.

Traditional Chinese Medicine

Herbs: The external use of herbs is common for corns and calluses. Purchase a powder form of the Chinese herb Ji Yian San. Soak the affected area in warm water until the corn or callus becomes soft. Cover the normal skin around the corns and put Ji Yian San on the top of the affected area. Cover the affected area with a dressing. Repeat this procedure once a day for seven days or until the corn is gone. Make sure Ji Yian San does not come into contact with unaffected skin. It should not be used around eyes or nose, and should never be taken orally.

Naturopathy

Footwear: The best way to treat corns and calluses naturopathically is by wearing shoes that fit properly, so as not to cause friction, are activity-appropriate, and are kept in good repair. Socks and stockings should not cramp the toes. Feet should be measured, while standing, whenever buying new shoes. It is best to shop for shoes late in the day, when feet are likely to be swollen. It is also important to buy shoes with toe-wiggling room and to try new shoes on both feet.

Moleskin pads: Placing moleskin pads over corns can relieve pressure, and large wads of cotton, lamb's wool, or moleskin can cushion calluses.

Topical remedy: Mix 1 tsp of lemon juice with 1 tsp of dried chamomile tea. Crush a clove of garlic and add it to the mixture. Rub this remedy directly on the corn once or more times a day.

Epsom salt soak: Soak your feet in a solution of Epsom salts and warm water for at least 10 minutes a day before rubbing the area with a pumice stone. This will remove part or all of your calluses. It is important to see a doctor if the skin of a corn or callus is cut or bleeds because it may become infected. If a corn discharges pus or clear fluid, it is infected.

Tip: HOT WATER SOAK

Soak your feet in hot water daily for 20 minutes before going to bed. This will help foot circulation.

Physical medicine: Standing and walking correctly can sometimes eliminate excess foot pressure. Several types of bodywork can help correct body imbalances. Bodywork is a term used for any of a number of systems, including Aston-Patterning, Alexander technique, rolfing, and Feldenkrais method, that manipulate the body through massage, movement education, or meditational techniques.

Herbs: Aloe vera cream is an effective skin softener. Two or three daily applications of calendula salve can also soften skin and prevent inflammation. Apply a paste made by combining 1 tsp of aloe vera gel with half that amount of turmeric and apply the paste to the affected area. Bandage overnight, soak in warm water for 10 minutes every morning, and then massage gently with mustard oil (available from health food stores). Repeat this treatment for seven days. Since turmeric can stain skin and clothing, put on an old pair of socks after applying this remedy. Any skin discoloration should wash off in about two weeks.

Homeopathy

Corns and calluses need to be treated by a chiropodist or podiatrist. The measures listed below can provide some temporary relief until the offending extra layers of skin have been removed and, following treatment, speed up the healing process.

Antimonium crudum: Used before treatment, this remedy can provide relief from pain that is caused by thickened skin under the soles of the feet, or sensitive corns that develop under the toenails or on the tips of toes. Nails (especially on the big toe) can be particularly susceptible to developing corns that look rather like warts.

Silica: Try Silica if feet have a tendency to be sweaty and smelly, with burning sensations developing in the feet and soles while in bed at night. Silica can also be effective if there is a tendency to develop hard, painful calluses, bunions, or corns (especially between the toes or under the toenails) that give rise to shooting pains.

Hypericum: Take if there is residual pain and discomfort in the feet or toes after a podiatry treatment. It helps soothe discomfort in areas that are especially rich in nerves, such as the toes, fingers, and base of the spine. Pains that respond well to this remedy are tender and sore, characteristically shooting away from the affected area, especially when touched.

Calendula: After treatments try applying Calendula cream daily to areas of hard or dry skin. This cream is a moisturizer, antiseptic cream, and healing agent all in one.

Herbalism

Greater celadine: This herb can be used to slowly dissolve a corn. Apply the fresh juice of greater celandine topically to the corn or callus. Alternatively, if the fresh plant is not available, make an infusion of greater celadine. Place 1 tbsp of the herb in a cup of freshly boiled water for 10 minutes. Strain the water and let it cool. Soak a cotton or linen cloth in the decoction and place it on the corn. Cover the affected area with a waterproof cover and tape this onto the skin. Leave the compress on overnight and wash it off in the morning.

Fig, papaya, and pineapple: These fruits all contain enzymes that break down skin growths. Patented formulas with extracts of these plants can be purchased and should be used according to instructions on the label. Sometimes a number of treatments are required to obtain the best result.

Willow: The bark of this tree is popular for its pain-relieving qualities, and the same constituent responsible for the pain relief also dissolves skin growths. Boil 1–2 tbsp of dried willow bark in strips or chunks in 1½ cups of water for 10 minutes, making sure that the water does not evaporate and the pan boil dry. Once it has cooled, apply it to the corn, holding the willow in place with a cloth or gauze for 10 minutes several times a day. Avoid contact with the skin around the corn as the salicylates in the bark can irritate unaffected areas.

Wintergreen: The essential oil of wintergreen contains salicylates that can be used to dissolve corns. Apply essential oil of wintergreen to the corn, preferably at night, and wash it off in the morning. Avoid contact with surrounding skin to avoid irritating it. Synthetic oils of wintergreen have been made and are sold as oil of wintergreen, but these oils do not have the same healing properties as the natural oil.

Plantar Warts

Diagnosis

Also known as a verruca, a plantar wart is found on the sole of the foot, and is particularly common in children. It is caused by a viral infection in the skin, which multiplies and spreads. A hard, black, horny swelling is produced, which is pushed under the skin by the pressure of walking. It manifests as a small, brown-black circle on a level with the surface of the skin. Sometimes you can also see tiny black spots, which are caused by bleeding in the plantar wart as a result of standing and walking on it.

Changing rooms and communal pools are a breeding ground for this type of infection—the wart virus is very contagious. It can take several months for plantar warts to develop after infection. Not everyone is susceptible to the virus. When children share bathrooms that contain wart viruses, some will contract plantar warts, while others seem to be immune. The reason for this variance in susceptibility is unknown.

Symptoms

- One or more circular lumps, which can be white, flesh-colored, or brown-black, on the sole of the foot, often no bigger than a pin prick
- Occasionally these may appear in clusters, known as a mosaic wart

Treatment Goal

To clear up the plantar wart and protect against further infections.

Conventional Medicine

Duct tape occlusion: Plantar warts that are not painful do not need to be treated, but can be removed through duct tape occlusion. Completely cover the area with duct tape for about one week. Remove the tape, soak the foot, and debride the area with a pumice stone. After a day, reapply the duct tape. Continue this treatment until the lesion is gone.

Topical treatment: Apply tretinoin cream before bed for several weeks. A 17% salicylic acid, obtained over the counter, can also be applied to a clean, dry foot twice a day. The area should be bandaged after treatment. Flourouracil cream (Efudex®), applied daily for three weeks, can also be applied to treat plantar warts. However, this treatment can lead to a darkening of the skin. If none of these treatments help, liquid nitrogen can be applied, or electrocautery can be performed. If all of these treatments fail, bleomycin, a chemotherapeutic agent, can be injected into the lesion.

Surgical and laser therapy: If the lesion is very large or does not respond to the above, the area may be cut off in the doctor's office using a scalpel or other surgical instrument such as a curette or an electrosurgical unit. For plantar warts that are painful, laser therapy can be used. This leaves a wound that takes four to six weeks to heal.

Traditional Chinese Medicine

Herbs: It is not generally necessary to take internal Chinese medicine to treat plantar warts. If there are many sores that spread quickly, the following formulas can be used to help the body clean out the virus.
• **Herbal decoction:** Mix 30 g of Ma Zhi Xian (dried purslane), 30 g of Yi Yi Ren (seeds of Job's tears), and 10 g of Da Qing Ye (woad leaf) in a ceramic or glass pot. Add 3 cups of water, bring the mixutre to the boil, and simmer for 30 minutes. Strain and drink 1 cup three times a day for three to five days.

• **Herbal body wash:** Boil 15 g of Ma Zhi Xian (dried purslane), 8 g of Chen Pi (tangerine peel), 15 g of She Chuang Zi (cnidium seed), 10 g of Ku Shen (sophora root), and 12 g of Dang Gui (Chinese angelica) in 5 cups of water. Strain the liquid and allow it to cool. Use the decoction to wash the affected area, or add it to bath water.

Diet: A healthy diet is recommended to avoid infection.

Naturopathy

Diet: Eat a diet based on whole foods to support your immune system. Avoid processed foods that are high in simple carbohydrates as they can weaken your immune system and reduce your body's effectiveness in fighting the virus that causes warts.

Supplements: The following nutritional supplements will support immune function and healing, which will help combat the viral infections that cause plantar warts. Take 500 mg of vitamin C twice a day. Take 400 IU of vitamin E and 100,000 IU of beta carotene a day. B complex vitamins (50–100 mg a day) will help to reduce the effects of stress, which can weaken your immune system. Taking 200 mcg of selenium and 15–30 mg of zinc a day is also recommended.

Herbs: Thuja has a caustic effect on warts as well as antiviral properties. Apply one drop of thuja tincture, available from health food stores, two to four times a day. Take 500 mg of olive leaf extract orally twice a day for its antiviral properties. Garlic also has antiviral properties, and 1 drop can be applied to the plantar wart two to four times a day. You can also use a raw garlic patch by covering the wart and surrounding skin with a thin layer of castor oil or olive oil and then taping a thin slice of fresh garlic in place. This patch should be left on overnight. To maximize the benefit, place 2–4 drops of greater celandine tincture on the wart before covering it with garlic. This application may need to be repeated nightly for up to three weeks. The wart will turn black as it begins to die.

> *Tip:* EAT FOR IMMUNITY
>
> A diet based on whole foods, such as vegetables, fruit, and whole grains, can support the immune system in fighting the virus. Avoid processed foods.

Homeopathy

When dealing with a well-established case of plantar warts you will need help from a homeopathic practitioner, who will treat the underlying imbalance. When this is successful, the current plantar wart should slowly be eradicated and the development of any future episodes discouraged. However, if a small plantar wart is showing early signs of emergence and there is no established tendency to this problem, one of the following remedies may encourage it to resolve itself.

Thuja: Use Thuja to treat a plantar wart that is uncomfortable when in contact with cold water. Skin quality may be poor with a greasy texture and a tendency to look sallow and dull. Burning and itchy sensations will be experienced in the plantar wart.

Causticum: To treat an itchy, painful plantar wart that has jagged edges and bleeds very readily, use Causticum. Skin may be cracked and sore, especially where there are folds of skin. Plantar warts are most likely to develop when the child is stressed and/or rundown.

Antimonium crudum: A possible choice of remedy where plantar warts emerge on soles of feet that have a marked tendency to produce calluses and hard skin. The feet may feel generally very tender, with the soles being especially sensitive when walking.

Silica: If the emergence of a plantar wart coincides with poor-quality nails or the development of soft corns between the toes, this remedy is worth considering. The soles of the feet may also itch, especially in the evenings.

Herbalism

Greater celandine: A herb restricted to practitioner use, the tincture can be applied topically to the warts. Fresh juice from plants can also be used topically, where available. Apply at least three times daily.

Thuja: This tincture may be applied topically, directly onto the warts three times daily. Warts can be very persistent, so it is important to persevere with applications. It is high in thujone, and has antimicrobial and antimitotic properties. May be used alternately with greater celandine. Using a variety of herbs in combination can often be most effective.

Echinacea: Consider taking something to support the immune system while treating the warts topically. Echinacea is a useful immune-modulatory herb. It may be taken in tincture form, 3 ml three times daily, or as a decoction. If making a decoction, add 1 tsp of the root to 1½ cups of water in a saucepan. Bring to a boil and simmer while covered for 10 minutes. Strain and drink three times daily.

2

Eyes
and
Mouth

Conjunctivitus

Diagnosis

Conjunctivitis is a common eye condition involving an inflammation of the thin membrane that covers the eyeball. It is not serious but can be very uncomfortable and irritating. It usually affects both eyes at the same time, although it may start in one eye then eventually spread to the other. If the whole eye is affected, the condition has probably been triggered by a bacterial or viral infection, which is the most common cause of conjunctivitis. It is a very contagious condition and stringent hand washing is required to prevent it from spreading. Newborn babies are also prone to this condition. If you have recurrent attacks, it is important to isolate the trigger. Triggers and irritants can include a foreign body in the eye, such as a piece of grit, dirt, or dust, an allergy or hayfever, an intolerance to dairy products or other food, or chlorine in swimming pools. Antibiotic drops or ointment, or antihistamines if the conjunctivitis is an allergic reaction, are usually prescribed.

Symptoms

- Sore, irritated eyes that feel gritty or sandy
- The white of the eye becomes pink or red and bloodshot
- Swollen eyelids
- Weepy eyes
- A thin, watery discharge
- A thick, yellow discharge that is sticky and causes crustiness and gumming together of the eyelashes
- Difficulty opening eyes in the morning as eyelids may be stuck together with pus
- Eye rubbing
- Impaired vision

Treatment Goal

Always seek medical advice if you develop conjunctivitis. Treatment aims to make the eyes comfortable, reduce inflammation, and eradicate any infection.

Conventional Medicine

It should not be assumed that "red eye" is conjunctivitis. Treatment depends on whether the cause is viral, bacterial, allergic, traumatic, or chlamydial. If any pain or eyesight changes occur, see your doctor as this indicates a more serious problem than conjunctivitis.

Artificial tears: Dry eyes are more prone to conjunctivitis. Artificial tears can be used to remedy this and protect against the condition.

Compresses: To help alleviate conjunctivitis at its onset, hold a moist, warm compress to the eye for about 20 minutes three times a day.

Antibiotic drops: Two drops of tobramycin, gentamicin, or a floxin ophthalmic solution can be applied to the eye every four hours for about a week. Sometimes betadine eye drops are prescribed. Avoid using eye drops that contain steroids (some antibiotic drops have a steroid in them) if an infection is present, as they will exacerbate the condition.

For allergic conjunctivitis: Chronic allergic conjunctivitis is treated with mast cell stabilizing medication such as Patanol, which is like an antihistamine for the eyes.

Traditional Chinese Medicine

Herbs:
• **Ginger compress:** Take one piece of fresh ginger, make a small hole in the middle, and place 1.5 g of Huang Lian (coptis root) inside. Bake the ginger and place it, while warm, on the Tai Yang acupoint. This point is located in the depression midway between the outer edge of the eyebrow and outer corner of the eye.
• **Herbal tea:** Mix 30 g of Ren Dong Teng (honeysuckle stem), 30 g Xia Ku Cao (common self-heal fruit-spike), 15 g of Pu Gong Ying (dandelion), and 15 g of Xuan Shen (ningpo figwort root) in a ceramic or glass pot. Add 3 cups of water, boil the mixture, and simmer for 30 minutes. Strain and give 2 oz to 1 cup of tea, three times a day for three to five days. Consult a TCM practitioner to ascertain the correct dose for a child.

Acupressure: Press the Hegu, Tai Chong, Tai Yang, and Cuan Zhu points. The Hegu point is located on the back of the hand between the thumb and index finger. The Tai Chong point is on the top of the foot in the depression between the first and second toes. The Tai Yang point is located at the temple, midway between the outer edge of the eyebrow and the outer corner of the eye. The Cuan Zhu point is on the inside end of the eyebrow. In a sitting position, close your eyes and place your index finger gently on the Cuan Zhu point. Press for one minute then press the Tai Yang point for one minute with your thumb. Press each point in turn for one minute. Wash your hands with soap and water before and after acupressure.

Diet: Eat foods with plain flavor, such as Chinese cabbage, celery, fresh lotus rhizome, mung bean sprouts, balsam pears, shepherd's purse, tomatoes, water chestnuts, and pears. Avoid wine, spring onions, garlic, pepper, and chilies.

Naturopathy

Diet: Maintain a diet that will strengthen the immune system so that your body is able to fight infections that can cause conjunctivitis. Eat fresh fruits and vegetables, whole grains, legumes, and quality protein such as fish, lean chicken, and beans every day. Eat plenty of green leafy vegetables for their high nutrient content, which will provide a base of nutrients required for a healthy immune system. Avoid foods that weaken your immune system, including processed foods that contain sugar and hydrogenated vegetable oils, store-bought baked goods, and all beverages other than tea, water, and freshly squeezed juices.

Supplements: A vitamin A deficiency has been reported in people that suffer from chronic conjunctivitis; take 10,000 IU of vitamin A a day. Take 250–500 mg of vitamin C a day to expedite the healing process and strengthen your immune system to fight toxins. Zinc also strengthens your immune system and helps you heal faster. Take 30–50 mg of zinc a day.

Herbs: The following herbs may be used as dried extracts (in the form of capsules, powders, or teas), glycerites (glycerine extracts), or tinctures (alcohol extracts). Compresses and eye washes are external

Tip: HERBAL EYEWASH

Mix 10 drops of goldenseal tincture with 1 tsp of boric acid in 1 cup of water. Use this mixture to wash the infected eyes.

treatments. A compress is made with a clean cloth, gauze pad, or cotton balls soaked in a solution and then applied over the eyes. Eye washes can be administered with an eye cup or a sterile dropper. Chamomile, fennel seed, marigold, and plantain help fight infection, soothe irritation, and have astringent and soothing properties. The fresh leaves are the most effective plant part. Make a soothing poultice with 28 g of bruised flaxseed steeped for 15 minutes in 4 fl oz of water. Strain the herbs, wrap them in a cheesecloth, and apply them directly to the affected eye. Grated fresh potato has astringent properties and can also be wrapped in cheesecloth and used as a poultice.

Hydrotherapy: Alternate using hot and cold compresses on the eye (three to four minutes hot, followed by 20–30 seconds cold). Use the compresses one to three times a day either by themselves or as part of a treatment program that includes an eyewash.

Homeopathy

It is sensible to confirm the diagnosis of conjunctivitis with your family doctor before beginning a course of homeopathic self-prescribing. A more established tendency to recurrent bouts of moderate to severe conjunctivitis will require treatment from a trained homeopathic practitioner.

Belladonna: Use this remedy at the first sign of inflammation, heat, and redness. When this remedy is appropriate, symptoms always develop quickly and dramatically. Pains feel throbbing and pounding, while the affected eye feels hot and dry. Discomfort is worse after jarring movement and exposure to bright light.

Apis: If the discomfort of conjunctivitis is noticeably increased by exposure to warmth, plus signs of pinkish puffiness and swelling around the eyes, consider this remedy. Symptoms include stinging, shooting pains, baggy swelling under the affected eyes, and great fussiness and fidgetiness when uncomfortable. Use this remedy for rapidly developing symptoms of allergic conjunctivitis, after seeking medical advice.

Pulsatilla: For more established symptoms, especially those that develop as a complication of the later stages of a head cold, use Pulsatilla. Symptoms include an irritating feeling of a film covering the surface of the affected eye or eyes, which makes you want to constantly rub or wipe the eyes. A thick, yellowish-green discharge may also be present, which becomes crusty and sticks the eyelids together in the morning, and you may feel weepy and tearful when in discomfort.

Herbalism

There are many dangerous conditions that can cause conjunctivitis, and these conditions can vary. Your health care practitioner should be involved in the diagnosis and treatment of conjunctivitis. The suggestions below are for mild conjunctivitis of a viral or allergic cause.

Eyebright: This plant is recommended for topical application in cases of conjunctivitis. Soak a clean piece of gauze or cotton in an infusion of eyebright and dab it on the infected area. Be aware of the possibility of introducing infection if tools are not kept sterile. Use a clean piece of gauze or cotton ball for each application and a fresh infusion of eyebright each time. If you notice the conjunctivitis worsening, or if it has not resolved after a few days, discontinue use and seek professional help.

Calendula: The flowers of this plant can be applied topically in the same manner as described for eyebright. Although there are very few contraindications or adverse reactions when used topically, applying calendula to the eye could cause more irritation. Discontinue use if this occurs.

Chamomile: Used topically chamomile can help to relieve irritation, soothe, and calm inflammation. Prepare an infusion by steeping 2 tsp in a cup of freshly boiled water and infusing while covered for 15 minutes. Strain and use cotton wool to apply as a compress. Repeat several times daily. As with all topical applications for eyes, use fresh preparations each time, and use separate preparations for each eye, if treatment for both is needed. A combination of chamomile with calendula and eyebright can be very useful.

Echinacea: Supporting the immune system can be useful. Take 3ml of tincture three times daily, or make a decoction of the root. 1–2 tsp can be boiled in a saucepan of 1¼ cups water for 10 minutes. Strain and drink three times daily. 🍵

> *Tip:* PREVENTION
>
> Viral and bacterial conjunctivitis are both very contagious. Family members should use separate towels and wash their hands often. Children with this condition should generally be kept home from school and nursery. If you wear contact lenses, keep them clean to avoid further irritation and any future infections. Do not wear lenses until your eyes have healed.

Glaucoma

Diagnosis

Glaucoma is one of the most common causes of blindness in the world today. It is an umbrella term for a range of conditions affecting the eye, where the pressure inside the eye becomes too high and the optic nerve at the back of the eye becomes damaged, which can lead to the loss of vision if left untreated. There are two main types of glaucoma. The most common form is chronic simple glaucoma, where loss of vision occurs slowly and is often irreversible, as people do not notice any problem until their vision has already been damaged. The second form is acute glaucoma, which comes on suddenly and causes painful red eyes and blurred vision.

Symptoms

Chronic
- Peripheral vision tends to be affected first so, to begin with, eyesight does not noticeably alter
- The loss of peripheral areas of visual field increases until the central vision is damaged, which can lead to blindness

Acute
- Eye suddenly becomes very painful
- Eye is usually red
- Vision becomes blurred
- You may notice a "halo" effect around lights
- Pupils become dilated
- Headaches
- Feelings of being unwell
- Nausea

Treatment Goal

Acute glaucoma is a medical emergency and treatment should be sought immediately. Treatment of chronic glaucoma aims to slow the deterioration of eyesight and relieve any discomfort.

Conventional Medicine

Glaucoma can be confused with allergies and with irritation from contact lenses, along with other more rare eye diseases, so treatment requires an accurate diagnosis. A diagnosis is made by using visual field examination and GDx nerve fiber analysis tests. The latter test measures the thickness of the retinal nerve fiber layer as those with glaucoma have been found to have thicker retinal layers. Blood tests are sometimes performed to rule out associated diseases.

Relieving pressure: Treatment aims to lower the pressure in the eye and to keep the pressure down. How this is carried out depends on how high the pressure in the eye is. Intravenous mannitol is sometimes given to bring down the pressure. An emergency treatment is an anterior chamber paracentesis, which is rarely necessary.

Medication: Eye drops containing pilocarpine, or a course of oral pilocarpine, beta-blockers, and Diamox® all lower intraocular pressure and they are sometimes prescribed for acute conditions to immediately lower the pressure.

Laser therapy: For chronic or long-term conditions there are new laser procedures that are effective. Iridotomy and trabeculectomy are traditional surgical procedures, which generally totally cure the elevated pressure so that no further treatment or medication is needed. Filter valves are sometimes placed surgically to prevent the recurrence of glaucoma after acute treatment is given. All of these procedures are done by an ophthalmologist. If your doctor diagnoses glaucoma, he or she will refer you to an ophthalmologist for treatment.

Tip: EXERCISE REGULARLY

Studies indicate that glaucoma patients who exercise regularly (at least three times a week) can reduce their intraocular pressure by an average of 20%. If they stop exercising for more than two weeks, pressure increases again. Talk to your doctor to determine an appropriate exercise program.

Traditional Chinese Medicine

Herbs:
• Herbal decoction: Combine 12 g of Di Huang (Chinese foxglove), 12 g of Bai Shao (white peony root), 10 g of Ye Ju Hua (wild chrysanthemum flower), 12 g of Gou Ji Zi (wolfberry), and 12 g of Gou Teng (stem and thorns of gambir vine) with 3 cups of water in a ceramic or glass pot. Bring to a boil and simmer for 30 minutes. Strain the liquid and drink 1 cup three times a day for three to five days. This formula nourishes the liver and kidneys, helping to promote energy flow in the eyes.

• **Herbal tea:** Add 3 g of Ye Ju Hua (wild chrysanthemum flower), 3 g of Bo He (field mint), 8 g of Gou Ji Zi (wolfberry), and 5 g of Cang Er Zi (cocklebur fruit) to a teapot of boiling water. Let the tea steep for five minutes before drinking. This formula has the gentle function of reducing the heat, and nourishing the eyes.

Acupressure: Wash your hands before this treatment. In a sitting position, close your eyes and place your index finger on the Cuan Zhu point (located on the inside end of the eyebrow) using medium pressure for one minute. Next press the Tai Yang point (located at the temple, midway between the outer edge of the eyebrow and the outer corner of the eye) for one minute with your thumb. Press the Chen Xi point (directly below the pupil between the eyeball and orbital ridge) for one minute. When you have finished open your eyes slowly. Perform this procedure twice a day to help circulation to the eyes.

Naturopathy

Diet: Eat a wholesome balanced diet based on whole grains and fresh fruit and vegetables. Include as many orange, yellow, and green leafy vegetables as possible. These contain pigments called carotenoids, which are essential for optimum eye health. Eat plenty of fruits such as blueberries and dark cherries, which contain anthocyanidin, a chemical that is also important for good eye health. Foods rich in magnesium and chromium, such as brewer's yeast, kelp, leafy greens, and apples, have beneficial effects on glaucoma.

Supplements: Some studies have shown that magnesium can dilate blood vessels and improve vision; take 250 mg twice a day. Taking 1,000 mg of vitamin C two to four times a day can significantly reduce elevated intraocular pressure in cases of glaucoma. Taking 150 mg of alpha lipoic acid a day for a month improves visual function in people with some types of glaucoma. Vitamin A may also have benefits for the eyes; take ½ tbsp twice a day. Chromium, zinc, and the B complex of vitamins, particularly thiamine, also appear to play a role in preventing and treating glaucoma. Those with elevated eye pressure have been found deficient in these elements. Anyone at risk should consider taking the following supplements: 100 mcg of trivalent chromium twice a day; 30 mg of zinc a day; and 50 mg of B complex a day.

Herbs: Bilberry contains flavonoids that support eye structure and function. Take 160 mg twice a day for 25% anthocyanosides (the active ingredient of the herb). Rutin has been found useful in restoring normal collagen metabolism and normalizing eye tissue, which is helpful in the prevention and treatment of glaucoma. Take 20 mg three times a day.

Homeopathy

Due to its potential seriousness unless managed by medical assessment and treatment, this condition is best left in the hands of conventional and complementary health professionals. An integrated approach to medical treatment is recommended rather than attempting to deal with the problem through self-prescribing.

Tip: USE SUNGLASSES

Glaucoma can cause the eyes to be very sensitive to light and glare and medications can aggravate the situation. Sunglasses solve this problem and are important in preventing cataracts. Protective sunglasses do not have to be expensive. Choose ones that block both UVA and UVB.

Herbalism

It is important to have regular health checks for this condition with eye care specialists, and to take measures to control any diabetes or high blood pressure, if relevant. The following herbs can offer additional support.

Ginkgo: Ginkgo can be taken as a tea or tincture two to three times a day; most scientific studies use standardized extracts once or twice a day. Ginkgo has few reported side effects, although care should be exercised for those who are also taking anticoagulant and antithrombotic drugs as there may be an added risk of bleeding.

Coleus: Coleus contains a compound called forskolin that may be helpful in lowering intraocular pressure (the pressure inside the eye), which is of primary importance when treating glaucoma. Coleus is not very easily available, and standardized extracts may be even harder to find, so a herbal practitioner may be able to help.

Bilberry: These berries help to support and strengthen capillaries, and are often used in cases of glaucoma. Standardized 80 mg extract capsules are available, and can be taken three times daily. This is also available in tincture form, and fresh bilberries may be eaten.

Stye

Diagnosis

A stye is a bacterial infection that develops at the root of an eyelash, causing an inflamed lump to form. After approximately seven days the stye will usually come to a head and burst. Styes can spread easily from eye to eye, and they are often recurrent. It is also common to get several styes at once because of cross infection. If you develop a stye it is important not to touch your eyes. Triggers include being rundown and having a depressed immune system, which lowers your body's resistance to infection. Some people are more susceptible to styes than others, and repeated flare-ups may sometimes indicate diabetes. See your family doctor if the stye is particularly large, if it seems to have developed on the inside of the eyelid, or if pain persists.

Symptoms

- Itchiness, soreness, and swelling of the eyelid
- A painful red lump that grows into a yellow head
- Inflammation along the rim of the eyelid
- Feeling that there is something in the eye; a gritty sensation

Treatment Goal

While irritating, styes cause no damage to the eye itself. Treatment aims to relieve the symptoms and keep the immune system strong to prevent recurrent attacks.

Conventional Medicine

A stye is known medically as a hordeolum. Treatment depends on the cause of the inflammation. About 80% are caused by the bacterium Staphylococcus aureus. The bacterium Streptococcus causes a few and a minority are caused by a mix of both organisms. Before treatment a doctor will determine that the stye is not another type of eye bump, such as an abscess of the eyelid, which must be taken seriously; chalzion (swelling due to a blocked lubrication duct), a contact dermatitis; or cellulitis of the eyelid. A herpes infection of the eye can also look like styes.

Eye compress: Good hygiene and warm compresses on the eye sometimes help to prevent and treat styes when they are in the early stages. Ideally the compress should be a sterile gauze pad soaked in water.

Antibiotics: Topical erythromycin ophthalmic ointment can be applied two to four times a day to the rim of the eye or the eyelid until the stye has cleared up, which usually takes about a week. If the redness and enlargement of the stye does not begin to resolve within 48 hours, oral antibiotics are used (usually a penicillin or analog to combat staphylococci).

Surgery: Very occasionally, surgical intervention is needed to treat repeated and progressive infections. This procedure involves making an incision and draining the stye, and should always be performed by a surgeon. Emergency treatment by an ophthalmologist is needed if there is a problem with eyesight or the movement of the eye.

Long-term prevention: If you suffer from chronic styes, an anti-inflammatory diet that excludes processed foods, sugar, dairy, and gluten, and immune-boosting protocol with the right nutrition and supplements should be followed.

Traditional Chinese Medicine

Herbs:
• Yin Qiao Jie Du Pian: This herbal pill is designed for clearing heat and infection. It is commonly used to treat upper respiratory infections, but it is also effective in the treatment of styes.
• Herbal decoction: Combine 12 g of Pu Gong Ying (dandelion),10 g of Jin Yin Hua (honeysuckle flower), 6 g of Bo He (field mint), 8 g of Huang Qin (baical skullcap root), and 10 g of Ye Ju Hua (wild chrysanthemum flower) with 3 cups of water in a glass or ceramic pot. Boil the mixture and let it simmer for 30 minutes before straining it. Drink 1 cup three times a day for three to seven days.

Acupressure: If the stye is on the upper eyelid, press the Yu Yao, Tai Yang, and Yang Bai points. The Yu Yao point is on the eyebrow, directly above the pupil. The Tai Yang point is at the temple between the lateral end of the eyebrow and eyelid, in the depression one finger behind. The Yang Bai point is also directly above the pupil, but 1 inch above the eyebrow. If the stye is on lower eyelid, press the Si Bai and Tai Yang points. The Si Bai point is directly under the pupil in the depression below the eye socket. Wash your hands thoroughly and, in a sitting position, apply gentle pressure with your index finger to each of these points for one minute two to three times a day.

Diet: Eat foods that are cooling, such as celery, spinach, lettuce, mung beans, tangerine, watermelon, and string beans. Avoid hot foods as they increase internal heat.

Naturopathy

Diet: The general idea of dietary therapy is to strengthen the immune system so that your body is able to fight infections that can cause styes. Make sure you eat a well-balanced diet that includes fresh fruits and vegetables, whole grains, legumes, and quality protein such as fish, lean chicken, and beans everyday. Eat plenty of green leafy vegetables for their high nutrient content, which will provide a good foundation of the nutrients required for a healthy immune system. Avoid foods that weaken your immune system, such as processed sugar, hydrogenated vegetable oils, baked goods, and all drinks other than tea, water, and freshly squeezed juices.

Supplements: Zinc strengthens your immune system and helps you heal faster. Take 30–50 mg per day. Take 25,000–50,000 IU a day of a betacarotene supplement for its antioxidant support. Recurring styes can be a sign of a vitamin A deficiency; take 25,000 IU daily. Pregnant women should not exceed 10,000 IU of vitamin A a day.

Herbs: Eyebright helps fight infection and dry up excess fluid; chamomile or fennel seeds also help fight infection; marigold soothes irritation; and plantain is astringent and soothing (the fresh leaves are the most effective plant part). To make a compress from any of these herbs dilute 5 drops of tincture in ¼ cup water, or steep 1 tsp of the herb in 1 cup of hot water for 5–10 minutes before straining. Soak a clean cloth or piece of gauze in the solution and apply it to the eyes for 10 minutes three to four times a day. To make a soothing flaxseed poultice wrap 28 g of bruised flaxseed steeped for 15 minutes in 4 fl oz of water in cheesecloth and apply it directly to the affected eye. Grated, fresh potato can also be wrapped in cheesecloth and apply to the affected area for its astringent properties. Another compress formula is diluted eyebright, goldenseal, and raspberry leaf. These herbs have antibacterial and antiviral properties and also work to support the immune system to prevent infections. Goldenseal is bright yellow and will stain fingers and worktops, so use it with care. You can also use this mixture as an eyewash to bathe both eyes or use a dropper bottle to place a few drops into each eye. Do this for 10–15 minutes four times a day.

Tip: BALANCED DIET

If a stye has developed after a period of high stress and pressure, make a deliberate point of taking adequate rest and include foods in your diet that have a reputation for boosting the immune system, such as fresh fruit, vegetables, whole grains, nuts, seeds, garlic, and green and/or white tea. Avoid sugary foods, which lower the immune system while also encouraging bacterial infection to develop.

Homeopathy

Any of the following homeopathic options can help to ease the inflammation and discomfort of a stye, encouraging it to resolve itself quickly. An underlying tendency to develop frequent or severe styes requires treatment from a homeopathic practitioner.

Hepar sulph: Consider this remedy to treat large, swollen styes that produce a thick, yellowish pus. Symptoms include discomfort and sensitivity to contact with the slightest draft of cold air. Pains in the affected area will be characteristically sharp and splinterlike. They are noticeably relieved by applying warm compresses or bathing in warm water.

Belladonna: This is a possible remedy if redness and throbbing sensations develop rapidly at the margin of the eyelid. Belladonna is helpful if the overall area affected is very sensitive, while the eyes feel dry and hot.

Pulsatilla: If styes affect the lower eyelid and produce a gluey, thick discharge that forms a crust in the morning, use Pulsatilla. Pain and sensitivity of the affected part of the eyelid is more intense for contact with warmth. Itchiness creates a constant desire to rub the eyes.

Apis: Apis is always suitable when puffy, baglike swellings develop around the eyes very rapidly and dramatically. The affected tissues feel as though they sting, and tears produced also feel painful. The discomfort becomes more intense if the affected area gets hot, while applying cool compresses brings relief.

Herbalism

The best treatment method is proper hygiene of the infected area and warm, wet compresses. There are a few herbs that can be added to the compress to augment healing.

Eyebright: This herb is recommended for topical application for styes. Make an infusion of eyebright by steeping a handful of the dried herb in a bowl of boiling water. Allow the infusion to cool to a warm temperature. Soak a clean washcloth in the infusion, wring out the excess liquid, and place it directly on closed eyes to help a stye resolve.

Chamomile: This herb has calming properties and anti-inflammatory effects. To treat a stye, make a chamomile compress by steeping approximately 2–5 g of dried flowers in ¾ cup of boiling water for 20 minutes. Cover while the flowers are infusing, strain the mixture, and allow it to cool. Soak a clean washcloth in the liquid, squeeze out the excess, and place it over your closed eyes for five to 10 minutes several times a day. If you begin to notice redness or irritation around the application site, discontinue use.

Calendula: Prepare an infusion as above, and apply as a compress several times daily, using a fresh preparation each time. Calendula may also be used in combination with eyebright and chamomile topically. If there is any increased irritation, discontinue use.

Gingivitis

Diagnosis

Gingivitis is an inflammatory condition of the gums that, if left unchecked, can eventually lead to the loss of teeth. It is primarily caused by a build-up of dental plaque in the mouth. Plaque is comprised of a damaging mix of food debris and bacteria, which causes the gums to become inflamed and pull away from the teeth. Women can be particularly prone to gingivitis, as hormonal changes during pregnancy and menopause can trigger the condition. The first sign of this condition is usually bleeding gums. Taking some types of medication can destroy protective bacteria in the mouth, leaving gums vulnerable. If left untreated, gingivitis can progress to periodontitis.

Symptoms

- Gums become red
- Gums become soft, shiny, and swollen
- Gums feel tender and sore
- Pain experienced when brushing teeth
- Bleeding gums, especially when brushing teeth
- Halitosis
- Painful to chew

Treatment Goal

If caught early, gingivitis is a reversible stage of gum disease. Treatment involves good dental hygiene, including regular brushing and flossing, plus frequent check-ups to prevent gingivitis from developing.

Conventional Medicine

Prevention: Gingivitis can occur mildly or as a more severe ulcerative form, known as trench mouth. It occurs more commonly with the hormonal shifts associated with conditions such as pregnancy. It is also associated with excessive use of alcohol and tobacco, a poor dental hygiene routine, and ill-fitting dentures. Treatment involves prevention by looking at and addressing any one of these situations. Regular flossing is the most important factor in good hygiene. Some drugs cause a condition known as hyperplasia of the gums, the symptoms of which are very similar to gingivitis. The most common of these drugs are phenytoin, an antiseizure medication, and nifedipine, which is a blood pressure medication. If you suspect any of these causes, see your doctor.

Dental treatment: Regular teeth cleaning together with professional plaque removal are essential. X-rays are usually taken to make sure the disease is not affecting the bones.

Changing your toothbrush every three months is also important as worn brushes do not remove plaque well.

Antibiotics: These are sometimes used to treat gingivitis in addition to plaque removal. Penicillin or clindamycin is the usual treatment.

Supplements: Make sure you take the recommended daily amount of vitamin C and D. Adults can take 500 mg of vitamin C and 400–1,000 IU of vitamin D to help improve gingivitis.

Traditional Chinese Medicine

To treat gingivitis effectively, a TCM diagnosis is important. If a patient with gingivitis also has an elevated temperature, bad breath, severely infected gums, and is thirsty, the pathogen is excessive heat.

Herbs:
• Herbal decoction: Combine 10 g of Jing Jie (schizonepeta stem and bud), 12 g of Lian Qiao (forsythia fruit), 12 g of Tian Hua Fen (trichosanthes root), 12 g of Fang Fen (ledebouriella root), and 10 g of Jin Yin Hua (honeysuckle flower) in a ceramic pot with 3 cups of water. Bring to a boil and simmer for 30 minutes. Strain the liquid and drink 1 cup two to three times a day for 10–15 days.
• Herbal decoction: To make this decoction, use the same method described above, but substitute the following herbs: 10 g of Huang Qin (baical skullcap root), 6 g Huang Lian

(coptis root), 12 g Dan Pi (cortex of tree peony root), 10 g Zhi Zi (cape jasmine fruit), and 12 g of Niu Bang Zi (great burdock fruit).

• **Chronic gingivitis:** If the infection in the gums is persistent and the patient is experiencing chronic bad breath, or yellowish-colored urine, this formula will help. Use the same method described above, but substitute the following herbs: 5 g of Huang Lian (coptis root), 12 g of Shu Di Huang (cooked Chinese foxglove), 12 g of Huang Bai (phellodendron), 15 g of Mu Gua (Chinese quince fruit), and 10 g of Zhi Zi (cape jasmine fruit).

• **Herbal tea:** Add 8 g of Jin Yin Hua (honeysuckle flower) and 6 g of Gan Cao (licorice root) to a teapot and add boiling water. Sip the tea throughout the day, but before swallowing swish the tea around and let it remain in your mouth for a few seconds to let the herbs clean the bacteria.

Acupressure: Pressing the Hegu and Di Chang points can be helpful as they are beneficial for dispelling heat and promoting local circulation. The Hegu points are located on the back of the hands between the thumb and first finger. The Di Chang point is found directly below the pupil of the eye beside the mouth. Press each point for one to two minutes twice a day.

Diet: Eat food that is cooling such as purslane, mung beans, lotus, lettuce, and mango.

Naturopathy

Diet: Avoid sugar and all refined carbohydrates. Sugar is known to contribute to gingivitis while weakening the immune system by decreasing white blood cell function. White blood cells are part of your body's "military" that defends against foreign substances. Eat a well-balanced diet that includes fresh fruits and vegetables, whole grains, legumes, and quality protein such as fish, lean chicken, or beans everyday. Eat plenty of green leafy vegetables for their high nutrient content, which will provide the nutrients required for a healthy immune system.

Tip: DENTAL HYGIENE

Take the time to brush teeth thoroughly and floss regularly. If you find dental floss difficult to master, try using slightly wider dental tape.

Supplements: Vitamin C with bioflavonoids can help check bleeding gums by contributing to the build up of collagen, a protein in the formation of gum tissue. In one study, administration of vitamin C plus flavonoids improved oral health in a group of people with gingivitis; there was less improvement, however, when vitamin C was given without flavonoids. Take 1,000 mg of vitamin C and 500 mg of flavonoids twice a day. Coenzyme Q10 (CoQ10) deficiency has been found in people that suffer from gingivitis. Some researchers believe this deficiency could interfere with the body's ability to repair damaged gum tissue. Take 60–100 mg of CoQ10 a day for at least eight weeks. Some studies have shown that a 0.1% solution of folic acid mouth rinse can reduce gum inflammation and bleeding caused by gingivitis. Use 5 ml of solution twice a day for 30–60 days, holding the solution in the mouth for one to five minutes before spitting it out. Zinc benefits oral health by stabilizing the gum membrane, increasing antioxidant activity, promoting collagen synthesis, inhibiting plaque growth, and numerous other immune activities. Take 15–30 mg of zinc in the picolinate form.

Herbs: Bloodroot contains properties that inhibit bacteria that breed in the mouth. Toothpastes and mouth rinses containing bloodroot should be used according to manufacturer's directions. A mouthwash combination that includes sage oil, peppermint oil, menthol, chamomile and myrrh tincture, clove oil, and caraway oil has been successfully used to treat gingivitis. Add 10 drops of some or all of the above to 1 cup of water to use as a mouth rinse two times in succession two to three times a day. Keep the solution in your mouth for 30 seconds when rinsing. Blueberries, hawthorn berries, and grapes are all rich sources of flavonoids and help repair gum tissue. Eat these as frequently as possible to supplement your diet.

Homeopathy

For the best outcome, the use of a homeopathic remedy must be combined with dental treatment. When neglected, gum disease can have serious consequences, eventually leading to the loss of teeth.

Prevention: Avoid sugary foods that can aggravate dental problems. Eat a minimum of five portions of fresh fruit and vegetables every day. Fresh, raw fruit and vegetables include antioxidant-rich nutrients that support the immune system in fighting infection.

Lycopodium: If gums are sensitive and there is an unpleasant taste in the mouth that may be bitter, musty, or sour, try using Lycopodium. The patient may experience cravings for sugary foods and drinks, and gums may bleed easily when touched or when the teeth are brushed.

Kreosotum: A useful remedy for treating spongy-looking, inflamed gums with a bluish tinge. When this remedy is indicated the teeth are likely to be of poor quality and breath may be sour. In addition, the lips may look inflamed and have a tendency to bleed easily.

Nitric ac: This remedy is helpful if the gums have taken on a swollen, flabby-looking appearance, while the teeth may be yellow-tinged and develop cavities easily. The tongue may also look furry and discolored, while the gums are subject to sharp, splintering pains.

Carbo veg: This is a possible choice if blood oozes slowly from the gums when the teeth are brushed. The action of chewing may also trigger pain, sensitivity, and discomfort, and this may be accompanied by a nasty taste in the mouth and bad breath. Teeth may also be sensitive to contact with hot and cold food or drinks.

Herbalism

Myrrh: Myrrh is often in tincture form. Because 90% alcohol is used to extract the resins in myrrh, the tincture is diluted in warm water before being used as a mouthwash. It has antiseptic and antibacterial properties, as well as being anti-inflammatory and vulnerary. Use as a mouthwash after brushing two to three times daily. Do not swallow, but do not rinse out of mouth after using.

Echinacea: This is also often used as part of a mouthwash. Use as a tincture, diluted in warm water three times daily, or prepare a root decoction by boiling 2 tsp in a mug of water for 10 minutes. Strain and use as a mouthwash after brushing two to three times daily. Echinacea may also be taken as capsules, decoction, or tincture to support the immune system.

Calendula: Again, as with myrrh, a 90% tincture contains the resin component, which is most useful to aid repair. This may most easily be available from your herbal medicine practitioner, as many health shops stock 25% tinctures. Use the tincture as a mouthwash by diluting 5–7 ml in ¼ cup of water and using after brushing (not before) three times daily. A blend may be made of calendula with echinacea and myrrh.

Periodontitus

Diagnosis

Periodontitis is a serious form of gum disease where severe inflammation of the gums is accompanied by erosion of the bone and ligaments that support the teeth. This can eventually lead to a tooth becoming loose in its socket and falling out. How quickly the disease progresses largely depends on the type of bacteria present and how well your body's natural defenses work against it. The main trigger for this condition is the build-up of plaque on teeth, so practicing good dental hygiene is the best way to avoid this particular type of gum disease. This includes cleaning your teeth regularly, flossing, and frequent check-ups at the dentist.

Symptoms

- Gums become red
- Gums become soft, shiny, and swollen
- Gums feel tender and sore
- Pain when brushing teeth
- Persistent bleeding from the gums, especially during brushing teeth
- Halitosis
- Painful to chew
- Toothache triggered by hot or cold foods or drinks
- Offensive taste in the mouth
- Wobbly, loose teeth

Treatment Goal

This condition is not easily cured. The aim of treatment is to prevent the disease from progressing further. Surgery may be required if the condition is advanced.

Conventional Medicine

Prevention: Good oral hygiene and a non-processed, sugar-free, relatively alkaline diet are essential in protecting against periodontitis. Adequate and high-quality dental work on a regular basis is also important. Keeping stress at bay by regular stress reduction techniques, such as meditation, lowers cortisol and enhances immune function; both of these are key in the prevention of periodontitis. Hormonal balance is also important, as periodontal disease is exacerbated during the premenstrual time. Smoking of any kind encourages periodontal disease. The severity and risk of the disease goes up in direct proportion with the number of cigarettes smoked. Poor antioxidant levels, particularly of vitamin C, is associated with the disease. At the first sign of disease, vitamin C should be supplemented in amounts of 500 mg a day. Coenzyme Q10 in amounts of 100 mg a day can slow periodontal disease, as does eating soy and avocado.

Treatment: Treatment depends on the progression of the disease. A focus on the bacteria that cause the problem is needed. For example, certain herpes viruses and varicella (chickenpox virus) are known causes of gingivitis, which precedes periodontitis. Treatment involves the removal of plaque in a dentist's office and a low dose of oral or topical antibiotics. Fluoride treatments discourage formation of plaque forming bacteria. Sometimes surgery is needed, which is done by a periodontist.

Traditional Chinese Medicine

Herbs:
• **Herbal decoction:** Mix 12 g of Huang Qin (baical skullcap root), 10 g of Jin Yin Hua (honeysuckle flower), 10 g of Da Qin Ye (woad leaf), 10 g of Chuang Xin Lian (green chiretta), 8 g of Lian Zi Xin (lotus flower), 10 g of Pu Gong Ying (dandelion), and 5 g of Gan Cao (licorice root) in 3–4 cups of water. Boil the combination in a ceramic pot for 30 minutes and then strain. Drink 1 cup of the liquid two to three times a day.

• **Qin Dai powder:** This patent formula reduces infection. Apply it to the inflammation area as indicated on the package, or consult the pharmacist about the usage.
• **Herbal powder:** Grind 6 g of dried ginger, 6 g of hard red dates, and 6 g of dried alum into a powder and apply over the affected area.

Acupressure: Press the Hegu points, located on the back of the hands between the thumb and first finger. Press the Di Cang point, directly below the pupil of the eye beside the nostril. Also press the Feng Chi point at the base of the skull 2 inches below the center point. Press each point for one to two minutes.

Diet: Foods that are good for this condition include purslane, mung beans, lotus, lettuce, mango, eggplant, spinach, strawberries, pears, red beans, flat beans, and coix.

Naturopathy

Diet: Avoiding sugar and all refined carbohydrates is extremely important. Sugar is known to contribute to dental problems, while weakening the immune system by decreasing white cell function. White blood cells help defend the body against foreign substances, such as bacteria. Eat a well-balanced diet that includes fresh fruits and vegetables, whole grains, legumes, and quality protein (such as fish, lean chicken, and beans) every day. Eat plenty of green leafy vegetables for their high nutrient content, which provides the foundation required for a healthy immune system. Blueberries, hawthorn berries, and grapes are all rich sources of flavonoids and help in repairing gum tissue. Eat these as frequently as possible.

Supplements: Vitamin C with bioflavonoids can help check bleeding gums by contributing in the build up of collagen, a protein involved in the formation of gum tissue. Take 1,000 mg of vitamin C and 500 mg of flavonoids twice a day. Some researchers believe that a deficiency in coenzyme Q10 (CoQ10) could interfere with the body's ability to repair damaged gum tissue. Take 60–100 mg a day for at least eight weeks. A 0.1% solution of folic acid in a mouth rinse is thought to reduce gum inflammation and bleeding. Use 5 ml twice a day for 30–60 days, rinsing the mouth with the solution for one to five minutes before spitting it out. Zinc stabilizes the gum membrane, increases antioxidant activity and collagen synthesis, and inhibits plaque growth; take 15–30 mg of the picolinate form.

Herbs: Bloodroot contains properties that inhibit oral bacteria. Use a toothpaste and mouthwash that contain bloodroot according to the manufacturer's directions. Make a mouthwash by combining 10 drops of some or all of the following: sage oil, peppermint oil, menthol, chamomile and myrrh tincture, clove oil, and caraway oil. Dilute these oils in 1 cup of water and rinse the mouth for 30 seconds twice in succession two to three times a day.

> *Tip:* BRUSH AND FLOSS
>
> Floss your teeth thoroughly twice a day. Studies show that an electric toothbrush can remove 98.2% of plaque; only 48.6% is removed through conventional brushing.

Homeopathy

Due to the nature of this condition, this is a problem that needs to be addressed by consultation with an experienced homeopath in combination with treatment from your dental specialist.

> *Tip:* MOUTH RINSE
>
> Make a mouth rinse with hydrogen peroxide (H2O2) in a 3% solution, mixed half-and-half with water, and swish it around your mouth for 30 seconds. Use this wash three times a week to inhibit bacteria, but do not swallow.

Herbalism

Due to the advanced nature of this disease, and the risk of permanent damage resulting in teeth removal, herbal therapy is not recommended as a first option for treatment. The suggestions listed below are beneficial as adjuncts to therapy provided by your dentist. It is also beneficial to support the immune system.

Myrhh: Use myrrh in tincture form. 90% alcohol is used to extract the resins in myrrh, which are particularly beneficial. Use the tincture diluted in warm water as a mouthwash after brushing two to three times daily. It has antiseptic and antibacterial properties, as well as being anti-inflammatory and vulnerary. Do not swallow, but do not rinse out of mouth after use.

Echinacea: This is also often used as a mouthwash. Use as a tincture, diluted in warm water three times daily, or prepare a root decoction by boiling 2 tsp in a cup of water for 10 minutes. Strain and use as a mouthwash after brushing two to three times daily. Echinacea may also be taken as capsules, decoction, or tincture, to support the immune system.

Calendula: Again, as with myrrh, a 90% tincture contains the resin component, which is beneficial to aid healing. This may most easily be available from your herbal medicine practitioner, as many health shops stock 25% tinctures. Use the tincture as a mouthwash by diluting 5-7 ml in ¼ cup of water and using after brushing (not before) three times daily. A blend may be made of calendula with echinacea, and myrrh.

Green tea: To treat periodontitis, prepare a strong infusion and use it as a mouthwash. Used in this manner there are virtually no side effects to green tea, although it does have the potential to further irritate the gums and can stain the teeth. Green tea is rich in polyphenol antioxidants which help to inhibit the growth of bacteria that cause periodontitis.

Oral Thrush

Diagnosis

Oral thrush, also know as candidosis or moniliasis, is an infection caused by the yeast fungus candida albicans. It establishes itself in the membranes that line the mouth and the throat. Many people have the candida yeast present in their mouths without necessarily suffering any ill effects. The condition does not manifest itself until there is a change in the delicate internal balance, making the environment ripe for infection. It is particularly likely to be present in those who wear false teeth, take antibiotics, suffer from diabetes, or have immune deficiencies as a consequence of poor nutrition. Newborns are also prone to outbreaks of oral thrush. The symptoms of thrush are similar to many other conditions, so it is important to have a thorough check-up by your doctor if you suspect you have oral thrush. Oral thrush is generally treated by antifungal medicines applied to the mouth. If whatever caused the thrush can be brought under control, the infection is likely to go away after a few days of treatment with a fungicide.

Symptoms

- Spots in the mouth that are white, cream, or yellow in color
- Occasionally, pale pinks spots on the lips
- A burning sensation in the mouth and throat
- Sensitivity in the mouth

Treatment Goal

To establish and remove the cause of the thrush to clear up the infection and prevent the condition from reoccurring.

Conventional Medicine

Oral thrush is caused by an overgrowth of the candida yeast, which is found normally on the skin and in the mouth. Certain environmental and physical factors can allow the colonization of the yeast to increase, resulting in an infection. This imbalance often occurs after taking certain antibiotics, as a side effect of using inhaled steroids (to treat asthma or an allergy), or in those with compromised immunity or who have experienced chronic trauma that has disrupted the body's delicate internal balance.

Prevention: Enhance the immune system by minimizing intake of sugar, yeasty foods, and high fructose foods such as fruit—substances upon which yeast thrives. Probiotics (at the billion or trillion colony-forming-unit quantity) and the probiotic saccharomyces boullardii

(which is found in Florastore) can discourage yeast. These may be taken daily by those prone to oral thrush, and should always be taken when prescribed antibiotics.

To treat an existing infection: Treat oral thrush with 1 ml of nystatin oral suspension (Mycostatin) four times daily or ketoconazole 2% cream (Nizoral) four times daily as a first step. Give 100 mg of systemic fluconazole (Diflucan) a day for 7–10 days or 200 mg of itraconazole (Sporanox) a day for 7–10 days if the oral suspension does not work. Liver enzymes should be taken if liver failure or incompetence is present, which is determined by a blood test.

Traditional Chinese Medicine

Herbal tea: Combine 8 g of Jin Yin Hua (honeysuckle flower), 5 g of Bo He (field mint), and 3 g of Gan Cao (licorice root) in a pot and add boiling water. Drink the tea three to four times a day, swishing it around and holding it in your mouth for a few seconds before swallowing. Young babies with oral thrush should drink 1–2 oz of tea two or three times a day.

Acupressure: Gently press the Di Cang point, which is found directly below the pupil of the eye above the cheekbone, and the Xia Guan

point, in front of the ear in the depression above the jawbone.

Diet: Mothers who are breastfeeding a baby with this condition should eat food that disperses dampness such as mung beans, red beans, flat beans, coix seeds, watermelon, and cucumber. Food that has a pungent flavor is also recommended, such as spring onions, garlic, pepper, and chilies. Hot and spicy foods should be eaten only in small amounts.

Naturopathy

Diet: To help control candida, eat chicken, eggs, fish, yogurt, vegetables, nuts, seeds, oils, and plenty of raw garlic. Increase your fiber intake to 1 tsp–1 tbsp of soluble fiber, containing guar gum, psyllium husks, flaxseeds, or pectin, mixed with 8 fl oz of water, drunk twice a day on an empty stomach. Eliminate refined and simple sugars, including white or brown sugar, raw sugar, honey, molasses, or grain sweeteners. The sugar substitute stevia is allowed. Avoid milk, alcohol, fruit or dried fruit, and mushrooms. Avoid foods that contain yeast or mold, including all breads, muffins, cakes, baked goods, cheese, dried fruits, melons, and peanuts.

Supplements: Take 1,000 mg of caprylic acid, a fatty acid that has been shown to have antifungal properties, three times a day.

> *Tip:* NEW TOOTHBRUSH
>
> Candida can collect on your toothbrush. Change your toothbrush monthly to avoid reinfecting yourself.

Vitamin C, taken at a dose of 1,000 mg twice a day, helps to enhance immune function. Take a high-potency multivitamin to obtain many nutrients that will help support immune function. Take probiotics with about four billion micro-organisms twice daily 30 minutes before each meal. These micro-organisms provide acidophilus and bifidus, which are friendly bacteria that prevent yeast overgrowth and fight candida. Take 200 mg of grapefruit seed extract two to three times a day for its anti-candida properties.

Herbs: Take 500 mg of garlic twice a day to fight the fungus and boost the immune system. Take 200 mg of grapefruit seed extract twice a day for its antifungal properties. Undecylenic acid, a derivative from castor bean oil, has been shown to have strong antifungal activity; take 200 mg three times a day. Drink 2 cups of Pau d'Arco tea a day, which also has strong antifungal properties. Take 250–500 mg of barberry a day for its antimicrobial and antifungal properties. Tea tree oil had anti-yeast properties and can be used as a mouth wash. Mix 15 drops in water and swish it around in your mouth two to three times a day.

Homeopathy

Any of the following homeopathic options can be helpful in speeding up recovery from a recently developing bout of oral thrush. In cases of an ongoing tendency to develop problems with oral thrush at regular intervals, more professional homeopathic support will be appropriate. The practitioner will be able to prescribe at a level that aims to eradicate the underlying tendency in the system that leaves it vulnerable to candida overgrowth.

Natrum mur: If oral thrush is accompanied by a tendency to develop dry, cracked lips and sore corners of the mouth, consider using Natrum mur. Contact with heat intensifies distress, while cool things are soothing.

Kali mur: When this remedy is appropriate, there is a "mapped," patchy appearance to the tongue, which is coated with a white or gray film. The gums of breastfeeding babies may

also take on a whitish tinge. Symptoms are worse during the night and for becoming overheated. Rubbing the affected area and contact with cool things provides temporary relief.

Mercurius: If oral thrush leads to noticeably bad breath and increased saliva to the point of drooling, use Mercurius. Confirmatory symptoms include a flabby-looking tongue that becomes imprinted by the teeth in older children.

Herbalism

Garlic: Fresh cloves of garlic are most effective in treating yeast infections. However, a garlic tincture, oil, or capsule may be recommended by your herbal expert.

Thyme: This is a potent antifungal, antibacterial, and anti-inflammatory herb that

also has antioxidant properties. A few drops of the essential oil diluted in ½ tsp of olive oil can be placed on the patches of thrush daily.

Oregano oil: This oil eradicates yeast on the membrane of the mouth. A few drops of the oil should be diluted with ½ tsp of olive oil. Oregano and thyme exhibit more potent antifungal activity when used together.

Goldenseal: The alkaloids berberine and hydrastine, which are effective against yeast and bacteria, can be found in goldenseal. This bitter herb has a healing effect on all mucosal tissues. A herbal medicine practitioner will advise on its usage. Choose cultivated goldenseal rather than goldenseal harvested from the wild, which is endangered.

> *Tip:* AVOID ACIDIC FOODS
>
> Since the mouth is likely to be sore and sensitive, especially in babies and toddlers who suffer from oral thrush, avoid giving any foods that are too hot or acidic. Instead give foods and drinks that are cool, bland, and as nutritious as possible. Let your child drink with a straw if possible as this can make drinking feel more comfortable.

Toothache

Diagnosis

Toothache usually indicates that something is wrong in your mouth, and the first thing to do is visit the dentist. The most common causes of toothache are an abscess, dental decay, inflammation of the tooth pulp, a damaged tooth, an exposed tooth root, or irritation following dental treatment. Other triggers include an ulceration or inflammation of the gum caused by conditions such as gingivitis, periodontitis, and sinusitis. The best way to prevent toothache is to make sure your teeth and gums are healthy. Try to reduce your intake of sugary foods and drinks, brush your teeth regularly using a toothpaste containing fluoride, and make sure you floss as often possible. Visit your dentist regularly so that any problems can be detected early.

Symptoms

- Continuous or intermittent throbbing pain
- Raised temperature
- Pain above and below the gum level
- Chewing becomes painful
- Swollen gums
- Earache and swelling on one side of the face
- Swelling in the neck
- Pain in the face
- Sinusitis
- Difficulty eating

Treatment Goal

To identify the cause of the toothache, relieve any immediate pain, and prevent any future problems from developing. Most cases of toothache require the attention of a dentist.

Conventional Medicine

Toothache is not a condition in itself, but a symptom of another disease. Conventional medicine aims at diagnosing the cause of the toothache and treating the underlying problem. In the interim, take pain relief, such as 800 mg of ibuprofen three times a day, as needed (but for a short period of time only).

Prevention Preventing toothache involves rigorous oral hygiene, including daily flossing, proper brushing, and avoiding sugar and processed foods in your diet. Maintaining good oral flora with probiotics is also helpful. Look for a product with colony-forming units of bifidus in the billions. Adequate amounts of vitamin C (500 mg a day) and CoQ10 (120 mg of an oil-based product a day) can help maintain gum health. To keep your teeth in good condition, regular dental examinations are also crucial, particularly during high-risk times such as childhood and middle age.

When should I see a dentist? A dentist should be your first port of call if toothache develops. The most common cause of toothache is tooth decay, which if not addressed can lead to further problems such as a bacterial infection of the tooth pulp and irritation of the nerve of the tooth. Treatment requires dental work. Other common causes are a fracture or crack in the tooth, gum disease, overuse (grinding or gum chewing), or a damaged filling. Ask your dentist for an examination to locate the problem. Generally, you can wait until the next available appointment unless there is an unpleasant-smelling discharge or fever accompanying the toothache, in which case you will need an emergency appointment.

Traditional Chinese Medicine

Herbs:
• Herbal decoction: Combine 15 g of Shi Gao (gypsum), 15 g of Sheng Di Huang (Chinese foxglove root), 6 g Sheng Ma (bugbane rhizome), 10 g Huang Qin (scutellaria root), 10 g of Dan Pi (cortex of tree peony root), and 5 g of Huang Lian (coptis root) in a ceramic or glass pot. Add 3–4 cups of water, bring to a boil, and simmer for 30 minutes before straining it. Drink 1 cup three times a day.
• Herbal tea: Place 12 g of Bai Zhi (angelica dahurica) and 10 g of Wu Zhu Yu (evodia fruit) in a teapot and add 3–4 cups of boiling water to make a herbal tea that will cleanse the mouth. Drink the tea throughout the day, but swish it around and hold it in your mouth for a few seconds before swallowing to let the herbs cleanse the bacteria.
• Ya Tong Shan (toothache powder) or watermelon frost: These two patent formulas are herbal mixtures in powder form. Apply the powder three to four times a day to the area

that is causing you pain. If after using these formulas for one to two days you do not get any relief from the pain or infection, see your dentist.

Acupressure: Press the Hegu points, located on the back of the hands between the thumb and first finger, and the Jia Che point, found on the cheek in the depression above the jawbone, with strong pressure for one minute two to three times a day.

Diet: Foods that cleanse heat, such as mung beans, red beans, flat beans, coix seeds, watermelon, and cucumber, are recommended. Avoid food that is hot and spicy.

Naturopathy

Clove oil: Make a compress of clove oil, which contains eugenol, a natural painkiller and antibacterial. Mix 2–3 drops of pure clove oil with ¼ tsp of olive oil and apply the mixture with a cotton wool bud two to three times a day. You can also saturate a cotton wool ball with the mixture and place it inside the mouth beside the tooth.

Tip: CHECK-UPS

To keep your teeth in good condition, regular dental examinations are crucial, particularly during high-risk times such as childhood and middle age.

Homeopathy

The following homeopathic remedies can be used in the short term to relieve pain until you can see your dentist.

Hepar sulph: Use this remedy if toothache is combined with an excruciating sensitivity to the slightest draft of cold air. Pains are characteristically sharp and splinterlike, especially when associated with abscess formation.

Belladonna: This remedy tends to be most helpful when given at the first twinge of discomfort. Signature symptoms are throbbing, shooting, and piercing pains, and inflammation and redness around the affected gum. This remedy is most effective in treating pains that appear suddenly, violently, and dramatically.

Hypericum: Consider this remedy to relieve toothache that feels so intense it's intolerable. Pains are characteristically shooting, are made more intense by sudden, jarring movements, and are temporarily eased by lying quietly on the affected side.

Arnica: Once dental work has been done, Arnica, which reduces swelling, pain, tenderness, and bruising, can be used to ease traumatized tissues. Do not use Arnica after a wisdom tooth extraction: It has a very powerful potential for promoting reabsorption of blood from damaged tissue and can leave the patient vulnerable to developing a dry socket.

Herbalism

As the causes of toothaches are manifold, a dentist should always be consulted to address any potential infection or medical condition. The herbs recommended below are primarily to decrease swelling and pain, and facilitate healing of the tissue surrounding the tooth.

Witch hazel: This soothing antibacterial agent heals inflamed and infected mucous membrane tissue and decreases inflammation, blood flow, and pain. Your herbal medicine practitioner may recommend swishing a tincture around the mouth and letting it sit for two minutes before spitting it out. As the tannins in witch hazel can be irritating, it does not tend to be used long term.

Hops: This bitter herb has sedative and pain-relieving properties. Many people unknowingly consume this herb in its most common form: beer. Hops will relax you and decrease tissue swelling. It is best used as a tincture in water.

Chamomile: This can soothe the gum and calm inflammation. It is also gently calming. Use the infusion to drink, or topically to swish around the mouth.

Cloves: Clove oil is readily available, as are whole cloves as a dried spice. A couple of drops of the oil can be applied to a cotton bud and quickly run through water to dilute, before applying directly to the affected area of the gum one to two times daily. Watch for any signs of irritation, and halt use if this occurs. Alternatively, hold 1 whole clove in affected area of the mouth, two to three times daily as needed. It can be chewed a little, but take care not to bite down on the clove too hard and cause pain or injury.

Teething

Diagnosis

Teething is the process whereby a baby's teeth break through the gums. Children have around 20 milk or primary teeth, and usually have a complete set by the age of two. Babies usually start producing teeth when they are about five months old. Although some lucky babies seem to be untroubled by the teething process, there are many others who find it a painful experience. A baby's sleep may be disturbed and there will probably be quite a high level of irritability during the daytime, too. As the teeth emerge, your toddler may find comfort in gnawing on a cold object, such as a stick of raw carrot from the fridge. Sometimes a fever can occur during teething, but if it lasts for longer than two days consult your doctor, as your child may have an unrelated infection.

Symptoms

- Redness on the cheek on the side the tooth is coming through
- Dribbling
- A rash around the mouth
- Biting on anything
- Putting fist in mouth
- Inflammation of the gums
- Crying and irritability
- Clinginess
- Disturbed sleep
- Fever
- Upset stomach
- Loss of appetite
- Diaper rash

Treatment Goal

Teething is an inevitable part of a child's development, but there are many things that can be done to help ease the painful symptoms.

Conventional Medicine

Teething is a normal process of development that all babies go through. A high fever is not usually a symptom of teething, but a slight temperature elevation can occur.

Non-pharmaceutical treatment: Try to comfort and reassure your baby. A cold teething ring can provide relief, as can cool drinks and gels that numb the gums. Do not use a pacifier dipped into honey, sweet drinks, or alcohol. Do not give your baby freezing items to suck on, as they can damage gum tissue.

Over-the-counter medications: Children's pain relief should always be given in the correct dosage as labeled.

When should I consult a doctor?: If your baby has a fever of over 100.5°F, severe diarrhea, lethargy, or unremitting screaming, and a complete loss of appetite such that fluids are not consumed for three or more hours during the day, speak to your doctor. These symptoms may indicate a more serious condition.

Traditional Chinese Medicine

Herbs: Chinese herbal medicine is not appropriate for treating teething.

Acupressure: Press the Hegu point, located on the back of the hand between the thumb and first finger, for one minute. Press the Xia Guan point, which is found in front of the ear in the depression above the jawbone, for one minute.

Diet: Mothers who are breastfeeding should avoid food that is warm and spicy such as ginger, pepper, chilies, cloves, leeks, mussels, beef, mutton, and coriander.

Naturopathy

Teething is a natural process and cannot be prevented, but pain can be minimized by following the remedies below.

Herbs: Chamomile helps relax the child's nervous system before going to bed. Give your child a cup of chamomile tea in the evening before bedtime. Do not use this remedy if your child is allergic to ragweed, the symptoms of which are a skin rash, watery eyes, and excess mucus in the nasal passages. Clove oil acts as a general anesthetic. Blend 1 drop of clove oil with 1–2 drops of olive oil. Using your fingertips or a cotton bud, gently massage the mixture onto your child's gums. This application should be used in moderation as directed above as excessive amounts can cause blistering.

Homeopathy

The results from treating teething homeopathically can seem miraculous. When an appropriate homeopathic remedy is given, your child should become calmer, less fractious, and less distressed very quickly. Since distress with teething tends to be intermittent, make sure you have the remedy that most often works for your child in the medicine cabinet, so it can be administered at the first signs of pain. The appropriate remedy should both reduce localized inflammation and pain, and have an emotionally soothing effect.

Belladonna: This remedy will help reduce pain and inflammation that occurs rapidly and dramatically, making your child hot and bothered and very irritable. Use Belladonna if there is a general state of feverishness and if your child's skin looks flushed, red, and dry, and feels very hot to the touch. Symptoms are also likely to be restricted to, or be more intense on, the right side, with possible associated earache.

Chamomilla: If your child is beside themselves and frantic with pain, and has one flushed and one pale cheek, consider Chamomilla as a possible remedy. Temper tantrums associated with teething pains reach such a crescendo that any toys offered in an effort to pacify the child get hurled to the floor.

Herbalism

Chamomile: An infusion may be made by steeping 1–2 tsp in a cup of freshly boiled water. Cover the cup and infuse for 10 minutes. Strain and soak a cloth in the infusion to dab on infant's gums. This infusion will help to sooth and calm the inflammation.

Tip: CHEWING RELIEF

Giving teething infants something hard to bite on, such as a rubber teething ring or a hard biscuit, helps to balance the pressure exerted by an emerging tooth. A cold flannel is also comforting for teething children to bite on.

Sensitive Teeth

Diagnosis

Sensitive teeth are a common problem. Teeth are covered by a protective layer of enamel. When this is eroded, the cavities underneath become exposed and sensitive. Tooth decay, an abscess, or gum disease—including conditions such as gingivitis (see p. 100) and periodontitis (see p. 105)—can leave the roots of teeth exposed, leading to pain and sensitivity. Another trigger could be a cavity that needs filling, or a filling that needs repairing. More general sensitivity is often triggered by everyday substances, such as hot and cold food or drinks. Aching teeth can also be caused by poor brushing technique, such as using a toothbrush with bristles that are too hard. If your teeth are causing you pain and discomfort, make an appointment to see your dentist to get checked out for any underlying disease that could be causing you problems.

Symptoms

- Sudden shooting pains in teeth when eating hot or cold food or drinking hot or cold drinks
- A dull aching sensation in teeth or gums

Treatment Goal

To determine the underlying causes of the pain and resolve them to bring relief from the discomfort.

Conventional Medicine

Sensitive teeth is not a disease in itself but a symptom of a larger problem. Conventional medicine aims to diagnose and treat the cause. For immediate alleviation of pain while the cause is being sought, non-steroidal anti-inflammatory drugs are prescribed, which can be obtained over the counter.

If an infection is present: The doctor will carry out a history, examination, and laboratory tests to determine whether the tooth pain is infectious and what is most likely to be the cause. Infections of the sinuses, inner ear, and teeth can all cause sensitivity in teeth. A sinus infection is treated with a 14-day course of antibiotics. An ear infection is treated with a seven-day course of antibiotics. A tooth infection should be treated by a dentist.

If headaches are present: Headaches can cause teeth pain, particularly migraines. Generally the migraine would have other symptoms as well, with head pain being the most obvious. To relieve pain in the teeth, treat the migraine (see p. 343).

If hypothyroidism is present: Hypothyroidism is another illness that can include among its symptoms generalized sensitivity of the teeth, although this is an unusual cause of dental pain. To treat sensitive teeth, treatment of the thyroid hormone deficiency is needed.

Treating children: Normal growth and development in children includes a stage of teeth eruption, which causes pain. This can be treated with symptomatic pain relievers, such as children's Tylenol® or Motrin®.

Traditional Chinese Medicine

TCM approaches sensitive teeth by treating pathogenic heat and wind. The condition is normally caused by excess stomach heat.

Herbs:
• Internal decoction: Add 15 g of Shi Gao (gypsum), 15 g of Sheng Di Huang (Chinese foxglove root), 6 g of Sheng Ma (bugbane rhizome), 10 g of Huang Qin (scutellaria root), 10 g of Dan Pi (cortex of tree peony root), and 5 g of Huang Lian (coptis root) to 3–4 cups of water in a ceramic pot. Bring to a boil, simmer for 30 minutes, and then strain the liquid. Drink 1 cup two to three times a day.

• Herbal tea: Combine 10 g of Bai Zhi (angelica dahurica), and 10 g of Wu Zhu Yu (evodia fruit) in a ceramic pot. Add 3 cups of water and boil for 20 minutes. Drink throughout the day, but before swallowing, swish the tea around your mouth for a while to allow the herbs to have the maximum effect.
• Watermelon frost: Safe to use in the mouth, watermelon frost cleans out the heat in the teeth and calms sensitivity. Spray the fine powder on the surface of the sensitive area.

Acupressure: Press the Xia Guan point, located in front of the ear in the depression above the jawbone, the Jia Che point, found on the cheek in the depression in front of where the jawbone turns at the back, and the Di Cang point, directly below the pupil of the eye beside the mouth angle, for one minute. Repeat two to three times a day, washing your hands before each treatment.

Diet: Eat foods that are cooling, such as mung beans, lotus, lettuce, mango, cucumber, aubergine, spinach, strawberries, and pears. Avoid foods that are hot and spicy.

TIP: EAT RICE PORRIDGE

If your teeth are highly sensitive to cold and hot, try eating rice porridge, which contains cooling properties and has a mild taste. Add 100 g of rice to 1,000 ml of water. Cook the rice in plain water until it is soft. Eat the porridge as part of a meal.

Naturopathy

Diet: Good dietary habits are the first step towards overall healthy teeth and treating sensitive teeth naturopathically. Avoiding sugar and all refined carbohydrates is important. Sugar is known to contribute to teeth and gum problems by feeding bacteria surrounding your teeth, which decrease white blood cell function. White blood cells are part of your body's "military" that defends you against foreign substances. Eat a balanced diet that includes fresh fruits and vegetables, whole grains, legumes, and quality protein (such as fish, lean chicken, and beans) every day. Eat plenty of green leafy vegetables for their high nutrient content to provide a base of nutrients required for a healthy immune system. Do not eat acidic foods or sweets. Lemons, tomatoes, and other foods with a high acid content can eat away at your tooth enamel and hinder your teeth's natural healing process. For some people, eating sweets causes a flare-up of pain. Serve hot or cold foods at temperatures close to room temperature, and try to avoid biting into foods of different temperature extremes at the same sitting.

TIP: ADOPT A GOOD BRUSHING TECHNIQUE

Brush your teeth using a gentle up and down motion, and be careful when brushing close to the gum line, which is where most sensitivity occurs. Bad brushing can not only cause hypersensitivity, it can undo all of nature's repair work. Use a soft-bristle brush, as stiff, hard brushes can scrape and strip away enamel and cause gums to recede, especially in those who use excessive pressure when brushing. Softer bristles are less likely to irritate sensitive teeth and will not expose underlying nerves.

Supplements: Nutritional supplements that help with periodontal problems can be helpful in treating sensitive teeth. Vitamin C with bioflavonoids can help treat gum disease by contributing to the building of collagen, a protein that is important in the formation of gum tissue. Take 1,000 mg of vitamin C and 500 mg of flavonoids twice a day. Coenzyme Q10 (CoQ10) deficiency has been found in people with gum disease. Some researchers believe this deficiency could interfere with the body's ability to repair damaged gum tissue. Take 60–100 mg of CoQ10 a day for at least eight weeks. Some studies show that folic acid in a 0.1% solution used as a mouth rinse has reduced gum inflammation and bleeding. Rinse the mouth with 5 ml of solution, available from health food stores, twice a day for one to five minutes for 30–60 days. Zinc stabilizes the gum membrane, increases antioxidant activity, promotes collagen synthesis, inhibits plaque growth, and performs numerous immune activities. Take 15–30 mg of the picolinate form a day.

Homeopathy

Your dentist should be able to identify the reason for undue sensitivity in your teeth. Once you have established the cause of the problem, one of the following homeopathic remedies may be helpful in easing pain and sensitivity when used in the short term.

Chamomilla: If teeth become sensitive to warm food and drinks, or when breathing in the cold night air, consider using Chamomilla. Pain and discomfort may cause a tantrumlike reaction, to the point of using abusive language to vent feelings.

Staphysagria: For poor-quality, sensitive teeth that show signs of decay, this remedy may be used. It is well indicated if hypersensitivity of the teeth is aggravated or brought on by eating or during a menstrual period. Applying heat and pressure helps to ease the pain.

Pulsatilla: This may be a helpful remedy if hot food and drinks make sensitivity more intense, and if pain is relieved by contact with cool things. Symptoms include a dry mouth without thirst and a white-coated tongue. Another key symptom is a tendency to burst into floods of tears when in pain and discomfort, with a need for sympathy and attention.

Coffea: Use this remedy if there is a huge intolerance to pain that feels insupportable. Sensitive teeth are soothed by the cooling sensation of ice water in the mouth.

> ### *TIP:* DAILY TOOTHPASTE
>
> If you know your teeth have a tendency to become sensitive, use a toothpaste that has been specially formulated with this problem in mind. However, you will need to use it on a regular basis in order to reap the cumulative benefits.

Herbalism

Cloves: These can be processed to extract an oil called eugenol, which can be used as a pain reliever and local anesthetic. Traditional therapies for teething babies have included clove oil due to these properties, but it is no longer recommended for use by those under 2 years of age. Apply 2 drops of clove oil to a cotton bud and use this to apply the oil directly on the sensitive tooth four to six times a day. If the oil causes a burning sensation, discontinue use. There is also the potential for an allergic reaction inside the mouth.

Chamomile: There is some suggestion that a chamomile tea gargle may work well to relieve sensitive teeth. A strong infusion may be recommended as a mouthwash.

3

Ears, Nose, and Throat

Common Cold

Diagnosis

Colds affect everyone at one time or another, especially during the winter months, and it is usual to get at least two a year. A cold, one of the most common ailments, can be caused by over 200 different types of virus. The cold virus is contracted by breathing in infected droplets that have been coughed or sneezed into the atmosphere, or by picking up germs on your hands then transferring them to your nose or mouth. The virus can survive outside the body for three hours, so it is easy to see why it is so virulent. The infection manifests in the mucous membranes in the nose and upper respiratory tract, causing them to swell and produce even more mucus. Older people and those who don't maintain a healthy diet are more at risk. Pre-schoolers with immature immune systems also tend to suffer repeated infections until they have built up a stronger immunity by being exposed to constant infections. Triggers and irritants include lifestyle issues, such as being rundown, tired, or stressed.

Symptoms

- Feeling under the weather
- Aching joints and feeling shivery
- Sore throat and swollen glands
- Runny nose
- Stuffed-up nose
- Sneezing
- Running watery eyes
- Difficulty breathing
- Tickly cough from mucus running down the throat
- Congestion and popping in the ears
- Slight fever
- Lack of appetite
- Tiredness and irritability

Treatment Goal

There is no cure for the common cold. Antibiotics are of no use in treatment, nor are there any effective antiviral drugs available yet. Treatment aims to alleviate the symptoms.

Conventional Medicine

The medical name for a cold is an upper respiratory tract infection and it is caused by something called a rhinovirus.

Prevention: Frequent hand washing is of paramount importance in preventing the virus from spreading. Vitamin C, zinc, and immune-stimulating plants such as echinacea, larch arabinogalactans, and reishi mushrooms are good daily supplements to give during the cold season.

Nasal decongestants: Use a saline nasal spray to prevent the build-up of mucus and nasal obstruction. Using a gentle decongestant such as Neo-Synephrine® or Afrin® for about three days can provide relief, but should be avoided by anyone with a history of cardiac or blood pressure problems, as well as anxiety disorders.

If a cough is present: Dextromethorphan may be effective for a limited period. This should not be taken by children less than five years of age or by anyone with asthma.

Traditional Chinese Medicine

Herbs:
• Gan Mao Lin: This Chinese patent herbal pill will help deal with the common cold. Three to four pills can be taken three times a day.
• Herbal decoction: To treat a severe cold, combine 12 g of Ban Lan Gen (isatis root), 12 g of Lian Qiao (forsythia fruit), 12 g of Niu Bang Zi (great burdock fruit seed), 8 g of Bo He (field mint), 10 g of Huang Qin (scutellaria root), and 6 g of Gan Cao (licorice root) in a ceramic pot. Add 3–4 cups of water and bring to the boil. Lower the heat and let the mixture simmer for 30 minutes. Strain the liquid and let cool. Drink 1 cup three times a day for three to five days or until symptoms subside.

Acupressure: Pressing the Feng Chi, Tai Yang, and Hegu acupressure points will help relieve symptoms such as headaches and congestion. The Feng Chi point is located at the back of the head at the base of the skull, 2 inches below the center point. The Tai Yang point is found at the temple, in the depression between the lateral end of the eyebrow and the eyelid. Press and release these points with your thumb, beginning with gentle pressure and gradually increasing, about 20 times. Use the tip of your thumb to press the Hegu point, located on the back of the hand between the thumb and first finger, with strong pressure for one to two minutes.

Diet: Soft and liquid foods such as watery porridge, noodles, lotus rhizome powder, and fresh vegetables are recommended. Avoid greasy food and seafood.

Naturopathy

Diet: It is important to stay hydrated by drinking plenty of water, freshly squeezed juices, and herbal teas to cleanse your body of toxins and keep the respiratory tract from drying out. Include in your diet lots of fresh fruit and vegetables, and light foods consisting of steamed vegetables, freshly made vegetable soups, and broth. Add garlic, ginger, and onions, which are tonifying spices that have antimicrobial and warming properties, to chicken soup. Avoid milky and mucus-forming foods such as cheese, yogurt, red meat, dairy, and simple carbohydrates.

Tip: NASAL RELIEF

Place peppermint oil or eucalyptus oil just under the nostrils several times a day to relieve nasal congestion.

Supplements: While symptoms last, take 500–1,000 mg of vitamin C every four hours to support the immune system. Take 1,000 mg of bioflavonoids a day in divided doses. Bioflavonoids work synergistically with vitamin C and have immune-enhancing properties. Take 25 mg of zinc in lozenge form every two waking hours for one week for its antiviral properties.

Herbs: Try drinking peppermint, eucalyptus, and chamomile tea three times a day. Add cayenne to stimulate the circulation, cinnamon for its gentle warming effect, or grated ginger root to induce sweating.

Aromatherapy: Steam inhalations can loosen thick mucus. Add 5–10 drops of eucalyptus, lavender, peppermint, pine, thyme, or tea tree oil, or a combination of these oils, to a bowl of steaming hot water. Cover your head with a towel, place it over the bowl, and inhale.

Homeopathy

A well-indicated remedy may shorten the duration of infection and prevent complications of sinus or chest infections.

Aconite: Useful for treating a cold that develops abruptly after exposure to dry, cold winds. Aconite is best taken at the first onset of symptoms. Try Aconite if you feel well when going to bed but wake in the early hours feeling restless, fearful, and feverish. The throat is likely to feel hot and dry with a marked thirst.

Belladonna: Most effective when taken in the earliest stage of a cold, Belladonna is useful when symptoms include feeling unwell with a high fever and flushed, dry skin that radiates heat. The throat will also feel hot and inflamed, making it uncomfortable to swallow liquids. Earache may also develop, often worse on the right side.

Nux vomica: If cold symptoms make you feel hungover, especially on waking, use Nux vomica. Symptoms include a runny nose during the day and an uncomfortably dry nose at night. Being indoors makes the nose feel uncomfortably stuffed up, while taking a walk in the open air makes it run.

Arsenicum album: Consider this remedy if there are generalized burning sensations in the nose and throat that are soothed by contact with warmth. Symptoms include scanty, clear, nasal discharge that makes the nostrils feel sore and raw, and a dry, tight cough that is more persistent while lying flat in bed.

Although exhausted when feeling ill, patients will be anxious if their surroundings aren't neat and organized.

Natrum mur: Where the nose alternates between being dry and blocked and running profusely, try Natrum mur. Nasal discharge is made worse by sneezing bouts. Cold sores and dry lips may also be present.

Herbalism

Andrographis: This bitter antiviral herb is high in antioxidants. Andrographis stimulates the immune system to fight the cold while improving digestion and detoxifying the liver, thus protecting the body from harmful toxins due to infection. Because of its cold, bitter properties, andrographis is best taken with "warm" herbs such as ginger and astragalus. Studies have been carried out that have focused on the reduction in length and severity of the common cold when it is used.

Elderflower: Where there is much catarrh, elderflower is indicated for its mucolytic properties. Steep 2 tsp of elderflowers in a cup of freshly boiled water. Cover and infuse for 10 minutes. Drink 3 cups daily. A syrup of elderberries is readily available from health food stores and herbal practitioners. Elderberry is naturally rich in vitamin C and helps to support the immune system.

Lemon balm: Effective for a cold that causes restlessness, anxiety, insomnia, and headache associated with stress, lemon balm's sedative, antiviral, antispasmodic, and carminative (soothing and anti-flatulent) qualities ensure healing and relaxation. Infuse 2 tsp of leaves in 1 cup of water and drink before bed.

Astragalus: The flavonoids, polysaccharides, and saponins in astragalus enhance immunity by increasing antioxidant activity and the destruction of the offending virus. Boil 2 tsp of root in 1 cup of water for 20 minutes. Drink this tea, or take 3 ml of tincture, once a day.

Thyme: Effective for colds due to its antiviral properties, thyme may be used as an infusion by steeping ½ tsp in a cup of freshly boiled water for 10 minutes. Drink ⅓ cup two to three times daily.

Ear Infection

Diagnosis

The middle ear is the most common place for an ear infection to occur. Colds, sinus conditions, and throat infections cause the eustachian tubes (drainage canals running from the ear to the nose and throat) to become blocked, meaning that mucus is unable to drain. Middle ear infections can result in intense earache and fever. Occasionally hearing is affected, and sometimes the eardrum will burst, releasing a thick yellow matter. This will eventually heal on its own. Known as swimmer's ear, the outer ear can also become inflamed causing pain, discharge, and loss of hearing. Inner ear infections are generally caused by a virus, usually related to a cold or flu.

Symptoms

- Pain in the ear
- Pulling or rubbing at the ears
- May feel dizzy
- Discharge from the ear
- Raised temperature and fever
- Loss of hearing on the affected side
- Swollen glands and tonsils

Treatment Goal

Treatment is aimed at easing the pain and clearing up any existing infection.

Conventional Medicine

An adult who has experienced more than one case of ear infection should ask their doctor to refer them for a specialist ear, nose, and throat (ENT) evaluation. Generally, most uncomplicated cases will resolve themselves without antibiotics.

Tip: CONSULT A DOCTOR

There are several different types of ear infection. Consult a doctor to diagnose the condition before beginning treatment. It is important to get a proper diagnosis if pain continues for more than 24 hours or if there is any loss of hearing.

General recommendations: Drink plenty of fluids to remain hydrated. Decongestants may be used to encourage the mucus to drain through the eustachian tube. Avoid any substance that may be contributing to the inflammation, such as smoke or specific individual allergens.

Antibiotics: If the infection does not resolve itself within two to three days, amoxicillin is prescribed. Some bacteria are resistant to amoxicillin, so if there is no improvement after three days, a broader spectrum antibiotic, such as augmentin, is prescribed. Treatment generally lasts for 10–14 days.

Traditional Chinese Medicine

Herbs: For each formula, mix the herbs in a ceramic pot and add 3–4 cups of water. Bring the mixture to a boil and simmer for 30 minutes. Strain the liquid and drink 1 cup two to three times a day.
• Acute stage of ear infection: Combine 10 g of Jin Yin Hua (honeysuckle flower), 12 g of Lian Qiao (forsythia fruit), 2 g of Jie Geng (balloon flower root), 6 g of Bo He (field mint), 12 g of Niu Bang Zi (great burdock fruit seed), 12 g of Lu Gen (reed rhizome), 10 g of Jing Jie (schizonepeta stem and bud), and 10 g of Xia Ku Cao (common self-heal fruit-spike).

• Acute ear infection with a ruptured ear drum: If symptoms such as ear discharge, fever, ear pain, and hearing loss occur, mix 10 g of Jin Yin Hua (honeysuckle flower), 10 g Ye Ju Hua (wild chrysanthemum flower), 10 g of Pu Gong Ying (dandelion), 10 g of Zi Hua Di Ding (Yedeon's violet), and 12 g of Zhi Zi (cape jasmine fruit).

• Chronic ear infection: If ringing in the ear or loss of hearing occurs, mix 12 g of Jin Yin Hua (honeysuckle flower), 12 g of Zao Jiao Ci (spine of the Chinese honey locust fruit), 12 g Dang Gui (Chinese angelica), 10 g of Chai Hu (hare's ear root), and 10 g of Bai Zhi (angelica dahurica).

Acupressure: The Xia Guan point is located in front of the ear, in the depression above the jawbone. The Yi Feng point is situated just behind the ear lobe. The Er Men point is found in front of the notch on the forward edge of the ear. Press these points using gentle to medium pressure to reduce the pain in the ear and assist healing.

Diet: Food that has clearing heat properties is recommended, such as mung beans, red beans, watermelon, cucumber, grapefruit, and bananas.

Naturopathy

Diet: Avoid common food allergens, including wheat, eggs, dairy foods, corn, citrus, and peanuts, especially with chronic cases of ear infection. While suffering from an ear infection, avoid simple carbohydrates such as sugar, honey, biscuits, sweets, ice cream, carbonated beverages, chocolate, dried fruits, and fruit juices. To help prevent babies from developing allergies, breastfeed for as long as possible. Breastfeeding mothers should also avoid food allergens. Introduce new foods carefully to babies, watching to see if a reaction occurs. Wheat, eggs, and dairy foods should not be introduced to babies in the first nine months of life. Babies can drink diluted fruit juices instead of milk or in conjunction with a non-dairy formula.

Supplements: Vitamin C supplementation reportedly stimulates immune function; take 500 mg and 1,000 mg a day in separate doses. Reduce the dose if you notice diarrhea. Zinc supplements have also been reported to increase immune function. Adults should take 25 mg per day, and children should take lower amounts. For example, a 30 lb child might be given 5 mg of zinc per day while suffering from an ear infection. Vitamin A supports immunity. You can give a child up to six years of age 2,000–5,000 IU of vitamin A a day to support immunity. You should be able to find this in liquid form.

Herbs: Larix enhances immune function and also has antimicrobial activity. Dissolve 1–2 tsp in a non-dairy formula, or in water for older children or adults. Echinacea and goldenseal enhance immune function and have antimicrobial properties. Children should take 2 ml four times a day or as directed on the bottle. Thymus extract supports immune function. Take 50 mg per pound of weight a day. Mix St. John's wort oil with garlic oil to relieve ear pain and reduce infection. Place two warm drops of oil in the affected ear twice a day then gently place a cotton ball in the ear. Do not use this treatment if the ear is perforated.

Homeopathy

An appropriate homeopathic remedy can reduce distress and pain, and encourage the healing process of a one-off, mild episode of ear infection. Recurrent ear infections (especially if they are severe in nature) will require treatment from a homeopathic practitioner.

Belladonna: Use this remedy at the first sign of inflammation. Belladonna is effective in easing localized inflammation accompanied by throbbing pains. Symptoms may be restricted to or worse on the right side, with the glands becoming inflamed and swollen in sympathy with affected ear.

Aconite: Use this at the first sign of inflammation that follows exposure to dry, cold, and windy weather. Pains come on suddenly and dramatically and wake the sufferer from sleep. When this remedy is well indicated there is a hypersensitivity to pain, with a tendency to react by becoming fearful and fractious. There may also be an uncharacteristic sensitivity to noise (music in particular), which feels painful to sensitive ears.

Hepar sulph: Use this remedy to treat a later stage of infection, where pains in the ears are characteristically sharp and splinterlike. The glands are also likely to be sensitive and swollen. There is a high sensitivity to cold drafts, which make pain and discomfort much more intense and distressing. Symptoms also include a marked tendency to be short-tempered and irritable when in pain.

Chamomilla: If ear infection in children is associated with a severe bout of teething, this is a potential remedy. Symptoms include one flushed and one pale cheek (the flushed one usually being on the painful side), and temper tantrums that are not easily comforted. Sharp, sticking pains in the ears are combined with a generally stuffed-up feeling.

Pulsatilla: Consider this as a possible remedy if an ear infection has set in as a later complication of a heavy head cold. Characteristic symptoms include swollen glands and a general sense of mucus congestion involving the ears, nose, sinuses, and/or the chest. Mucus is thick, bland, and yellowish-green in color. Signature symptoms include a strong tendency to be clingy, weepy, and in need of a lot of sympathy and attention when in pain or feeling ill. Although chilly, being in stuffy surroundings feels unbearable.

Herbalism

Ear infection can be classified in several different categories: acute infection due to a virus or bacteria; chronic inflammation in the middle ear; and inflammation and/or infection in the external ear canal. Consult a doctor to diagnose the condition before beginning treatment.

Garlic and mullein: Garlic oil and mullein oil can be used to decrease pain, infection, and swelling in the ear canal in both acute and chronic infections. Place 3–5 drops of warm oil in the ear and cover with a soothing, warm towel. Before using this therapy, please check with your doctor to confirm there are no ruptures to the ear's membrane, which makes this treatment inadvisable.

Yarrow: Yarrow is excellent for easing the quick onset of fever, discharge, reddish complexion, hot, dry skin, and restlessness. An infusion or tincture might be recommended by your herbal expert. This works especially well in conjunction with elderflower and peppermint for fever.

Galium: Galium is a gentle lymph mover, good for dispelling heat, swelling, and stagnation. This assists the body in directing much-needed nutrients and immune cells to the affected areas, while stimulating the kidneys to detoxify and remove infectious agents. Taking a tincture may be recommended. Calendula is an alternative and may be used as an infusion of the flowers, or a 25% tincture.

Seek Professional Advice if Pregnant
Unless otherwise specified, the treatments recommended are for use by adults. Pregnant women should always consult a qualified health professional before using any treatments recommended in this publication.

Swimmer's Ear

Diagnosis

Swimmer's ear is the common name for the condition otitis externa. It is an infection of the ear canal caused by bacteria or fungi, and is associated with any pastime that involves repeatedly immersing the ear canal in water. It may also occur if water is trapped in the ear after bathing or showering, particularly if there is a significant amount of ear wax or the climate is very humid. Symptoms include swelling or redness of the skin of the external ear canal, fluid draining into the ear canal, and tender lymph nodes near the ears. To help keep your ear canal dry when swimming, try to limit your time exposed to water and thoroughly dry your ears after. You can also use a cotton wool ball covered with a layer of petroleum jelly to keep water out of your ears.

DANGER: Some people can develop a severe form of this condition known as malignant otitis externa that requires immediate hospitalization for treatment with intravenous antibiotics. If you have diabetes or another condition that makes you more susceptible to infections, contact your doctor immediately if you develop symptoms of swimmer's ear.

Symptoms

- Itchiness in the ear canal
- Redness of the skin in the ear canal
- Discharge from the ear canal that is often yellow or green
- Pain, when touching the ear or moving the jaw while talking or eating
- Hearing is affected

Treatment Goal

To relieve symptoms and resolve the infection. Call your doctor if the symptoms worsen, or any new symptoms develop, or if there is no improvement after two to three days.

Conventional Medicine

Swimmer's ear has many different names, including otomycosis, acute diffuse otitis externa, furunculosis, and eczematious otitis externa.

Prevention: Practice good hygiene and use a topical acetic acid (such as white vinegar) or isoprpyl alcohol (rubbing alcohol) if you are prone to swimmer's ear.

Topical treatment: Generally, a topical corticosteroid along with acetic acid or some other mild acidifying agent is used. If the condition is more severe, a topical antibiotic is also prescribed. Most commonly, ciprofloxin or neomycin mixed with polymixin sulfate is used.

Antibiotics: If there is redness that has spread to the skin or enlarged lymph nodes, an oral course of antibiotics geared to treat staphylococcus is prescribed.

Irrigation: In some cases, cleaning and debridement (using irrigation or suction) are necessary to remove debris, pus, and other material from the ear canal so that medication can be applied.

Traditional Chinese Medicine

Herbs: Place 3 g Jin Yin Hua (honeysuckle flower), 3 g of Ye Ju Hua (wild chrysanthemum flower), and 3 g of Bo He (field mint) in a teapot and add boiling water. Let the tea steep for five to six minutes and drink the tea throughout the day, which may help speed up your recovery time.

Acupressure: The Yi Feng and Ting Hui acupressure points are recommended for this condition. The Yi Feng point is situated just behind the ear lobe. The Ting Hui point is on the face, just in front of the lower notch of the ear. Use your thumbs to apply gentle pressure

to these, and gradually increase the pressure. Press and release about 20 times.

Diet: Avoid hot and spicy food, including dried ginger, chilies, hot radishes, and mustard. Eat plenty of fresh fruit and vegetables.

Naturopathy

Diet: Avoid the most common food allergens, including wheat, eggs, dairy foods, corn, citrus fruit, and peanut butter, especially for chronic cases of swimmer's ear. Also avoid simple carbohydrates, including sugar, honey, cookies, candy, ice cream, sodas, chocolate, dried fruits, and fruit juices.

Supplements: Zinc gluconate lozenges have both antiviral and immune-stimulating effects. Adults should take 25 mg per day; children should take a lower dosage. For example, a 30 lb child can be given 5 mg of zinc per day while suffering from swimmer's ear. Take 500 mg and 1,000 mg of vitamin C a day in separate doses to stimulate immune function. Reduce the dosage if you notice diarrhea. Vitamin A supports immunity. Give children up to six years old 2,000–5,000 IU of vitamin A a day, usually available in liquid form, to support immunity; adults should take 10,000–25,000 IU a day. Pregnant women should not take more than 10,000 IU of vitamin A a day.

Herbs: Mullein oil can be used to treat minor inflammation. To ease the discomfort of swimmer's ear, place 1–3 drops of a mullein preparation in the ear every three hours. Larix enhances immune function and has antimicrobial activity. Dissolve 1–2 tsp in a non-dairy formula or in water for older children or adults. Echinacea and goldenseal also enhance immune function and have antimicrobial properties. Children should take 2 ml four times a day, or as directed on the bottle. Mix St. John's wort oil with garlic oil and place 2 warm drops in the affected ear twice a day to relieve ear pain and kill infection. Do not use this treatment if the eardrum is ruptured.

> *Tip:* SESAME OIL
>
> One traditional remedy to help prevent swimmer's ear is to put 1 drop of sesame oil into the ears before going into the pool.

Homeopathy

The remedies listed below can be given along with conventional treatment if necessary. Recurrent infections will require treatment from a practitioner.

Belladonna: Use this remedy at the first sign of inflammation. Belladonna is effective in easing localized inflammation accompanied by throbbing pains. Symptoms may be restricted to or worse on the right side, with the glands becoming inflamed and swollen in sympathy with the affected ear.

Hepar sulph: Use this remedy to treat a later stage of infection, where pains in the ears are characteristically sharp and splinterlike. The glands are also likely to be sensitive and swollen. There is a high sensitivity to cold drafts, which make pain and discomfort much more intense and distressing. Signature symptoms also include a marked tendency to be short-tempered and irritable when in pain.

Pulsatilla: If there is an established history of mucus production and congestion that affects the ears, nose, or chest, this remedy is useful. The mucus produced is characteristically thick and yellowish-green in color. The affected ears feel stuffed up, with the sensation being mildly relieved only when traveling in a car. The external ear may become swollen and inflamed, with a sense of pressure as though something were pushing itself out of the ear.

Herbalism

Most treatments for swimmer's ear are topical. However, only use topical treatments once a ruptured eardrum has been ruled out by your doctor. All of the herbs listed may be combined to treat swimmer's ear, blend together and add 3–5 drops of the blend to the ear.

St. John's wort: Studies show this herb to be effective as an antiviral and antibacterial agent. Its ability to heal wounds is thought to be due to its high flavonoid and procyanidin content. Place 3–5 drops of oil into the affected ear(s). Cover with a warm, moist towel to ease discomfort.

Calendula: The flowers of this herb have been shown to be antiviral, anti-inflammatory, antiseptic, and to inhibit the growth of bacteria. Place 3–5 drops of calendula oil into the affected ear to soothe and promote healing of the ear canal.

Garlic: Garlic can inhibit the growth of a number of bacteria. The active compound, allicin, has antimicrobial properties. Place 3–4 drops of garlic infused oil into the affected ear.

Mullein oil: Place 2–3 drops of warmed mullein infused oil into the ear to soothe and relieve irritation.

Lavender essential oil: 1–2 drops of lavender essential oil can be rubbed externally around the ear to help soothe and relax. Lavender is one of the safest herbs to use neat, but you can seek advice from a practitioner for more information. In case of any irritation, dilute it in a base oil. Lavender essential oil may also be added to a blend of the above oils to use as ear drops.

Tinnitus

Diagnosis

Tinnitus is a condition that causes you to hear noises in your ears, most commonly ringing or buzzing. Tinnitus can vary in intensity and it is often linked with hearing loss. It is often caused by exposure to extreme noise, but it can also be triggered by a variety of conditions affecting the ear; an obstruction in the ear canal; a perforated eardrum; and inflammation of the middle ear. Rarely, it can be caused by a benign tumor on the acoustic nerve.

In some cases, tinnitus disappears without treatment. It can be successfully treated, although there is no cure for tinnitus caused by extreme noise.

Symptoms

- Buzzing, ringing, hissing, or whistling noises in the ear
- Intensity and loudness of noise can vary
- Noises are constant or intermittent

Treatment Goal

To identify the cause of the tinnitus and relieve the symptoms where possible.

Conventional Medicine

Also known as ringing in the ears, tinnitus is a false perception of sound without any acoustic stimulus present. It has multiple causes and these must be determined before deciding on a treatment plan. To determine the cause, an audiological evaluation is done. Sometimes brain imaging is carried out and blood tests performed to check for infection and other abnormalities, such as tumors on the acoustic nerve.

Prevention: Avoid drugs associated with tinnitus, such as non-steroidal anti-inflammatories and asprin. Also make sure you wear ear protection whenever you are likely to be exposed to loud noise to prevent any further hearing impairment.

Medication: Several medications have been tried for tinnitus with some success: antiarrhythmic drugs, benzodiazepines, anticonvulsants, and certain antidepressants. The herb ginkgo biloba has also been used.

Tinnitus retraining programs: These involve counseling and using broadband noise exposure, a type of wavelength that we are commonly exposed to on a daily basis, to habituate a person to tinnitus.

Traditional Chinese Medicine

Traditional Chinese medicine categorizes tinnitus into two common types: the first is due to excess heat in the liver and the second is due to deficiency in the kidney.

Herbs:
• **Excess heat in the liver:** Symptoms of this type of tinnitus are ringing in the ear, headaches, flushed face, yellow urine, and constipation. Combine 10 g of Jin Yin Hua (honeysuckle flower), 10 g of Huang Qin (baical skullcap root), 12 g of Zhi Zi (cape jasmine fruit), 10 g of Ye Ju Hua (wild chrysanthemum flower), 10 g of Long Dan Cao (Chinese gentian root), 10 g of Xia Ku Cao (common self-heal fruit-spike), and 5 g of Gan Cao (licorice root) in a ceramic pot. Add 3 cups of water, bring to a boil, and simmer for 30 minutes. Strain into a glass container and drink 1 cup twice a day. You can also purchase Long Dan Xie Gan Wan (patent herb pills) to treat this condition. Take the pills as the package indicates.
• **Kidney deficiency:** Symptoms may include a ringing in the ears that intensifies in the night or during exertion, or dizziness, insomnia, lumbago, and weak knees. To tonify the kidney, add 12 g of Di Huang (Chinese foxglove), 10 g of Shan Zhu Yu (Asiatic cornelian cherry), 15 g of Zhi Mu (anemarrhena rhizome), 12 g of Sang Shen Zi (mulberry fruit-spike), 12 g of Ji Shen

(jilin root), 15 g of Niu Xi (achyranthes root), and 8 g of Da Zhao (Chinese jujube) to 3 cups of water. Bring to the boil, simmer for 30 minutes, and strain the liquid. Drink 1 cup twice a day. Er Ming Zhuo Ci Wan and Zhi Bai Di Huang Wan patent herbal pills may also be helpful.

Acupressure: In sitting position, use your index fingers to apply medium pressure to the Er Men, Tin Hui, and Yi Feng points for one minute each twice a day. The Yi Feng point is located just behind the ear lobe. The Er Men point is in front of the notch on the forward edge of the ear. The Ting Hui point is on the face just in front of the ear.

Naturopathy

Diet: Eat plenty of foods that contain zinc, as zinc deficiency is associated with tinnitus and certain kinds of hearing loss. Good sources of zinc include spinach (the best), papaya, collards, brussels sprouts, cucumbers, string beans, endive, cowpeas, prunes, and asparagus. It is difficult to get the recommended daily amount of zinc (60 mg) from diet alone, but make a point of taking more zinc from your food while trying other herbal treatments for tinnitus. You can also take a 60–120 mg zinc supplement a day.

Supplements: Magnesium deficiency may cause tinnitus, and magnesium supplements (1,000 mg a day) may relieve tinnitus associated with Meniere's disease and protect the ears from damage. A manganese deficiency may be the cause of some cases of Meniere's disease, so if you have been diagnosed with this condition take 5 mg of manganese a day. The B vitamins have shown positive benefits for those suffering from hearing loss, and taking a high-potency complete B-complex capsule is recommended. Alternatively, take 500 mg of vitamin B1, 250 mg of B6, and 500 mcg of B12. Vitamin C has also been shown to relieve the symptoms in some patients with Meniere's. Take 1,000 mg three times a day. Make sure you take a formula that contains at least 250 mg of bioflavonoids.

Herbs: Fenugreek tea (fenugreek steeped in cold water) stops cricket noises and ringing in the ears, while chamomile tea promotes relaxation and may help the patient to sleep. If you suffer from tinnitus, do not take aspirin or aspirin-like herbs, including willow bark, meadowsweet, and wintergreen. High doses of aspirin may cause ringing in the ears. Other herbs, such as cinchona, black haw, and uva ursi, have been linked with tinnitus.

Homeopathy

As tinnitus tends to be an on-going, chronic problem, it is best managed by consulting a homeopathic practitioner, rather than attempting self-help.

Herbalism

Tinnitus can be caused by many conditions. The herbs listed below focus on treating tinnitus relating to allergies and decreased circulation.

Ginkgo biloba: Research has shown that ginkgo is an effective treatment for tinnitus, especially when the condition is related to poor circulation. It is thought that the active constituents in ginkgo, the ginkgolides, prevent metabolic damage from poor blood flow by increasing small arterial circulation. The ginkgolides also decrease the blood's ability to clot, thereby assisting circulation. Because of this ability, ginkgo should not be used by individuals on blood-thinning medication.

Gotu kola: Also known as hydrocotyle, this herb is rich in glycosides and flavonoids. It is useful for soft tissue and wound healing, and has anti-inflammatory properties. It is of great use in treating tinnitus, and works especially well alongside ginkgo. Drink as an infusion by steeping 1 tsp of the leaves in a cup of freshly boiled water. Strain and drink 2 cups daily.

Stinging nettle: One study of those suffering from tinnitus demonstrated that 33% of people tested had tinnitus related to allergies. Nettle leaf has anti-inflammatory and anti-allergic qualities as its key constituents, which act as antihistamines while significantly decreasing pro-inflammatory chemicals within the body. Take 4 g of dried leaf or 6 ml of tincture a day.

Tip: STRESS MANAGEMENT

If you notice that tinnitus increases in intensity when stress levels rise, investigate proactive ways of stress management. These may include stress counseling, taking up T'ai chi or yoga, or making relaxation techniques a regular part of your daily routine.

Allergic Rhinitis

Diagnosis

Rhinitis is the inflammation of the mucous membrane lining the inside of the nose. Triggers and irritants include pollen, pets' fur and dander, the house dust mite, molds, certain foods, and chemicals in household products. The inhalation of airborne irritants prompts an exaggerated response of the immune system, which forms antibodies to fight against invaders. This triggers the release of histamine, which causes inflammation and mucus production in the nasal passages. Perennial sufferers will experience a reaction throughout the year, and it is often very hard to identify the exact allergen. Hay fever sufferers can be affected from spring right through to fall, with tree pollen acting as an irritant in the spring, grass pollen in summer, and weed pollen in the fall, but the condition generally tends to peak in the summer months.

Rhinitis is a common complaint. The condition runs in families, and is more common in those with a history of asthma or eczema.

Symptoms

- Constantly runny nose
- Copious clear mucus
- Sneezing, particularly on first waking
- Blocked-up nose
- Breathing through mouth
- Snoring
- Itchy nose
- Stuffy head

Treatment Goal

To relieve the symptoms and identify the irritants. If you are suffering badly, allergy testing can be carried out to identify the exact trigger for the attacks.

Conventional Medicine

Avoid allergens: Avoid outdoor exposure and use HEPA filters indoors during the pollen season. Exposure to dust mites can be minimized by encasing pillows and bedding in plastic and using a dehumidifier. Shampoo pets on a regular basis to reduce pet dander. Humidifiers can be used in a dry climate, since they will help to moisturize the respiratory system. Too much humidity however, can actually cause more problems. The optimum level is about 35%.

Nasal washes: Using saline (saltwater) made from 1 tsp of salt to each pint of distilled warm water is an inexpensive and effective treatment. Sniff a small amount of the saline water into the nostrils one at a time and blow your nose. A syringe can also be used, as can a nasal spray.

Supplements: Take 1,000 mg of quercetin (eucalyptus flavonoid) three times a day. Take 500 mg –1 g of vitamin C a day, and add zinc and vitamins A and E to your diet. Take 4 g of EPA DHA (an omega-3 fat) fish oil a day in a 3:2 ratio.

Diet: Eliminating dairy products from your diet usually decreases the symptoms of the allergic reaction. Other common allergens are spices, yeast products, and gluten.

Medication: Topical nasal steroids such as Flonase®, oral antihistamines, topical azelastine, or cromolyn sodium in combination with mucolytics (guaifenesin) and decongestants are usually prescribed. Although they do mask symptoms, they do not alleviate the actual cause.

Traditional Chinese Medicine

Traditional Chinese medicine practitioners will classify the particular type of allergic rhinitis to focus treatment. Patients may be diagnosed for lung deficiency, lung and spleen deficiency, or lung and kidney deficiency.

Herbs: To bring relief to sinus congestion and a runny nose, use the following decoction. Add 2 g of Niu Bang Zi (great burdock root), 12 g of Cang Er Zi (cocklebur), 12 g of Fang Fen (ledebouriella root), 10 g of Jing Jie

Tip: NASAL WASH

Pound an adequate amount of green onion stalks and collect the juice. Wash the nasal cavity with a saline solution at night and then apply the green onion juice to both nasal cavities with a cotton wool ball. This will help to open the nasal pathways.

(schizonepeta stem and bud), and 5 g of Shen Gan Cao (raw licorice) to 3–4 cups of water in a ceramic pot. Bring to a boil, simmer for 30 minutes, and then strain. Drink 1 cup of the liquid two to three times a day.

Acupressure: The Ying Xiang point is located just to the side of, and slightly above, the lower border of the nostril. The Yin Tang point is in the depression midway between the eyebrows. Use your thumb or fingertip to gently press these points for about one minute.

Diet: Eat fresh vegetables such as carrots, squash, kale, Chinese cabbage, and broccoli.

Naturopathy

Diet: Look at your nutrition to work out strategies for mucus reduction, elimination of allergenic pathogens, and immune support. Choose non-mucous-forming foods, including gluten-free whole grains (brown rice, quinoa, and buckwheat), fresh fruit and vegetables, cold-pressed oils, and raw seeds and nuts. Eat a well-balanced diet that includes fresh fruits and vegetables, legumes, and quality protein (fish, lean chicken, and beans) every day. Eat plenty of green leafy vegetables for their high nutrient content. This will provide a good base of the nutrients required for a healthy immune system. Make sure you get enough anti-inflammatory essential fatty acids (omega-3s) in the form of fatty fish, walnuts, flax seeds, cod liver oil, fish oil, and flax seed oil. Also make sure you drink plenty of water— aim for at least eight glasses a day. Identify aggravating substances, including food dyes and colorings, artificial preservatives, and additives, and eliminate them from your diet. Avoid dietary sources of arachidonic acid (found in animal products), which contributes to inflammation.

Supplements: Vitamin C has natural antihistamine effects. Take 1,000 mg three to five times a day (reduce the dosage if diarrhea occurs). Take 250 mg of quercetin three times a day to control inflammation by reducing the release of histamine and other mediators of allergic reactions from cells. Quercetin also works by stabilizing cell membranes so they are less reactive to allergens. Take 3 g of fish oils a day to relieve inflammation associated with allergic rhinitis and allergies in general. Probiotics have been shown to be beneficial for allergies. Take a product that contains four billion organisms of Lactobacillus acidophilus

Tip: COOL WATER

Bathing the eyes with cool water tends to be universally soothing to irritated, itchy eyes.

and bifidus. Protease enzymes assist in decreasing inflammation; take 2 capsules twice a day on an empty stomach. Digestive enzymes along with Betaine hydrochloride assist in the digestion of food and reduce the chances of food sensitivities. Take one or two of each with each meal.

Herbs: Take 300–500 mg of freeze-dried stinging nettles. They have been shown to be beneficial for allergic rhinitis and hay fever. Butterbur is a traditional herbal remedy used for seasonal allergies and asthma. Research has shown it to be as effective but less sedating than commonly prescribed antihistamines for treating seasonal allergies over a two-week period. Consult a practitioner regarding an appropriate dosage.

Homeopathy

A chronic condition, rhinitis is best treated by a practitioner. Acute remedies can be used in the short term, but they will not discourage symptoms from recurring.

Allium cepa: Use Allium cepa if there is an acrid nasal discharge that burns the skin of the upper lip. Although the eyes water profusely, the tears feel bland in contrast to the nasal discharge. Symptoms tend to be more intense in the evening and in humid weather, and contact with cool, fresh air feels soothing.

Euphrasia: Use Euphrasia when tears feel hot and burning, while the nasal discharge is profuse and bland. As a result, the eyes look red, inflamed, and sore. Symptoms tend to be at their worst when indoors and are relieved by walking in cool, fresh air.

Apis: This remedy can help if allergic symptoms build rapidly, making the eyes look pink, swollen, and puffy. Stinging, itching sensations are marked in the eyes and throat and the eyelids look noticeably swollen. If these symptoms become intense, or there is any sign of swelling of the lip, seek emergency medical attention. The eyes are likely to feel light sensitive and produce tears that sting. Contact with heat feels awful, while cool compresses bring temporary relief.

Pulsatilla: Consider using Pulsatilla if mucus discharges are thick, bland, and yellow-green in color. Symptoms are worse when resting at night, and especially uncomfortable if you are in stuffy, overheated surroundings. Due to a general sense of congestion in the ears, nose, throat, and chest, there is likely to be a reduction in, or complete loss of, hearing, smell, or taste. You are also likely to cough up mucus when you first get up in the morning. Nasal congestion may cause you to breathe through the mouth during the night, leading to a dry mouth and tongue in the morning.

Herbalism

It is important to begin treatment four to six weeks prior to the time when your symptoms of allergic rhinitis first appear. If you are currently symptomatic, you can begin the herbal therapies mentioned below, but it may take several weeks for your symptoms to improve.

Plaintain: Plantain leaf is used in tincture and infusion form. In allergic rhinitis, it helps to dry up excessive mucous secretion, but is also soothing to nasal mucous membranes. Take 2–4 ml of tincture in a little water three times daily.

Ephedra: Available from herbal practitoners only, this herb has strong antihistamine properties. It is used in small amounts, and is not used in cases of prostate enlargement, cardiovascular conditions, anxiety, glaucoma, thyroid conditions, diabetes, and more. Consult a practitioner before use.

Nettle leaf: Take either 10 g of dried nettle, 3–6 ml of a 1:2 liquid extract, or a freeze-dried standardized extract a day to help with allergy symptoms. Some practitioners prefer the standardized extract because they feel it is more effective and because of its use in clinical trials, but also because it is the most convenient form to take. Although there is a lack of scientific evidence for the effectiveness of stinging nettles on allergies or allergic rhinitis, many experts have found it very useful for their patients.

Tip: AROUND THE HOME

Vacuum mattresses and carpets and dust surfaces with a damp cloth regularly to keep house dust mites at bay. Using a humidifier can soothe nasal passages.

Sinusitis

Diagnosis

Sinusitis is a condition that can suddenly flare up (acute sinusitis) or recur for months or even years (chronic sinusitis). Acute sinusitis is much more common than chronic, but both types can be very painful. The sinuses, small air-filled cavities located at the front of the skull in the cheeks and forehead, and between the eyes and nose, are lined with a membrane that is lubricated with mucus. Infection results when the tube that runs from the nose to the sinus becomes blocked and the lining of the sinuses becomes inflamed. Infection can also spread from an abscess on the root of a tooth. Symptoms include pain in the cheeks, forehead, or the bridge of the nose. There may be partial nasal blockage and a lot of green mucus. Acute sinusitis is usually the result of a cold or other tract infection. Rarely, a CT scan or chest X-ray may be done in order to make the diagnosis of chronic sinusitis.

Symptoms

- Blocked or runny nose
- Bad breath
- Loss of sense of smell
- Swelling and pain around the eyes
- Headaches and the sensation of a build-up of pressure in the head
- Abscess

Treatment Goal

Sinusitis often resolves itself. Treatment involves preventing fluid from accumulating in the sinuses, and clearing up an existing infection.

Conventional Medicine

Identify allergens: Environmental and dietary allergens can trigger sinusitis. Dairy products commonly cause mild, chronic respiratory congestion in individuals who are susceptible to sinusitis. Try eliminating dairy products from your diet for 21 days and see if there is any improvement.

Enhance your immune system: Good nutrition, especially making sure you get enough zinc and vitamin C, can help you avoid infection. Exercising regularly and keeping stress levels low are also vital to a healthy immune system.

Clear your sinus passages Peppermint oil, Afrin™ nasal spray, and steam inhalation can all reduce inflammation and encourage mucus to drain from your sinuses. Nasal washes and rinses can improve symptoms. Afrin™ should be used sparingly to prevent dependence.

Antibiotics: Amoxicillin, Septra™, erythromycin, or ceftin can be used to treat sinusitis. If there is no improvement after one week, try a more potent antibiotic such as augmentin or levofloxin. Antibiotics should be used for at least 14 days. A four- to eight-week course is sometimes prescribed in chronic cases.

Warning: A complication of sinusitis called periorbital cellulitis requires immediate medical attention. Infection can sometimes spread to the brain, and this condition requires immediate hospitalization for treatment. Medical attention is also needed if the infection spreads to the bone.

Traditional Chinese Medicine

Herbs: There are two types of acute sinusitis that can be treated by herbal remedies. The first is due to wind-cold attacking the sinuses, which leads to nasal congestion, sneezing, chills, a runny nose, and headache. The second type is caused by wind with heat, resulting in nasal congestion with yellow mucus, fever, and a dry mouth.
• To treat type one: Combine 12 g of Chuan Xiong (Szechuan lovage root), 10 g of Jing Jie (schizonepeta stem and bud), 6 g of Bo He (field mint), 10 g of Bai Zhi (angelica dahurica), 6 g of Gan Cao (licorice root), 10 g Xin Yi Hua (magnolia flower), and 12 g of Fang Fen (ledebouriella root) in a ceramic pot. Add 3–4 cups of water, bring to the boil, simmer for 30 minutes, and strain the liquid. Drink 1 cup two to three times a day.
• To treat type two: Take the patent herbal pill Yin Qiao Jie Du Pian.

Acupressure: Press the Ying Xiang point, located to the side of and slightly above the border of the nostril, and the Yin Tang point, found in the depression between the eyebrows. This will relieve congestion and help open the nasal pathways.

Diet: Patients with sinusitis should eat foods that clear away heat such as balsam pear, mung bean sprouts, eggplant, persimmon, loquat, pears, banana, and Chinese chives. Avoid fatty, pungent, or irritating foods and do not drink wine.

Naturopathy

Diet: Avoid dairy, oranges, white sugar, and foods containing white flour because they promote the formation of mucus. Sugar inhibits the immune system from clearing bacteria. Eliminate wheat, soya, fermented foods, and eggs from your diet for a couple of weeks to see if sinus symptoms improve, and then re-introduce them to see if symptoms temporarily worsen. In general, a diet that is rich in vegetables, whole grains, and beans, and low in saturated fat (meat and dairy), sugar, mucus-forming, and allergenic foods will be beneficial to the sinuses. Adding cayenne, garlic, ginger, horseradish, and onions to dishes will aid mucus drainage and ease the pressure in your sinuses. Drink plenty of fluids, six to eight glasses of water a day, particularly during a cold or times of stress. If you are taking antibiotics, consume plenty of non-dairy sources of probiotics such as yogurt, sauerkraut, or kefir.

Supplements: Vitamin A and vitamin C can help with a sinus infection. Vitamin A thins the mucus, promotes the growth of healthy mucus-promoting cells, and strengthens the immune system. Take 10,000 IU of vitamin A and 1,000–2,000 mg of vitamin C a day. Take 500 mg of bioflavonoids a day with the vitamin C to improve its benefits.

Aromatherapy: Steam inhalations work directly on the sinuses, loosening thick mucus and fighting infection. Pour 5–10 drops of eucalyptus, lavender, peppermint, pine, thyme, or tea tree oil, or use a combination of some or all of these, in a bowl of hot, steaming water. Lean over the bowl with a towel over your head and inhale two to three times to complete one set. Complete three to four sets three times a day. The oils will fight the virus, ease congestion, and stimulate circulation.

Tip: PRESS THE NOSE

Pressure on the sides of your nose can relieve pain. Press the top of your nose on either side between two fingers for a few minutes and release.

Herbs: Take ½–1 tsp of a liquid extract of echinacea every three to four hours to stimulate the immune system and fight against bacteria. Echinacea can also be taken in capsule form (500–1,000 mg every three to four hours) or as a standardized extract 3.5% echinacoside (150–300 mg every three to four hours). Goldenseal has broad antibacterial activity and can stimulate the immune system against infections of the mucous membrane. Take ½–1 tsp of a liquid extract, 500–1,000 mg in capsule form, or as a standardized extract (8–12% alkaloid content) every three to four hours. Grapefruit seed extract can be used in a nasal spray four times a day.

Homeopathy

Any of the following remedies can help ease the pain of recently developed bouts of sinusitis. If the condition is chronic, consult a homeopathic practitioner.

Kali bich: Use this remedy if sinus pain and pressure is lodged at the bridge of the nose and accompanied by an unpleasant smell in the nasal passages. Pain and congestion affect the sinuses above the eyes, and the mucus produced is stringy, sticky, and greenish in color. Discomfort and pressure are aggravated by stooping and bending forward, while applying warmth and firm pressure brings relief.

Hepar sulph: If there is sensitivity to cold drafts of air and a tendency to swollen glands, and if a thick yellowish mucus and sharp, splinterlike pains are present, consider this remedy. When it is well indicated there is sneezing and nasal obstruction, with pains and discomfort radiating to the bones of the face.

Phosphorus: This remedy is helpful in treating sinus pains that tend to be one-sided. The yellowish mucus produced is often streaked with blood when the nose is blown. The eyes may be especially affected, feeling heavy and tired, and the eye sockets may also feel very tender. The nasal passages feel generally swollen and congested and the sense of smell is strong.

Pulsatilla: If sinusitis develops at the end of a very heavy head cold, if a yellowish-green, thick mucus is produced, and if there is a marked aversion to rooms that are overheated and stuffy, consider using Pulsatilla. The nose feels uncomfortably stuffed up at night and flows more freely during the day. Pains and discomfort lead to weepiness and a noticeable need for sympathy and attention.

Herbalism

Sinus oil blend: Create a cooling decongestant for the sinuses using antimicrobial and anti-inflammatory oils. Place 1 drop each of peppermint, thyme, and eucalyptus essential oils into slightly steaming water and breathe in deeply. Do not take internally.

> ### *Tip:* USE A HUMIDIFIER
>
> Use a cool-mist humidifier. Moist air can help clear the mucus in your nasal passages. Also try resting a towel or washcloth that has been wrung out with hot water over your face for a few minutes. It can stimulate blood circulation, loosen mucus, and relieve pain.

Echinacea and goldenseal: To treat a bacterial sinus infection, echinacea and goldenseal combined have a powerful antimicrobial effect. Capsules or a combined tincture might be recommended. Choose cultivated goldenseal rather than that harvested from the wild.

Thyme and licorice: These are effective in combination to fight the virus that may have caused the sinusitis. They can be taken combined as a syrup, or tincture. Dried herbs can also be prepared as thyme infusion and licorice root decoction.

Nosebleeds

Diagnosis

Nosebleeds can be worrying but often look worse than they are. Causes include a direct blow, bump, or other injury to the area; an infection of the mucus membrane that lines the nose, such as sinusitis; or the drying out of the nose due to cold weather. Other triggers include upper respiratory tract infections such as colds, flu, or coughs, allergic rhinitis or hay fever, abscesses, and nasal polyps. If you have a cold or are congested and blow your nose too hard, the delicate lining to the nose can easily become damaged. If the nosebleed follows a blow to the head or has not stopped after half an hour, always seek medical advice. Frequent nosebleeds can be a symptom of anemia.

If suffering from a nosebleed take the following steps:

- Sit and lean forward to prevent blood going down your throat
- Using your fingertips, pinch the soft part of your nose just above the nostrils and breathe through your mouth
- Hold this position for 5–15 minutes until the bleeding stops
- If bleeding does not stop, go to your nearest emergency room

Treatment Goal

To stop the nosebleed, determine the cause, and treat any underlying condition.

Conventional Medicine

Non-drug-based treatment is usually successful in treating nosebleeds. However, in more serious cases the source of the bleeding is from the lungs, esophagus, or tracheal/larynx area. The doctor can determine the source by examining the patient. If the patient has had many episodes or has unstable vital signs such as low blood pressure, the doctor may carry out tests to determine if the red cells and clotting cells are adequate.

Stop the bleeding: Leaning forward and breathing through the mouth, pinch the lower part of the nose for 10–15 minutes, or stay the blood with a cotton ball or tissue. Apply an ice pack to the bridge of the nose to try to constrict the blood vessels and stop the bleeding.

Pharmaceuticals: If these treatments fail, the doctor will apply a lidocaine and epinephrine cotton swab to the nostril, or a lidocaine and Afrin™ plug. This helps to constrict the blood vessels and stop the bleeding. Failing this, cocaine 4% is applied to a nasal tampon and inserted in the nostril by a physician. Cauterizing, or sealing the blood vessels, with silver nitrate is also an option.

Nasal packing: If the above options fail, gauze is layered into the nostril from the front nasal cavity to the back of the nose, or anterior chamber. This is done under local anesthetic, as pressure must be applied to pack the gauze. A catheter balloon or a nasal sponge can also be packed into the back of the nose.

To treat chronic nosebleeds: A procedure can be carried out to cauterize the vessels, a simple procedure that involves sealing them using heat.

Warning: Caution should be taken to prevent high blood loss during a nosebleed as this is life threatening. Also, blood loss can be so rapid as to cause cardiac instability.

Traditional Chinese Medicine

If nosebleeds do not stop by using the self-help methods recommended here, go to the hospital immediately.

Herbs:
• To treat all kinds of nosebleeds: Place 10 g of Bei Mao Gen (wooly grass rhizome) and 5 g of Jin Yin Hua (honeysuckle flower) in a teapot and add boiling water. Let the herbs steep for five minutes before drinking.
• To treat chronic nosebleeds: Make a decoction using 12 g Han Lian Cao (eclipta), 15 g of Xuan Shen (ningpo figwort root), 15 g of Zhi Mu (anemarrhena rhizome), 12 g of Di Gu

Pi (cortex of wolfberry root), 12 g of Dan Pi (cortex of tree peony root), and 12 g of Mai Men Dong (ophiopogon tuber). Place these herbs in a ceramic or glass pot and add 3–4 cups of water. Bring to the boil, simmer for 30 minutes, and strain. Drink 1 cup two to three times a day. Do not use if you have loose bowel movements or diarrhea.

Acupressure: Apply an ice pack to the Yin Tang point, located in the depression midway between the eyebrows. You can also very gently press the Yin Tang point with your index finger, while in a seated position and with your head tilted back.

Diet: Eat foods that are cooling such as purslane, mung beans, lotus, lettuce, mango, eggplant, spinach, pears, and cucumber. Avoid foods that assist heat, such as mutton, chicken, black pepper, chives, clove, fennel, ginger, red pepper, and sword bean.

Naturopathy

Diet: Eat two to three servings of green leafy vegetables a day. These have many of the nutrients that help your blood to clot.

Supplements: Vitamin C deficiency is associated with nosebleeds. Adults should take 2,000 mg with 500–1,000 mg of bioflavonoids; children should take 250–500 mg with 100–200 mg of bioflavonoids. Bleeding problems can occur because of a vitamin K deficiency. Take 15 mcg of vitamin K a day to help the blood to clot. Apply vitamin E, squeezed from a gel capsule, to the inside of the nose to lubricate dry airways. Vitamin E may increase the risk of bleeding in some patients and you should not take to more than 200 IU a day. Zinc is a natural wound healer and low levels can improve healing; take 15–30 mg a day.

TIP: KEEP YOUR NOSE LUBRICATED

Use a humidifier in the dry winter months, or year round if you live in a dry climate (especially at night while you are sleeping). Using a saline (saltwater) spray for your nose three to four times a day also prevents nosebleeds by keeping the mucous membranes in your nose from drying out.

Herbs: Agrimony, yarrow, and witch hazel are astringent herbs that can be used topically to decrease or eliminate bleeding. Bilberry decreases the fragility of small blood vesels. Take 120–240 mg of an extract standardized to contain 25% anthocyanosides, the herb's active ingredient, twice a day. Nettle tea contains vitamins A and C, both of which work to strengthen the mucous membrane in the nose. The tea also provides an easily absorbed form of iron. It has a strong "planty" taste so you can add it to orange or apple juice to encourage children to drink it. Adults should drink 2–3 cups of tea a day. Do not use ginkgo biloba if you are experiencing nosebleeds as it can increase the risk of bleeding.

Homeopathy

Any of the following suggestions can be helpful in stopping a mild nosebleed. Persistent, regular nosebleeds are best treated by a homeopathic practitioner, who will prescribe to treat the underlying problem.

Arnica: Use this remedy if a nosebleed has been triggered by a minor accident. It will relieve the physical trauma, and encourage the body to recover from the psychological shock of an accident.

Ipecac: If nosebleeds tend to gush bright red blood, and the bleeding is accompanied by nausea and cold sweats, use Ipecac. There is also a profound queasiness made unbearably intense by movement of any kind.

Phosphorus: This remedy is especially helpful in stopping nosebleeds that result from blowing the nose repeatedly and violently during a cold. Characteristic symptoms also include noticeable anxiety and a need for reassurance when bleeding.

Carbo veg: This is a potential candidate for nosebleeds that result in steady, oozing blood loss (unlike the gushing blood loss that calls for Ipecac). Symptoms include a marked sensation of faintness and dizziness during a nosebleed. Burning sensations are common with a noticeable craving for contact with cool, fresh air, or a strong desire to be fanned if indoors.

Herbalism

Chronic bleeding typically reflects a lack of blood vessel strength and nasal mucosa irritation. The goal of treatment is to improve integrity of the blood vessels and to reduce inflammation and irritation in the nasal passages.

Cinnamon: This herb can be used to stop bleeding, whether applied locally or taken internally. It also relieves pain and tonifies tissue. Place 1–2 drops of tincture on a cotton swab and place against the bleeding area within the nose, or drink a tea made from 1 tsp of bark steeped for 30 minutes in 1 cup of hot water.

Calendula: Antiseptic, anti-inflammatory, and demulcent, calendula is ideal for healing traumatized tissue, especially wounds and skin conditions that are slow to heal. Infuse 2 tbsp of calendula flowers in 1 cup of hot water. Apply it directly to the nasal tissue until bleeding resolves. For a more potent topical extract, a dilute 90% calendula tincture may be used instead. A 90% tincture is useful as it extracts the resins from the flowers, that aid healing.

Horse chestnut: This herb may be taken as a tincture 1–2 ml two or three times daily, in a little water. One of the phytochemical components is cin, which helps to decrease the permeability of venous capillaries and strengthen vessel walls. Suitable for short-term use. Consult a practitioner if there are other health complications, or medication is being taken.

Grape seed: Studies on grape seed extract have shown its ability to increase blood vessel integrity and to prevent damage by toxins and chemical and environmental irritants. Take 300 mg daily for three weeks, then decrease the dosage to 75 mg a day to prevent future nosebleeds.

Blueberries and bilberries: These closely related berries contain high levels of antioxidant flavanoids and phenolic acids, which promote and ensure vessel strength. A tincture may be used, or they may be included as part of a healthy diet, by eating 1 cup of the mixed berries a day.

Laryngitis

Diagnosis

Laryngitis is a painful condition that results in inflammation of the voice box, or larynx. This causes hoarseness and the distinctive croaky voice associated with laryngitis. In the acute form, this condition appears suddenly and is usually caused by an infection, such as a cold, flu, or bronchitis. The chronic type of laryngitis recurs on a regular basis. It can be triggered by shouting, loud singing or excessive use of the voice, or smoking. Your throat may need investigating to see if there are polyps on the larynx, which could be causing problems. Laryngitis usually clears up once the voice has been given a rest. If the hoarseness continues for more than two weeks, you lose your voice after a head or neck injury, or your voice disappears suddenly for no apparent reason, see your doctor.

Symptoms

- Difficulty speaking
- Sore throat
- Hoarse and throaty, or whispering, voice
- Dry coughing
- Occasionally, loss of voice completely
- Painful and tender larynx
- Sometimes, fever and a feeling of being generally under the weather

Treatment Goal

To ease symptoms of pain and discomfort in the throat and to encourage the voice to return to normal.

Conventional Medicine

Treatment of laryngitis depends on whether it is in an acute or chronic stage. Acute laryngitis usually develops after an upper respiratory tract infection. If the laryngitis does not resolve in three weeks, it is considered chronic. Chronic laryngitis may be due to a lesion present on the larynx, chronic sinusitis, or hypothyroidism.

Rest and hydrate your voice: Drink plenty of water, maintain a healthy diet, and completely rest your voice. Using a humidifier may also help the laryngitis to resolve.

Mucolytic: A mucolytic, such as guaifenesin, can be used to provide lubrication and encourage any thick mucus stuck on the larynx, which exacerbates an irritation, to resolve.

Antibiotics: Occasionally, laryngitis results from a bacterial infection. If this is the case penicillin or erythromycin is prescribed to resolve the condition.

To treat chronic laryngitis: An ear, nose and throat (ENT) specialist may do a scope to identify any potential lesions on the larynx. These will need to be surgically removed. Speech therapy is sometimes helpful after a prolonged bout of chronic laryngitis.

Traditional Chinese Medicine

Herbs:
• **Herbal decoction:** To treat wind and heat, combine 10 g of Jin Yin Hua (honeysuckle flower), 8 g of Jing Jie (schizonepeta stem and bud), 12 g of Jie Geng (balloon flower root), 12 g of Niu Bang Zi (great burdock fruit), 8 g of Bo He (field mint), 10 g of Zhu Ye (bamboo leaves), 6 g of Gan Cao (licorice root), and 12 g of Lian Qiao (forsythia fruit) in a ceramic pot. Add 2–4 cups of water, bring to a boil, and simmer for 30 minutes. Strain the liquid and drink 1 cup twice a day.
• **Herbal decoction:** To treat cold wind, running nose, and chills, mix 12 g of Fang Fen (ledebouriella root), 6 g of Bo He (field mint), 10 g of Jing Jie (schizonepeta stem and bud), 10 g of Zi Su Ye (perilla leaf), 12 g of Jie Geng (balloon flower root), 5 g of fresh ginger, and 3 g of Gan Cao (licorice root). Follow the directions above to make a decoction.
• **Herbal tea:** To treat yin deficiency, place 5 g of Mai Men Dong (ophiopogon tuber), 3 g of Gan Cao (licorice root), and 3 g of Bo He (field mint) in a teapot and add boiling water. Let the herbs steep for five minutes before drinking. Sip this tea throughout the day.

Acupressure: Use the tip of your thumb and press the Hegu point, located on the back of the hand between the thumb and first finger, with strong pressure for one to two minutes. Apply similar pressure to the Nei Guan point, which is found in the center of the wrist on the palm side, about 2 inches below the crease. These acupressure points can be pressed a couple of times during the day as needed.

Diet: Eat foods that are juicy and mild such as lettuce, bok choy, Chinese broccoli (found in Chinese groceries), daikon radish, pears, strawberries, mango, grapes, cantaloupe melon, and watermelon. Hot, spicy foods should be avoided.

Naturopathy

Diet: Eat light foods consisting of steamed vegetables, freshly made soups, and broths. Add garlic, ginger, and onions to soup for their tonifying, antimicrobial, and warming properties. Cut out all milky and mucus-forming foods such as cheese, yogurt, red meat, dairy, and simple carbohydrates. Drink plenty of water, freshly squeezed juices, and teas to cleanse your body of toxins. Herbal teas will assist your body's ability to heal itself. The most beneficial kinds of herbal teas are listed in the herbal section of this entry. Take 1 tbsp of honey and lemon juice with a pinch of cayenne pepper twice a day. The mixture helps coat your larynx, which can relieve laryngitis.

Supplements: To support the immune system take 500 mg–1,000 mg of vitamin C every four hours until symptoms subside. Bioflavonoids work synergistically with vitamin C and have immune-enhancing properties of their own. Take 1,000 mg a day in divided doses. Zinc supports the immune system and may have antiviral properties. Take 25 mg of zinc in lozenges several times a day for one week.

Herbs: Drink a tea made from peppermint, eucalyptus, and chamomile three times a day. Add cayenne to the tea to stimulate the circulation, or cinnamon for its gentle, warming effect. Grated ginger root can also be added to induce sweating. Elderflower and elderberry is an effective, natural antiviral that can be used to ease symptoms of laryngitis. Adults can take 10 ml of tincture and children 5 ml three times a day. Echinacea and goldenseal enhance the immune system and have antiviral properties. Take 2–4 ml of a tincture that combines the two, four times a day. Lomatium dissectum has strong antiviral effects; take 500 mg in capsule form or 2–4 ml of tincture four times a day. Take plenty of raw garlic or 300–500 mg in capsule form a day to fight and prevent infection.

Hydrotherapy: Try applying compresses to help speed up the healing process. Use a piece of an old sheet that's long and wide enough to wrap around your throat, and a similar-sized piece of cloth. Soak the sheet in cold water, wring it out, and wrap it once around your throat. Cover the sheet with the dry cloth and secure it with a safety pin. As your body heat warms and dries the compress, circulation will increase. Change the compresses every six to eight hours.

Aromatherapy: Carefully pour about 4–6 cups of boiling water into a large bowl and add 3 drops of eucalyptus oil. Hold your head over the bowl and cover both with a towel, making sure that you do not put your face too close to the hot water. Close your eyes and breathe slowly and deeply, continuing the treatment for about 15 minutes. If you start to feel overheated or uncomfortable, remove the towel. Repeat the steam inhalation for 5–10 minutes every hour over the course of a day. Inhaling eucalyptus oil presents an extremely low level of risk to most people. However, prolonged exposure (perhaps an hour or more) to relatively high levels of essential oil vapor (undiluted oil directly inhaled from the bottle) could lead to headache, vertigo, nausea, and lethargy. In certain cases, serious side effects such as incoherence or double vision may be experienced.

Warning: Those with serious heart problems and nervous disorders such as epilepsy, and pregnant women, infants, children, and the elderly may not be able to respond appropriately to this type of heat treatment.

Homeopathy

The remedies below can be helpful in speeding up recovery from a recently developed, acute episode of laryngitis. They will be most effective if used in combination with practical measures such as avoiding overusing the voice and drinking plenty of fluids. Repeated episodes of severe laryngitis are best treated by a practitioner.

Aconite: If symptoms come on very rapidly and dramatically, consider using Aconite. Overexposure to dry, cold winds trigger sensitivity to pain and restlessness. Symptoms

Tip: USE THROAT LOZENGES

If your throat feels dry and raspy, sucking throat lozenges can provide temporary, soothing relief by providing lubrication. Avoid lozenges that contain substances that may interfere with homeopathic remedies, such as eucalyptus, menthol, or peppermint.

tend to emerge most strongly when waking from sleep in the early hours.

Phosphorus: Use this remedy to treat hoarseness and complete loss of voice that is accompanied by a furry, raw sensation in the larynx and pain that is worse for speaking. If the voice has not been lost altogether, it is likely to sound very low. Symptoms are the most intense and distressing in the evening.

Causticum: Think of this remedy if the throat feels burning, raw, scraped, and constricted so that there is a need to swallow continuously. Efforts to cough up mucus are ineffectual, which prompts more swallowing. There is also a tendency to swallow the wrong way because of sensitivity and inflammation in the throat.

Herbalism

Yerba santa: A warming, aromatic, sweet herb, yerba santa fights infection while opening the bronchioles in the lungs and encouraging mucus expectoration. Infuse 1 tsp of leaves in 1 cup of hot water, or take 30 drops of tincture, and drink three times daily.

Sage: Place 2 tsp in a cup of boiled water, and cover to infuse for 10–15 minutes. Strain and use as a gargle when needed. Sage has anti-inflammatory and antiseptic properties that help to soothe the throat and fight infection.

Garlic: Crush a clove of fresh garlic and take with meals. Garlic contains allicin and ajoene, which offer great antibacterial properties, and help to fight off infection. Alternatively, take in capsule form, 500 mg three times daily.

Sore Throat

Diagnosis

A sore throat, also known as pharyngitis or tonsillitis, occurs when the pharynx or tonsils become inflamed. Sore throats are common all year round, not just during the winter months, and generally last for around two to three days. The infection is passed on through airborne droplets, which are breathed in, or by physical contact, particularly with hands, with a person carrying the infection. Sore throats can be caused by either a virus or a bacteria. In cases of a bacterial sore throat, the patient has swollen, coated tonsils, runs a temperature, has sour breath, and may feel quite ill. If the cause is bacterial, the condition can be treated with antibiotics. A sore throat can also be a side effect of other conditions, such as flu, glandular fever, and earache, and often clears up as soon as the underlying illness resolves. Occasionally the following complications may arise: a secondary infection in the middle ear or sinuses; occasionally a throat abscess; and in very rare cases diseases such as rheumatic fever or kidney disease.

DANGER: Always call your doctor if you have any type of throat discomfort that lasts for more than two weeks.

Symptoms

- Fever
- Bad breath
- Generally feeling unwell
- White spots on the tonsils
- Painful throat
- Difficulty swallowing
- Swollen tonsils
- Pain may spread to the ears
- The throat is red, and may be coated
- Possibly a high temperature
- Swollen lymph nodes

Treatment Goal

To establish the cause of the sore throat, whether it is viral or bacterial, and bring relief.

Conventional Medicine

Treating a sore throat depends on an accurate diagnosis. It can be caused by a viral or bacterial infection, by a chemical inflammation, or as a side effect of medications, and is known as pharyngitis in conventional medicine. The remedies below aim to alleviate pain, stop the infection, and prevent the secondary complications associated with bacterial infections.

To treat viral infections: Acetaminophen (Tylenol®), or ibuprofen (Motrin®) may be used as directed to alleviate pain. Saltwater gargles (1 tsp of salt mixed in 2 cups of distilled water) may also be helpful. Eating cool fruit that feels good to the throat for a couple of days may be more comfortable. Some plants, such as larch taken at 1 g twice a day in powder form, may boost the immune system and decrease the length of the viral infection.

To treat bacterial infections: Streptococcus A (see Strep Throat, p. 170) is the most common bacterial infection and is primarily treated with antibiotics. A course of antibiotics can be started before the results of throat cultures are received. The use of a five-minute, in-office "rapid-strep" test is now common practice. If a patient has a history of rheumatic heart disease, treatment is started immediately even before the doctor's evaluation. Penicillin and its derivatives are prescribed to treat strep throat. Erythromycin is used if a patient is allergic to penicillin. Some strains of the bacteria have become resistant to penicillin and erythromycin. If no improvement occurs after 48 hours, or if the culture indicates a resistance, an alternative such as clarithromycin (Biaxin®) is used.

Other causes: More rarely, yeast infections, herpes, diphtheria, gonococcus, syphilis, and chlamydia, as well as tuberculosis, can cause a sore throat. Treatment is specific to the organism causing the infection.

Traditional Chinese Medicine

Herbs:
• Acute sore throat: In the acute stage, chills, fever, and a cough often accompany a sore throat. Take the patent herbal pill Yin Qiao Jie Du Pian or make the following herbal tea. Combine 10 g of Jin Yin Hua (honeysuckle flower), 10 g of Ye Ju Hua (wild chrysanthemum flower), 8 g of Shen Gan Cao (raw licorice), 10 g of Ge Geng (kudzu root), and 8 g of Huang Qin (scutellaria root) with 3 cups of water. Bring to a boil, simmer for 30 minutes, and strain. Drink 1 cup twice a day.
• Chronic condition: If you develop a sore throat regularly—usually due to yin deficiency—

make the following herbal tea: Place 6 g of Mai Men Dong (ophiopogon tuber), 3 g of Gan Cao (licorice root), 6 g of Da Zhao (Chinese jujube), and 3 g of Bo He (field mint) in a teapot. Add boiling water and let the herbs steep for five to six minutes. Drink the tea throughout the day. This tea is safe for long-term use.

Acupressure: The Shao Shang point is on the corner of the thumb, ½ inch from the outside of the fingernail. The Chi Ze point is found on the inside bend of the arm, just off center. The Hegu points are located on the back of the hands, between the thumb and first finger. The Qu Chi point is 3 inches from the nostrils, in the depression below the cheekbone. Press these points with medium pressure for one minute at a time.

Diet: For acute sore throats eat foods that are light and mild in flavor, such as olives, persimmons, figs, turnips, peppermint, and honeysuckle. For chronic sore throats, pears and water chestnut are helpful. Avoid pungent and spicy foods.

 ## Naturopathy

Diet: Allicin, the compound responsible for garlic's pungent odor, has antibiotic and antifungal properties that can heal many types of sore throat. Take two or more cloves, crushed or whole, at the first sign of a sore throat and continue eating two cloves a day until your symptoms clear up. An ice-cold fruit juice popsicle can be an effective temporary anesthetic for a sore throat. Reduce your intake of dairy and simple carbohydrates, such as fruit, and stick to a diet that consists primarily of vegetables and whole grains. Drink fluids through the day consisting of water, teas, and soups. Chicken soup and miso soup are great for this condition.

Tip: SAGE, CIDER VINEGAR, AND HONEY GARGLE

Infuse sage by adding 1 tsp of the dried herb to a large cup of hot water. Let it steep for one minute before straining the liquid and adding 1 tsp each of cider vinegar and honey. Let the mixture cool to a comfortable temperature and gargle in the morning and evening.

Supplements: Vitamin C supports the immune system. Take 500–1,000 mg every four hours, until symptoms subside. Bioflavonoids work synergistically with vitamin C and have immune-enhancing properties of their own. Take 1,000 mg in two 500 mg doses a day. Take 25 mg of zinc a day in lozenges for one week. Zinc supports the immune system and may have some antiviral properties.

Herbs: Rub lavender, eucalyptus, thyme, or tea tree essential oil gently on the chest and around the front side of the neck. Only use the oils externally, and always dilute them in a carrier oil such as olive, apricot, or almond oil. This serves as an anti-infective and helps to loosen and shift sticky mucus. Elderflower and elderberry are effective natural antivirals and have been effectively used to treat sore throat symptoms. Adults can take 10 ml and children 5 ml three times daily. Take a combination of echinacea and goldenseal tincture, using 2–4 ml of each, four times a day for their immune-enhancing and antiviral properties. Lomatium dissectum also has strong antiviral effects; take 500 mg in capsule form or 2–4 ml of tincture four times a day.

Homeopathy

The remedies below can help shorten the duration of a recently developed sore throat, ease the pain, and speed up recovery. Recurrent, severe sore throats are best treated by a practitioner.

Aconite: Consider this remedy if a sore throat develops abruptly after exposure to dry, cold winds. Aconite can ease a sore throat that emerges early in the morning when you wake feeling fearful and agitated. The throat feels dry, tingly, or numb, with a sensation of acute pain and constriction when swallowing.

Belladonna: Opt for this remedy at the first twinge of a sore throat, especially if it is accompanied by a sense of being feverish with hot, flushed, dry skin. Symptoms include a dry sensation in the throat with burning and throbbing pains that make it very difficult to swallow even liquids.

Hepar sulph: If there is a sharp pain that feels as though a splinter were sticking into the sore throat (often worse on the right), try Hepar sulph. Glands may also be swollen and painful, while any mucus present is likely to be thick and yellowish. Contact with cold air intensifies pain and irritability. Warmth feels comforting.

Herbalism

Sage: Taken internally, this herb is pungent and tonifying, and has a strong antimicrobial effect. It reduces throat irritation upon contact, but should not be used long-term due to its thujone content. An infusion or tincture may be gargled and swallowed.

Myrrh: Myrrh may have antimicrobial effects and serve as an astringent for irritated tissues. You may be advised to gargle a tincture in water two to four times per day. Do not swallow.

Licorice: Prepare a decoction of the root and drink up to three times daily to help relieve a sore throat. Licorice has antiviral properties, and has a high mucilage content, making it soothing on contact with the mucous membrane of the throat. This herb is avoided in cases of high blood pressure, so speak to a herbal practitioner for advice.

Ginger: A warming and anti-infective herb, this may be used fresh, dried, or as a tincture. Fresh ginger is often seen as more potent, but the dried root (often in powder form) has a high shogaol content, which helps to calm coughing and is antimicrobial and anti-inflammatory. Gingerols are also a very active phytochemical component of ginger. To use fresh, cut a 1-inch slice, chop into smaller pieces and infuse in freshly boiled water for 10 minutes. Keep warm and sip throughout the day when required ❧

Tip: SOOTHING GARGLE

Herbal combinations typically have a stronger medicinal effect than one herb alone. This synergistic formula soothes and heals the throat, relieves discomfort and swelling, and actively treats infection. Combine peppermint, calendula, thyme, and licorice in equal parts and add a little ginger. Use 2 tsp of herbs per cup of water to make a tea, or use 5 ml at a time of tincture diluted in water. Gargle for 30 seconds four to six times a day, and drink 3–4 cups daily.

Strep Throat

Diagnosis

This is a common bacterial infection of the throat caused by group A streptococcus, which gives the condition its common name. It can be quite serious if not treated, and can lead to rheumatic fever, kidney disorders, ear infections, and sinusitis. Strep throat can spread quickly and easily, and is especially prolific during late winter and early spring. A strep infection also has the potential to spread within the body, resulting in pockets of pus in the tonsils and abscesses in the soft tissue around the throat.

DANGER: Call your doctor immediately if you have a sore throat that prevents you from drinking or is accompanied by pain when swallowing, labored breathing, excessive drooling, or a temperature above 100°F.

Symptoms

- Throat pain
- Fever
- Coating on the tonsils and tongue
- Pain on swallowing
- Loss of appetite
- Hoarseness and coughing
- Runny nose
- Swollen glands
- Headache
- Generally feeling unwell
- Children can also experience nausea, vomiting, and abdominal pain

Treatment Goal

To identify if strep is the causitive organism of the sore throat and treat with antibiotics; also to alleviate painful symptoms associated with the infection.

Conventional Medicine

Strep throat is differentiated from other sore throat conditions by the presence of swollen lymph glands around the neck, thick exudate of pus on the tonsils, absence of cough, and a fever of greater than 100°F. When all these symptoms are present, antibiotics may be taken without first taking a bacteria culture. It is important to start antibiotics immediately if you have a history of rheumatic heart disease.

Antibiotics: Penicillin V is the first choice for treating strep throat. An intramuscular shot of penicillin G may be prescribed if it is suspected that the full course of antibiotics may not be taken, for more rapid response to symptoms, or if the patient prefers a single-dose treatment. Medications related to penicillin such as amoxicillin are generally used to treat cases of strep throat in children because they taste better. Erythromycin can be used by those who are allergic to penicillin. If there is no improvement after 24–48 hours, the strep bacteria may be resistant to the type of antibiotic and a different one may be prescribed. Cephalosporins and newer macrolides, which are alternative antibiotics, are reserved for treating unresponsive cases.

Complications: It is important to treat strep throat with antibiotics, as it can lead to complications such as muscle infections, toxic shock syndrome, and rheumatic fever. Other less common complications include serious kidney conditions, sinusitis, mastoiditis, meningitis, infection of the blood stream, and pneumonia.

Traditional Chinese Medicine

Herbs:
• **Patent herbal pills:** Yin Qiao Jie Du Pian and Chuan Xin Lian Pian are patent Chinese medicines available from Chinese pharmacies or groceries. Take both pills three times a day for one week (refer to the dosage as indicated on the package).

• **Herbal decoction:** Combine 10 g of Jin Yin Hua (honeysuckle flower), 15 g of Ban Lan Gen (isatis root), 10 g of Da Qing Ye (woad leaf), 5 g of Shen Gan Cao (raw licorice), and 10 g of She Gan (belamcanda rhizome) in a ceramic or glass container. Bring to a boil and simmer for 30 minutes. Strain the liquid and drink 1 cup twice a day. If you have a severe case of strep throat, you can take this decoction together with one of the pills mentioned above.

Acupressure: Use the tip of your thumb to press the Hegu point, located on the back of the hand between the thumb and the first finger, with strong pressure for one to two minutes. Beginning with gentle pressure and gradually increasing, use your thumb to press the Feng Chi point, which is located at the back of the head, at the base of the skull, about 2 inches from the center. Press and release about 20 times.

Diet: Eat foods that are mild and cooling, such as cucumber, mango, eggplant, spinach, strawberry, pears, and lettuce.

Naturopathy

Diet: Take two or more cloves of garlic, crushed or whole, at the first sign of a sore throat and continue eating two cloves a day until your symptoms clear up. Garlic contains allicin, which has antibiotic and antifungal properties. Your diet should consist primarily of vegetables, whole grains, lots of soups (particularly chicken and miso soup), and water. Dairy products and simple carbohydrates, such as fruit, should be avoided. An ice-cold fruit juice popsicle can be an effective temporary anesthetic.

Supplements: Take 500–1,000 mg of vitamin C every four hours until symptoms subside to support the immune system. Take 1,000 mg of bioflavonoids in two 500 mg doses a day. Bioflavonoids work synergistically with vitamin C and have immune-enhancing properties. Zinc also supports the immune system and may have some antiviral properties. Take 25 mg in lozenges every day for one week.

Herbs: Dilute lavender, eucalyptus, thyme, or tea tree essential oil in olive, apricot, or almond oil and rub it gently on the chest and the front of the neck. These should only be used topically. These oils are anti-infective and will help to loosen and shift sticky mucus.

Tip: FLUSH OUT FLUIDS

Keep your fluid intake up to encourage the body to flush out infection and to keep the body temperature down.

Homeopathy

If you have a severe sore throat (especially if there is difficulty in opening the mouth or swallowing), your doctor will want to establish whether a streptococcal infection is present. If this is the case, conventional treatment will be prescribed to treat the infection. Homeopathic treatment can be used in a complementary fashion to ease pain. Once the immediate problem has been dealt with, consider more long-term homeopathic treatment from a practitioner in order to discourage recurrence. Also see Sore Throat (p. 168).

Gelsemium: If there is an overwhelming feeling of exhaustion when feeling ill, Gelsemium may help. Symptoms that respond well to this remedy characteristically come on slowly over a few days. There may be a nasty taste in the mouth, with severe pain in the throat and ears that is made worse when swallowing. As a result, the patient may be unwilling to drink.

Mercurius: When a severe sore throat is combined with swollen, tender glands, increased amounts of saliva, and an unpleasant sweetish or metallic taste in the mouth, use Mercurius.

Phytolacca: Try this remedy if there is a characteristic pain at the root of the tongue, which becomes more severe when sticking the tongue out when being examined.

Herbalism

The following herbs may be used in addition to antibiotics to relieve the symptoms of strep throat and treat infection.

Myrrh: Myrrh can be used in tincture form and has effective anti-inflammatory and antimicrobial properties. Use the tincture dilute in warm water as a gargle four to six times daily. This is particularly effective in combination with goldenseal.

Ginger: This pungent, hot herb is used to treat cold conditions. Normally regarded as a soothing digestive remedy, it may also have antimicrobial activity against streptococcus. Your herbal medicine practitioner might suggest taking fresh or dried root in a capsule, tea, or tincture.

Goldenseal root: This herb may inhibit the streptococcus bacteria, as well as other types of bacteria. A tea or tincture in water might be taken three to four times daily. Choose cultivated goldenseal, or substitute Oregon grape root, which has similar effects due to the berberine content.

Tonsillitis

Diagnosis

Tonsillitis occurs when the tonsils become infected and swell, becoming red and inflamed. The condition manifests with flu-like symptoms, including a sore throat and trouble swallowing. It spreads from person to person by airborne droplets that are breathed in, hand-to-hand contact, or through kissing. Tonsillitis is usually caused by the bacteria streptococcus, but it can also occasionally be caused by a virus. Other triggers include congestion, a cold, flu, laryngitis, or being rundown. If you suffer from recurrent tonsillitis, it is important to start assessing the cause so that it can be resolved. Always seek the advice of your doctor if you have a fever with a sore throat and swollen glands.

Symptoms

- Sore throat
- Difficulty swallowing
- Red and swollen tonsils
- Swollen glands
- Fever and chills
- The adenoids can also be affected, resulting in snoring
- Poor appetite and lethargy
- Voice loss or changes to the voice
- Cough
- Earache

Treatment Goal

To treat and relieve symptoms in acute cases, and to determine and remove the cause in chronic cases. The standard treatment is a course of antibiotics. Surgery to remove tonsils is still used occasionally to treat recurrent and acute tonsillitis, particularly if linked with breathing problems.

Conventional Medicine

Tonsillitis can be bacterial or viral in origin and should be treated accordingly. (Also see Sore Throat, p. 166, and Strep Throat, p. 171.) A medical emergency exists if there is an abscess surrounding the tonsils. Also if the tonsils remain very enlarged following treatment, referral to an ear, nose, and throat (ENT) specialist is usual.

To treat viral infections: Acetaminophen (Tylenol®), or ibuprofen (Motrin®) may be used as directed to alleviate pain. Saltwater gargles (1 tsp of salt mixed in 2 cups of distilled water)

Tip: REST AND RECUPERATE

Get as much rest as possible, maintain a stable temperature to avoid getting chilly or overheated, and keep fluid intake up. Stick to food that is easily digestible.

may also be helpful. Eating cool foods that feel good to the throat for a couple of days may be more comfortable. Some plants, such as larch taken at 1 g twice a day, may decrease the length of the viral infection.

To treat bacterial infections: Penicillin and its derivatives are prescribed to treat tonsillitis. Erythromycin is used if a patient is allergic to penicillin. Some strains of the bacteria have become resistant to penicillin and erythromycin. If there is no improvement after 24–48 hours, the bacteria may be resistant to the antibiotic and an alternative, such as clarythromycin (Biaxin®) or a cephalosporin (Keflex®), is prescribed.

Recurrent tonsillitis: This is generally a reason for surgical removal of the tonsils.

Traditional Chinese Medicine

Chinese medicine is effective in treating both acute and chronic tonsillitis. If you have tried antibiotics without success, and before you resort to surgery, try comprehensive TCM treatment.

Herbs:
• Acute tonsillitis: Combine 5 g of Ye Ju Hua (wild chrysanthemum flower), 3 g of Gan Cao (licorice root), and 5 g of Jin Yin Hua (honeysuckle flower); or 5 g of Bo He (field mint), 8 g of Ban Lan Gen (isatis root), and 8 g

of Jie Geng (balloon flower root); or 5 g of Pu Gong Ying (dandelion) and 5 g of Bai Hua She She Cao (heydyotis). For all formulas, place the raw herbs in a teapot and add boiling water. Steep for three to five minutes and drink throughout the day.

• **Chronic tonsillitis:** Combine 10 g of Pi Pa Ye (loquat leaf), 3 g of Chen Pi (tangerine peel), 8 g of Wu Mei (mume fruit), and 3 g of Gan Cao (licorice root); or 10 g of Xuan Shen (ningpo figwort root), 10 g of Mai Men Dong (ophiopogon tuber), 10 g Jie Geng (balloon flower root), and 5 g of Gan Cao (licorice root). Add 3 cups of water to the herbs from either formula and boil for 6–10 minutes. Drink throughout the day.

Acupressure: Use the tip of your thumb to press the Hegu and Tai Yang points for one to two minutes. The Hegu points are located on the back of the hands between the thumb and first finger. The Tai Yang point is on the temple in the depression next to the lateral end of the eyebrow and eyelid.

Diet: Rice porridge is comforting if you are suffering from tonsillitis. Place 1 cup of washed rice in a pot and add 5 cups of water. Bring the rice to a boil and cook just under the boil until rice is soft and creamy.

Naturopathy

Diet: Drink fluids throughout the day consisting of water, teas, and soups, particularly chicken soup and miso soup. Reduce the amount of dairy and simple carbohydrates (found in fruits and processed foods, and in anything with refined sugar added) you are consuming. Your diet should consist primarily of vegetables, whole grains, some fresh fruit and lots of soup and water.

Supplements: Take 500–1,000 mg of vitamin C every four hours to support the immune system until symptoms subside. Children should take 250 mg of vitamin C three times a day. Bioflavonoids work synergistically with Vitamin C and have immune-enhancing

properties of their own. Take 1,000 mg in divided doses a day; give children 100–200 mg three times a day. Zinc also supports the immune system and may have antiviral properties. An aggressive dose of zinc is needed to treat tonsilitis, so consult a practitioner. Zinc depletes the body's store of copper so also take copper alongside zinc supplements.

Herbs: Echinacea and goldenseal enhance the immune system and have antiviral properties. Take 2–4 ml of a combination tincture four times a day. Astragalus is excellent for treating and preventing tonsillitis and infections in general. Take 500–1,000 mg in capsule form or

4–6 ml of tincture three times a day. Take plenty of raw garlic or 300–500 mg in capsule form to fight infection or as a preventive measure. Drink slippery elm and marshmallow root tea two to three times a day. Place 25 g of slippery elm root and 25 g of marshmallow root in 5 cups of cold water. Boil the mixture for 30 minutes and strain the liquid. Let it cool before drinking. It is very soothing to the tonsils and throat. Shiitake and reishi mushrooms are effective for viral and bacterial tonsillitis. Once fever has resolved, take 2–6 g of the extract a day. Teas and baths prepared with peppermint and thyme assist in reducing fever. Drink peppermint or thyme tea, or use 10 drops of peppermint or thyme oil in a warm bath, as needed.

Homeopathy

Any of the following homeopathic remedies can be helpful in easing pain and inflammation, and speeding up recovery, from an isolated bout of tonsillitis. However, a recurrent condition should be treated by a homeopathic practitioner. See the suggestions given for sore throat (p. 168) and strep throat (p. 173) in addition to the following.

Arsenicum album: If burning pains are present in the throat that cause great anxiety, distress, and restlessness, especially in the night or the early hours of the morning, try Arsenicum album. The body is likely to feel incredibly chilly, while the head feels better from contact with cool, fresh air (ideally while the body is kept very warm). Taking small sips of warm drinks temporarily soothes the burning sensations in the throat.

Lycopodium: Consider this remedy if symptoms arise when feeling anxious and stressed. Symptoms characteristically start on the right side and move to the left, or may remain more painful and inflamed on the right side. Pain and distress is made more severe by contact with cold drinks, and eased by warm liquids.

Herbalism

The herbal approach to tonsillitis is to support the immune system, while fighting infection.

Andrographis: This herb has several active constituents that impart antiviral, immune-stimulating, and antioxidant properties that may successfully treat tonsillitis. Because Andrographis is very bitter, some people may find it easier to take in capsule form. A preventive adult dose is 2–3 g or 4–6 ml of tincture a day. During infection, take up to 6 g or 12 ml of tincture a day. Do not take during pregnancy.

Astragalus: Although astragalus has demonstrated a potent ability to enhance immunity, inhibit viral infections, and improve fatigue, it should not be used to treat an acute infection. Astragalus is best taken to treat chronic tonsillitis or as a preventive measure. Boil 10 g of root in 1 cup of water and drink, or take 6 ml of tincture per day.

Echinacea: Although several species of echinacea are used medicinally, Echinacea purpurea is the most widely cultivated due to the fact it can be easily grown and the whole plant (flower, leaf, seed, and root) can be taken. Studies have shown that echinacea has immune-stimulating, antibacterial, mild antiviral, and anti-inflammatory properties. Take 2–3 g of dried root as a decoction, or 3–6 ml of tincture a day until the infection resolves. 🌿

Tip: THROAT SPRAY

Combine 20 ml each of licorice, sage, echinacea, and thyme, and 10 ml of ginger tincture to create a soothing, antimicrobial, antiviral, and immune-stimulating blend. Spray this mixture directly into the throat throughout the day as needed.

4

Digestive System and Urinary Tract

Diabetes

Diagnosis

Diabetes mellitus is a condition in which the amount of glucose (sugar) in the blood becomes too high because the body cannot process it properly due to insufficient levels of insulin or cellular resistance to insulin.

There are two main types of diabetes. Type 1 develops when the body is unable to produce insulin. It is treated by insulin injections, and a diet overhaul and regular exercise are also recommended. With Type 2 the body can still produce some insulin, but not enough. This condition is often linked to being overweight and usually appears in people over the age of 40. Recently, more children are being diagnosed with the Type 2 condition. Type 2 diabetes is treated with lifestyle changes such as a healthier diet and weight loss.

Symptoms

- Frequent urination
- Excessive thirst
- Extreme tiredness
- Weight loss
- Smell of nail polish (acetone) on the breath
- Thrush
- Blurred vision

Treatment Goal

To maintain blood glucose, blood pressure, and cholesterol levels as near to normal as possible. Together with a healthy lifestyle, this will help protect against long-term damage to the body's major organs.

Conventional Medicine

To treat Type 1 diabetes: Those with Type 1 diabetes require insulin as none is produced by the pancreas. The amount of insulin needed varies and must be administered several times a day. The insulin pump has been a major advance in improving glucose control in Type 1 or brittle diabetics. The prevention of both low and high blood sugar levels is very important to avoid the complications of diabetes, and blood glucose levels must be checked at least once a day with insulin-dependent diabetes, preferably before each dose of insulin. The dose is adjusted according to exercise levels and food intake, as both of these factors affect the blood sugar. Monitoring the diet for calories, carbohydrates, fat, and protein is also essential. The body's requirements vary according to height, weight, and age, but generally calorie requirements are between 15 and 25 calories per pound of body weight per day. Your diet should be made up of 55% carbohydrates (as whole grains, fruits, and vegetables, not processed food), 25% fat (monounsaturated), and about 20% protein, such as fish, chicken, and vegetable proteins.

To treat Type 2 diabetes: This condition initially results when the insulin produced by the body does not work appropriately (known as insulin resistance). It is associated with obesity, and the illness can be prevented by modifying your lifestyle. Studies show that, compared to managing the condition through medication, lifestyle modification more successfully controls sugar levels and the complications of diabetes. Following the diet above, keeping the body mass index under 28, exercising, reducing stress, and keeping alcohol intake to a minimum are usually enough to ensure prevention. At the first signs of insulin resistance, begin a weight-loss program, swap carbs for complex, low glycemic index foods (whole grains and fruits and vegetables), and exercise (for example, fast walking) at least 20 minutes a day. The minerals chromium and vanadium are helpful for this condition as are several herbs, fenugreek and cinnamon in particular. Medications used for Type 2 diabetes include several groups of blood-sugar-lowering drugs, such as the sulfonylureas, the biguanides, the glucosidase inhibitors, the thiaxolidinediones, and the meglitinides. Each medication acts in a different way and a doctor will choose the most appropriate one according to the history of illness, other medications being taken, and other diseases suffered. Type 2 diabetes is monitored by family physicians.

Complications of diabetes: Each type of diabetes predisposes a person to complications, including cardiac, renal, and neurologic problems, infections, retinal damage in the eyes, and high cholesterol and triglycerides. Those with diabetes should be regularly checked for these complications and referred to a specialist as needed. Most of the associated problems can be prevented by keeping the blood sugar level in a normal range.

Traditional Chinese Medicine

Diabetes often occurs in those who have a deficiency of yin. Consult with a Chinese medicine doctor before using the suggested formulas. For severe cases of diabetes TCM treatment can be used alongside Western medicine, but it is not a replacement for conventional medication. Consult your doctor before integrating treatments.

Herbs:
• **Formula one:** This can be used to treat either Type 1 or Type 2 diabetes. Symptoms of dryness in the mouth and on the tongue, thirst, frequent urination, dizziness, and vertigo usually indicate an insufficiency of kidney yin. Combine 12 g of Bei Mao Gen (wooly grass rhizome), 10 g of Yu Mi Xu (corn silk), 12 g of Xuan Shen (ningpo figwort root), 12 g of Di Huang (Chinese foxglove), 10 g of Shan Zhu Yu (Asiatic cornelian cherry), 12 g of Tian Men Dong (asparagus tuber), and 12 g of Wu Wei Zi (schisandra fruit) with 3–4 cups of water in a ceramic or glass pot. Bring to a boil and simmer for 30 minutes. Strain and drink 1 cup two to three times a day.
• **Formula two:** This can be used to treat either Type 1 or Type 2 diabetes. Symptoms include overheating and emotional disturbance, fever,

perspiration, anxiety, irritability, anger, constipation, strong thirst, and a yellow, dry tongue. Place 12 g of Zhi Zi (cape jasmine fruit), 12 g of Yu Zhu (atractylodes rhizome), 10 g of Huang Qin (baical skullcap root), 12 g of Tian Hua Fen (trichosanthes root), 10 g of Chai Hu (hare's ear root), 12 g of Zhi Mu (anemarrhena rhizome), and 12 g of Dan Pi (cortex of tree peony root) in a ceramic pot and add 3–4 cups of water. Bring to a boil, simmer for 30 minutes, and strain. Drink this decoction twice a day.

Acupressure: Use a moderate pressure on the Nei Guan, San Yin Jiao, and Tai Xi points. The Nei Guan point is in the center of the wrist on the palm side, 2 inches below the crease. The San Yin Jiao point is on the inside of the leg, 3 inches above the anklebone. The Tai Xi point is on the inside of the leg in the depression between the Achilles tendon and the anklebone.

Diet: Recommended foods include spinach, turnip, millet, Chinese yam, and water chestnuts. Avoid fatty food, alcohol, and spicy food, along with foods high in sugar.

Naturopathy

Diet: The most important therapy for diabetes is a healthy diet. Eat plenty of vegetables, beans, nuts, seeds, and whole grains. The high fiber in these foods helps balance blood sugar.

Ground flaxseeds should be eaten on a daily basis as well. Sprinkle 2 tbsp on your cereal or salad. Do not expose the flaxseeds to too much heat. Focus on good fats found in foods such as salmon and sardines. Use extra virgin olive oil and flaxseed oil on your salad. Refrain from eating large meals throughout the day. Instead, frequently eat small meals that consist of some good quality protein. Do not go for longer than three hours without eating. Avoid eating simple sugars, including junk foods like sweets, cookies, and carbonated drinks. These foods contribute to blood sugar instability. Avoid cow's milk. Some studies show a link between cow's milk and diabetes in children. Use stevia or xylitol as a sweetener, which are safe for diabetics and are healthier choices.

Supplements: Take a high-quality multivitamin as directed to obtain many of the nutrients involved with blood sugar metabolism. Take 200–400 mcg of chromium a day to improve glucose metabolism and balance blood sugar levels. Take 300–600 mg of alpha lipoic acid a day to improve insulin sensitivity and reduce the symptoms of diabetic neuropathy. Vanadyl

sulfate improves glucose tolerance; take 100–300 mg a day. Take 3 g of fish oils a day to support the nervous system and assist in proper insulin function. B-complex vitamins are involved in glucose metabolism, and should be taken at 50 mg a day. Biotin, taken at 7,000–15,000 mcg a day, reduces the changes of diabetic neuropathies. This is a B vitamin so consider the amount included in your B-complex vitamin and adjust the dosage accordingly. You can also take 500 mg of magnesium, involved in insulin production and utilization, a day. Reduce the dosage if your stools soften.

Herbs: Bitter melon helps balance blood sugar levels. The typical dosage of bitter melon is one small, unripe, raw melon a day, or about 50–100 ml of fresh juice, divided into two or three doses over the course of the day. Bitter melon tastes unpleasant to some, and can be taken in capsule form at 200 mg three times a day. Billberry helps prevent problems with the retinas caused by diabetes. The standard dosage of bilberry is 120–240 mg of an extract standardized to contain 25% anthocyanosides twice a day. Taking 15–30 g of defatted fenugreek three times a day with meals stabilizes blood sugar. Fenugreek seeds are bitter so the herb is best taken in capsule form. Banana leaf has also been shown to lower blood sugar levels. Take 16 mg in capsule form twice a day.

Tip: EXERCISE REGULARLY

Exercise regularly to maintain optimal blood sugar levels. Exercise helps reduce weight and lowers blood sugar. It improves insulin sensitivity, the immune system, and circulation. It lowers blood pressure and LDL ("bad") cholesterol, raises HDL ("good") cholesterol, and reduces the risk of heart disease. Find an exercise that you like and try to do at least four sessions a week.

Homeopathy

Diabetes is a condition for which it is inappropriate to suggest self-help homeopathic prescribing, since both Type 1 and Type 2 diabetes are chronic conditions. As such, any homeopathic treatment that is given will be of a constitutional nature and needs to be provided by an experienced homeopathic practitioner.

Herbalism

Herbal medicines used to treat diabetes generally aim to lower blood sugar, protect vascular integrity, and preserve the function of the pancreas. Insulin and other diabetic agents may need to be adjusted if herbal remedies are used in a complementary manner, because of many herbs' hypoglycemic effect. All recommended herbs are safe for both Type 1 and Type 2 diabetics but it is advised to monitor blood sugar and work with a practitioner to adjust dosages as necessary.

Gymnema: This woody plant was traditionally used to treat diabetes long before its positive results were discovered in clinical trials. Gymnema discourages sugar consumption by inhibiting the taste of sugar placed on the tongue. Studies have also shown that Gymnema effectively lowers blood sugar when taken at 400 mg per day. Current research shows that Gymnema increases insulin levels

or decreases insulin sensitivity, possibly indicating that it regenerates pancreatic beta-cells (insulin-secreting cells). Take 400 mg in capsule form or 5 ml of tincture daily.

Bilberry: These berries have been shown to decrease hyperglycaemia in trials. It is a generally useful herb in diabetes, as it may also prevent against glaucoma and cataracts, and also supports blood vessels. Standardized extract capsules of 25% anthocyanidins are available, and the berries can also be decocted or taken as a tincture.

Fenugreek: This herb slows carbohydrate absorption, delays gastric emptying, and increases insulin receptors, all of which have blood sugar lowering effects. In most clinical trials, patients took 50 mg per day to achieve significant effects.

Acid Reflux

Diagnosis

Acid reflux is caused when the sphincter (ring of muscle at the lower end of the throat or esophagus) becomes abnormally relaxed, allowing the acidic contents of the stomach to flow back or "reflux" into the throat. The condition is typically triggered by eating large or rich meals, drinking alcohol, or smoking. The reflux tendency increases when the stomach is overfull, leading to increased pressure. Obesity also increases pressure on the stomach, as does pregnancy. Prolonged exposure to refluxed acid results in the serious condition esophagitis (inflammation of the esophagus), which can eventually lead to difficulties swallowing and in some cases a condition called Barrett's esophagus, which may lead to esophageal cancer. This complication is rare, but persistent symptoms require medical investigation.

Symptoms

- Painful burning sensation in the chest
- The acid reflux may reach the throat and mouth
- Sour taste in the mouth
- Occasionally, breathing difficulties occur
- Hoarseness due to irritation of the larynx
- Belching

Treatment Goal

To relieve the symptoms and identify the cause of the acid reflux to prevent further problems from occurring. This may involve lifestyle changes as well as medications.

Conventional Medicine

Antacids: These can be taken on an intermittent basis according to the instructions on the packet. Antacids can reduce the absorption of certain vitamins, especially B vitamins, so it is a good idea to take a multivitamin with extra B vitamins when on this kind of medication. The multivitamin should be taken at a different time in the day than the antacid.

Lifestyle modification: Try raising the head while sleeping by elevating the head of the bed. Avoid alcohol and nicotine, and any foods that aggravate the condition. Spicy foods such as onions, peppers, tomatoes, and peppermint may stimulate reflux. Obesity is a contributing factor, and in these cases weight loss can also help. Stress reduction techniques are important as the hormone released when stressed (cortisol) affects the acid level of the stomach as well as the muscle tone of the stomach, making acid reflux worse.

H2 blockers: If the above techniques do not work, medications that block acid receptors in the stomach (H2 blockers) such as cimetidine, ranitidine, famotidine, and nizatidine can be tried. These do bring relief from symptoms, but can also affect the body's absorption of B vitamins. Be sure to take extra B vitamin supplements if you are taking these medications.

Proton pump inhibitors: This class of drugs helps by reducing the secretion of acid in the stomach. They are stronger than antacids and acid blockers and are usually reserved for severe diseases.

Surgery: If the reflux becomes very severe and the esophagus is damaged, then surgery may be required, some of which may be done through new endoscopic procedures.

Traditional Chinese Medicine

Herbs: If your condition worsens, consult your doctor immediately.
• **To relieve heartburn and other symptoms caused by acid reflux:** Combine 10 g of Mu Xiang (costus root), 5 g of Sha Ren (cardamom), 12 g of Bai Zhu (white atractylodes rhizome), 15 g of Shan Yao (Chinese yam), 12 g of Fa Ban Xia (pinellia rhizome), 30 g of Dai Zhe Shi (hematite), 12 g of Lian Qiao (forsythia fruit), and 3 g of Gan Cao (licorice root) in a ceramic pot. Add 3 cups of water, bring to a boil, and simmer for 30 minutes before straining the liquid into a container. Drink 1 cup twice a day for 10 days as one course of treatment. Take three to five courses of treatment.
• **To treat a deficient digestive system:** Combine 12 g Tai Zi Shen (pseudostellaria), 10 g of Huang Qi (milk-vetch root), 12 g Bai Zhu

(white atractylodes rhizome), 8 g of Zhi Ke (bitter orange), 15 g of Fuling (poria), and 3 g of Gan Cao (licorice root) in a ceramic pot with 3 cups of water. Bring to a boil, simmer for 30 minutes, and strain. Drink 1 cup of the liquid twice a day for 10 days as one course of treatment. Take three to five courses of treatment.

Acupressure: Apply gentle pressure to the Nei Guan, Susanli, and San Yin Jiao points for one to two minutes. The Nei Guan point is located in the center of the wrist on the palm side about 2 inches below the crease. The Susanli point is on the lower leg, 1 inch to the outside of and 3 inches below the kneecap. The San Yin Jiao point is on the inside of the leg, about 3 inches above the anklebone.

Diet: Eat food that is nourishing to the spleen and stomach such as sweet rice, beef, honey, corn, celery, spinach, lettuce, and potatoes. Avoid fruits (especially oranges, lemons, pineapple, and apricots) and acidic food such as tomato and chilies.

Naturopathy

Diet: Cut common trigger foods, including coffee, chocolate, fried and fatty foods, alcohol, and spices, out of your diet. Increase the amount of high-fiber foods to help your body absorb excess acid and gas, and rid itself of toxins more quickly. Eat plenty of whole grains and fresh fruit and vegetables. Drink at least eight glasses of water each day to allow your body to expel acid naturally. Herbal teas containing chamomile, ginger, licorice root, and catnip, as well as green tea, help the stomach lining repair itself. Steep these herbs in water overnight and drink 1 cup of tea, diluted to taste, after dinner to reduce acid reflux. Do not drink any kind of mint tea. This may worsen the symptoms.

Herbs: Take 500–1,000 mg of slippery elm three times a day to soothe the gastrointestinal (GI) tract. Deglycyrrhizinated licorice (DGL) capsules can also bring quick relief and may help heal the damaged lining in the stomach. Take two DGL licorice tablets (380 mg) three or four times a day between meals as needed. Aloe vera juice is another fast-acting supplement that frequently helps soothe an irritated esophagus. Take ½ cup of aloe vera juice three times a day between meals. Make sure it contains 98% aloe vera and no aloin or aloe-emodin. To treat chronic acid reflux, take 150 mg of gamma-oryzanol three times a day on an empty stomach. This rice bran oil extract can help repair the entire digestive system and improve the central nervous system's digestive control. Choline, pantothenic acid, and thiamine are B-complex vitamins that can have long-term digestive benefits. If you suffer from chronic acid reflux, try them in combination for a month or so to see if they help.

Supplements: Medications used to treat acid reflux deplete the body of vitamin B12, folate, and various minerals. Take a multivitamin/multimineral supplement to compensate for this problem. Take 500 mg of choline, sold as plain choline or phosphatidylcholine, three

times a day. To treat chronic acid reflux, take this in combination with 1,000 mg of pantothenic acid twice a day and 500 mg of thiamine first think in the morning for one month to see if symptoms resolve. Digestive enzymes, such as lipases, proteases, and amylases, help to speed the digestive process, often helping eliminate acid reflux altogether. Take two to three capsules with every meal. You can also take papaya enzyme as a chewable capsule after each meal.

Homeopathy

Choosing the most appropriate of the remedies listed below may help ease the discomfort of a mild case of acid reflux that is due to a specific cause. Chronic conditions will benefit most from professional homeopathic treatment.

Arsenicum album: This remedy can be helpful in easing symptoms that develop in the night or early hours of the morning. Sipping on warm drinks temporarily soothes gastric uneasiness. Any nausea that is present causes a disproportionate amount of anxiety and distress. Other symptoms include feeling more

comfortable for lying slightly raised on two or three pillows.

Lycopodium: If there is a noticeable amount of noisy gurgling and rumbling combined with acid reflux, use Lycopodium. Symptoms are aggravated or triggered by stress. Dietary factors can also trigger the condition, with very high-fiber foods having an adverse effect on digestion. Appetite is irregular, with a tendency to start a meal feeling very hungry, but becoming quickly satisfied.

Bryonia: Use this remedy if there is a heavy feeling in the stomach that develops almost immediately after eating, and if a bitter-tasting liquid washes up into the mouth. Symptoms are aggravated by moving around, pressure to the stomach, and by eating quickly.

Nux vomica: This is a leading remedy for acid reflux. It is especially useful when used by those who are irritable, impatient, competitive, and prone to anger fits. Symptoms may be worse after eating a large amount of rich or spicy food, or drinking coffee or alcohol.

Herbalism

Herbs can help with reflux in several different ways. Demulcent herbs coat the skin and can soothe and protect the inflamed mucous membranes in the oesophagus and stomach that may occur with reflux. Anti-inflammatory herbs can improve acid reflux symptoms and help the damaged tissue to heal. Anti-anxiety herbs are part of an herbalist's overall healing approach to a patient with acid reflux.

Slippery elm root bark powder: Stir 1–2 tbsp of this demulcent powder into a glass of water and drink after meals and before bedtime. Begin with a smaller amount of powder until you become accustomed to it; if too much powder is mixed in the water, the preparation can be very thick and difficult to tolerate. Slippery elm is safe, though some of the compounds contained in it can bind medications that are taken at the same time and decrease their absorption. Do not take slippery elm within one to two hours of taking any other medication.

Marshmallow: This demulcent herb can relieve acid reflux symptoms. Make a cold infusion overnight with 5–6 g of marshmallow root and

drink throughout the day. As with slippery elm, medicines taken at the same time may not be absorbed as well.

Chamomile: This herb has an anti-spasmodic effect on the intestines and acts as an anti-inflammatory to treat acid reflux. Make a tea from 1–3 g of chamomile flowers and drink three to four times daily.

Anti-anxiety botanicals: Anxiety and acid reflux can be linked in some people. Common anti-anxiety plants recommended as part of an acid reflux prescription are valerian and skullcap; see Anxiety (p. 448) for more information. Diet should also be considered for intolerances and triggers.

Heartburn

Diagnosis

Heartburn occurs when harsh stomach acid flows up (know as reflux) and comes into contact with and irritates the delicate lining of the esophagus. This generally occurs when the lower esophageal sphincter (LES), the natural valve that keeps stomach acid in the stomach, does not do its job properly. Various lifestyle and dietary factors, as well as certain medications, can contribute to heartburn. Foods that are problematic for heartburn sufferers include citrus fruits, tomatoes, onions and garlic, vinegar, and anything fatty or spicy. Large meals and eating just before bedtime can also cause irritation, as can caffeinated and carbonated drinks. Episodes of heartburn can also be triggered by body position, certain movements, or exertion. Heartburn commonly occurs during pregnancy.

Symptoms

- Burning chest pain moving up toward the throat
- Sensation that food is coming back into the mouth
- Bitter taste at the back of the throat
- Difficulty swallowing
- More painful when lying down or bending over

Treatment Goal

To relieve any immediate symptoms and put into practice lifestyle changes that will help ease the problem of heartburn.

Conventional Medicine

If left unchecked, heartburn can result in more serious conditions, such as damage to the esophagus with bleeding, ulceration, and even cancer. Sometimes the upper airways can become involved, resulting in asthma, chronic cough, and chronic laryngitis. Conventional medical treatment provides relief for the symptoms and discomfort associated with heartburn, while preventing further complications.

Antacids: Over-the-counter antacids, which consist of aluminum hydroxide, magnesium carbonate, and magnesium trisilicate preparations, are usually taken five or six times a day between meals. Dissolving 1 tsp of sodium bicarbonate in a glass of water is also effective; however, excessive amounts of sodium bicarbonate can interfere with the acid base balance of the body and add excess sodium to the system, which can contribute to hypertension. Many antacids inhibit the body's ability to absorb minerals, so take vitamin and mineral supplements.

Lifestyle changes: Try raising the head of the bed so that acid does not reflux while you are sleeping. Avoid smoking, as this irritates acid reflux. Eating a diet of plain, natural organic foods usually leads to an improvement of symptoms. Taking herbs such as aloe and mallow root can also be beneficial. Studies show that stress contributes greatly to acid reflux, so managing stress levels is important. Weight loss should be considered if you are overweight.

Medications: A class of drugs that blocks acid in the stomach, known as H2 receptor antagonists, is used to treat heartburn. It includes medications such as cimetidine, ranitidine, and famotidine. Proton pump inhibitors such as omeprazole and lansoprazole also reduce gastric acid secretion and tend to be more effective than the H2 blockers.

Traditional Chinese Medicine

TCM identifies two types of heartburn: an excessive or deficient condition. A diagnosis from a conventional doctor is helpful, as Chinese medicine can then be used in a complementary manner.

Herbs: Combine the ingredients of either of the herbal remedies below in a ceramic pot. Add 3 cups of water, bring to a boil, and simmer for 30 minutes.
• **Excessive heartburn:** Usually due to improper diet and irregular eating patterns,

or a cold or fever. Mix 10 g Zhi Shi (immature fruit of bitter orange), 10 g of Mu Xiang (costus root), 10 g of Zhu Ru (bamboo shavings), 15 g of Fuling (poria), 10 g of Xuan Fu Hua (inula flower), 30 g of Dai Zhe Shi (hematite), 8 g of Shen Qu (medicated leaven), 10 g of Huo Xiang (agastache), 5 g of Sha Ren (cardamom), 5 g of fresh ginger, and 5 g of Gan Cao (licorice root). Drink 1 cup two to three times a day for three to five days.

• **Chronic condition:** Symptoms include weakness, fatigue, poor appetite, and indigestion. Combine 12 g of Dan Shen (salvia root), 15 g Bai Zhu (white atractylodes rhizome), 15 g of Fuling (poria), 15 g of Shan Yao (Chinese yam),10 g of Mu Xiang (costus root), 6 g of Bai Kou Ren (round cardamom fruit), and five pieces of Da Zhao (Chinese jujube). You can use this formula for 7–10 days, or consult a practitioner about long-term use.

Acupressure: Use the tip of your thumb to apply medium pressure to the Nei Guan, Hegu, and Tan Zhong points for one minute and repeat. The Nei Guan point is located in the center of the wrist on the palm side, about 2 inches above the crease. The Hegu points are located on the back of the hands, in the depression between the thumb and the first finger. The Tan Zhong point is found on the midpoint between the nipples.

Diet: Foods that are good for this condition are corn, rice, tofu, spinach, celery, bamboo shoots, Daikon radishes, carrots, cherries, pomegranates, pears, fish, and water chestnuts. Avoid acidic food, such as tomatoes, oranges, and grapefruit, and hot, spicy food, such as black and white pepper, green and red peppers, chilies, dried ginger, and star anise.

Naturopathy

Diet: Eat a whole food diet and eliminate unnatural refined foods. Whole grains, raw vegetables, and raw nuts and seeds are rich in fiber and contain essential nutrients important in relieving gastric symptoms and healing gastric mucosa. Bananas seem to be particularly beneficial for relieving heartburn. You may also use ground, dried banana. Drink 8–10 glasses of water a day to maintain good digestive health and neutralize the excess acidity in the stomach. Some foods, including

wheat, citrus fruits, and corn, can aggravate the condition. Pay attention to see if symptoms flare up when eating these foods. Avoid foods that contain saturated fats, hydrogenated oils, and partially hydrogenated oils, such as fried and greasy foods, processed foods, heavy sauces, and red meats, as they can lead to acid reflux. Caffeine, alcohol, chocolate, and minty and spicy foods can make symptoms worse and should be avoided. White wine, especially dry young whites from Germany, may cause heartburn as they are very acidic. Avoid overeating and take small meals regularly throughout the day to help soothe the digestive tract. Also avoid eating three hours before bedtime, as sleeping on a full stomach tends to aggravate symptoms.

Supplements: Calcium carbonate is a well-known heartburn reliever and the principal active ingredient in antacid tablets such as Tums®. It can provide immediate relief and may be particularly effective for treating sporadic heartburn. Take 250–500 mg of calcium carbonate three times a day with food. Chewable tablets provide the quickest relief. Avoid brands that include peppermint, which has been shown to relax the low esophageal sphincter, the muscle at the base of the esophagus that normally keeps food and digestive acids in the stomach.

Herbs: Drinking aloe vera juice between meals is another fast-acting method of soothing an agitated esophagus. Make sure the juice contains 98% aloe vera and no aloin or aloe-emodin. Take 500 mg of mastic gum three times a day to heal stomach mucosa and for its antibacterial benefits. Gamma-oryzanol, also known as rice bran oil, can help repair the entire digestive system. Take 150 mg three times a day for one month.

Homeopathy

If symptoms occur suddenly, with no obvious cause, see a physician. Seek professional medical attention to treat more established, severe, or recurrent heartburn.

Lycopodium: If acid washes into the gullet from the stomach when anxiety levels are high, or when you eat high-fiber foods such as pulses and beans or indigestible foods such as onions, use Lycopodium. You may feel ravenous but become full quickly, or lack an appetite during the day, only to wake up from hunger at night.

Arsenicum album: Heartburn and acidity with burning pains in the stomach and severe nausea may be eased by this remedy. There is a marked anxiety and restlessness when feeling ill, distraction and warmth feel soothing, as well as lying propped up on two or three pillows. Lying too flat aggravates symptoms.

Herbalism

Slippery elm: Your herbal expert may suggest drinking root bark powder mixed with water after meals and before bedtime. If too much powder is mixed into the water, the liquid can be very thick and difficult to drink, so use small amounts until you get used to making it. Slippery elm is very safe, though some of its compounds can prevent medications from being absorbed by the body, which your herbal expert will be able to advise you on.

Marshmallow: An overnight cold infusion made from marshmallow root, a demulcent herb, can be drunk throughout the day. As with slippery elm, medicines taken at the same time as marshmallow may not be absorbed well, so take advice from your herbal practitioner.

Chamomile: This anti-inflammatory herb is a popular mild sedative, but it also has anti-spasmodic and soothing effects on the intestines. An infusion of chamomile flowers might be drunk three to four times daily. Chamomile is generally well tolerated, although people who are allergic to other plants in the daisy family may notice that their allergy symptoms worsen; it is best to avoid chamomile if this happens.

Tip: EAT BANANAS

Eating bananas seems to be particularly beneficial for relieving heartburn, since they have a natural antacid effect in the body.

Indigestion

Diagnosis

Indigestion, also known as dyspepsia, is the term used to describe pain or discomfort in the upper abdomen or chest that develops after eating. The stomach produces a strong acid that helps digest food. A layer of mucus that lines the stomach acts as a barrier against this acid, but if this lining becomes damaged the acid irritates the tissues underneath, causing indigestion. The condition tends to occur after eating heavy meals, eating late at night, or eating irregularly. Indigestion can also be triggered by drinking too much alcohol, smoking, stress and anxiety, drugs such as aspirin and anti-inflammatory medication, pregnancy, and stomach ulcers. Indigestion is sometimes accompanied by heartburn, a burning sensation in the chest (see p. 192).

Symptoms

- Pain, often in the upper part of the abdomen or chest
- Heartburn, a burning pain caused by reflux of the stomach's contents up the gullet
- Loss of appetite
- Nausea and vomiting
- Flatulence or belching

Treatment Goal

To introduce lifestyle changes to reduce the long-term occurrence of indigestion, and to relieve any immediate symptoms of burning or discomfort.

Conventional Medicine

Indigestion is often a symptom of peptic ulcer disease or results from using non-steroidal anti-inflammatory drugs (NSAIDs). Treatment is determined by identifying the cause, which can involve a procedure called an endoscopy, where a tube is inserted through the mouth to view the esophagus and the stomach. This is part of the treatment for patients over 45 years old who have severe and unremitting indigestion. Patients under 45 are often tested for the bacteria associated with ulcers, H. Pylori. If the test is positive, treatment involves eradication therapy, where two antibiotics and a proton pump inhibitor are given simultaneously for a three-week period.

To treat acute indigestion: Treatment usually involves using an H2 blocking agent or a proton pump inhibitor. These drugs block the H2 receptor cells in the stomach and the proton pump in the cells to decrease acid production. If these do not work, Reglan® (metoclopramide), which increases stomach motility, is tried. Carafate® may also be used, as well as over-the-counter products such as Maalox®, Mylanta®, and Gaviscon®.

Modify your lifestyle: Eliminating wheat and dairy products from your diet may be beneficial. Biofeedback, a treatment that trains your body to listen to its own signals, can also be helpful, as are stress reduction techniques such as breathing and meditation.

Traditional Chinese Medicine

Herbs:
• To treat indigestion due to overeating or stomach bloating: Mix 12 g of dried Shan Zha (hawthorn fruit) with 12 g of Bin Long (betel nut), 30 g of Yi Yi Ren (seeds of Job's tears), and 8 g of Shen Qu (medicated leaven). Make a decoction by placing the herbs in a ceramic or glass pot and adding 3½ cups of water. Bring to a boil and simmer for 30 minutes. Strain the liquid and drink 1 cup twice a day.
• To treat indigestion with food retention due to deficiency of spleen and stomach: Combine 12 g of dried Shan Zha (hawthorn fruit) with 12 g of Mu Xiang (costus root), 15 g Fuling (poria), 12 g of Bai Zhu (white atractylodes rhizome), 10 g of Shen Qu (medicated leaven), 12 g of Bai Shao (white peony root), and 12 g Fa Ban Xia (pinellia rhizome) in a glass or ceramic pot. Add 3 cups of water, bring to a boil, and simmer for 30 minutes. Strain and drink 1 cup twice a day.
• To treat indigestion with strong abdominal pain: Mix 12 g of Shan zha (hawthorn fruit), 8 g Qing Pi (immature tangerine peel), 10 g of Zhi Shi (immature fruit of bitter orange), 12 g of Lian Qiao (forsythia fruit), 12 g of Long Dan Cao (Chinese gentian root), 8 g of Huang Qin (baical skullcap root), 10 g of radish seeds, 8 g of Chai

Hu (hare's ear root), and 12 g Bai Shao (white peony root). Place the herbs in a ceramic or glass pot, add 3½ cups of water, and bring to a boil. Simmer for 30 minutes and strain the liquid. Drink 1 cup twice a day.

Acupressure: To treat indigestion, press the Nei Guan, Hegu, and Tian Shu points. The Hegu point is located on the back of the hand in the depression between the thumb and the first finger. The Nei Guan point is located in the center of the wrist on the palm side about 2 inches above the crease. The Tian Shu point is found on the middle of the abdomen 1 inch to the side of the navel.

Tip: MANAGE STRESS LEVELS

Unmanaged stress makes indigestion symptoms worse. Exercising regularly is an effective method of reducing stress. Vigorous exercise works for some people, while gentler exercises such as yoga and T'ai chi work well for others.

Naturopathy

Diet: Eat a whole food diet, eliminating unnatural refined foods. Whole grains, raw vegetables, and nuts and seeds are rich in fiber and the essential nutrients important in relieving symptoms of indigestion and should be staples in your diet. Some natural foods, however, such as wheat, citrus fruits, and corn can aggravate symptoms. Avoid overeating, and eat small meals throughout the day. Drink 8–10 glasses of water a day to maintain good digestive health and neutralize excess acidity in the stomach that can cause indigestion. Saturated fats, hydrogenated oils, and partially hydrogenated oils lead to acid reflux, another potential cause of indigestion. Avoid foods that contain these substances, such as fried and greasy foods, heavy sauces, and red meat. Avoid caffeine, alcohol, chocolate, and minty or spicy foods, as they make symptoms worse. Stop eating three hours before bedtime as sleeping with a full stomach can aggravate symptoms.

Supplements: If using antacids, avoid brands that include peppermint, as this can relax the low esophageal sphincter. This muscle, at the base of the esophagus, keeps food and digestive acids in the stomach. If relaxed, it can release stomach acid, leading to indigestion. Instead, take 250–500 mg of calcium carbonate three times a day with food. Chewable tablets provide the quickest relief. To restore friendly bacteria to the gut, take a probiotic product in the lactobacillus family that contains at least four billion active organisms twice daily with meals or 30 minutes after meals. Digestive enzymes help you digest food more effectively so that less irritation is caused. The enzymes include lipases that digest fat, proteases that digest proteins, and amylases that digest starch. Take 2 capsules or tablets of a full spectrum enzyme product with each meal. Also take 1–2 betaine hydrochloride capsules to support stomach acid levels.

Herbs: De-glycyrrhizinated licorice (DGL), which is safer than other types of licorice, may help to heal damaged mucous lining in the stomach. Take two 380 mg DGL licorice tablets three or four times a day between meals as needed. Slippery elm serves as a demulcent to soothe the digestive lining of the stomach. Take 3 ml of tincture or 500 mg of a capsule three times a day, or lozenges if preferred. Marshmallow is another demulcent that soothes the digestive lining and reduces inflammation in the stomach. Take 300 mg in capsule form or 3 ml of tincture three times a day. Mastic gum has been shown to heal stomach mucosa and has antibacterial benefits. Take 500 mg three times a day. Gamma-oryzanol, also known as rice bran oil, can help repair the entire digestive system. Take 150 mg three times a day for one month.

Homeopathy

Any of the remedies suggested below should help a one-off bout of indigestion. Indigestion that sets in for no obvious reason, especially if recurring, should not be ignored or suppressed temporarily with conventional antacids. Instead, consult your usual doctor.

Lycopodium: If symptoms of indigestion, such as burping, bloating, or acid rising into the gullet, occur as a result of eating a lot of high-fiber foods, try using Lycopodium. Symptoms may also set in when feeling stressed and anxious. Rumbling and bloating in the belly are so severe that it becomes necessary to loosen the waistband in order to get comfortable. Cold food and drinks aggravate the condition, while warm food and drinks are generally soothing.

Carbo veg: To treat trapped gas in the belly accompanied by a heavy, nauseous feeling, and bloating in the stomach, use Carbo veg. Symptoms include feeling discomfort after eating even the smallest amount when feeling gassy, or while being in stuffy, overheated surroundings. Contact with cool air and being fanned provides relief.

Pulsatilla: Use this remedy if indigestion occurs after eating rich or fatty foods. Uneasiness and discomfort in the stomach is aggravated by jarring movements, such as walking very quickly. The mouth is dry without thirst, and food eaten tends to "repeat." Lying down makes the uneasiness in the stomach worse, while taking a stroll in the open air gives relief. 🍂

Herbalism

The two main classes of herbs used to treat indigestion are carminatives and bitters. Carminative plants stimulate the stomach lining, increase stomach secretions, and promote the flow of bile. Bitter herbs increase the flow of saliva and stomach secretion, and promote the motility of the stomach.

Peppermint: This carminative plant is a hybrid of spearmint and water mint. When used in tea form, peppermint leaf may ease upper intestinal tract gas, spasm, and indigestion. It may be more effective if you cover the cup as the leaf is steeping to capture as much of the essential oil (primarily menthol) from the leaf as possible—it can otherwise can be volatile and disperse in the air. Sometimes peppermint tea can worsen heartburn, and it isn't recommended for those with hiatus hernia.

Chamomile: This carminative has anti-inflammatory, antispasmodic, and soothing effects on gastrointestinal tissue. The beneficial effects of chamomile are probably due to two main classes of compounds, the volatile oils (such as bisabolol) and the flavonoids (such as apigenin). To treat indigestion, steep 1 heaped tbsp of chamomile flowers in 1 covered cup of hot water for 10 minutes to extract the medicinal flavonoids and some of the volatile oils. This tea can be taken several times a day to help with symptoms.

Fennel: Another common carminative, fennel seeds can simply be eaten after a meal to aid digestion, calm the stomach and intestines, and dispel gas. Alternatively, ½ tsp of the seeds can be crushed a little, then infused with hot water and consumed throughout the day.

Gentian: Roots and rhizomes of this bitter herb have a long history of use as a gastrointestinal "tonic." Its effects are due to several different medicinal compounds; one of them, amarogentin, a glycoside compound, provides much of the bitter taste. Gentian can be consumed in several different forms. Boil 1 g in 1 cup of water for five minutes to make a liquid decoction that should be taken 30 minutes before meals, up to three times daily. Alternatively, an alcohol-based tincture of gentian can be made and similarly used before meals. Some people may develop a headache after using gentian, or find the bitter taste intolerable. It is also not used in those with gastric ulcers.

> ### *Tip:* AVOID TRIGGERS
>
> Certain combinations of food tend to trigger indigestion. With this in mind, it may be helpful to avoid protein-based foods, such as red meat, combined with starchy side dishes, such as potatoes, and followed by a sweet dessert; or fatty foods, such as cheese, combined with bread or crackers.

Colic

Diagnosis

Colic is a common condition in babies, affecting around one in five newborns. It is characterized by a gripping pain in the abdomen, thought to be caused by trapped gas or intestinal spasms. It affects both breast- and bottle-fed babies. The baby becomes very uncomfortable and will cry continually unless rocked, walked, carried in a baby sling, or otherwise comforted. Some babies feel comforted when wrapped in a blanket or held tightly. Gently massaging the baby's tummy also helps in some cases. When all else fails, some parents find their baby is comforted by a car ride. The condition usually first manifests itself within two to four weeks after birth and mostly occurs in the first 12 weeks of life. Happily, it often resolves after about three months of age.

Symptoms

- Drawing legs up to stomach
- Clenched fists
- Baby out of sorts, particularly in the evenings
- Flushed or red face
- Baby wants to feed constantly
- Intense crying, sometimes for hours
- Abdomen feels hard
- Discomfort after feeding
- Poor sleep

Treatment Goal

Treatment aims to relieve symptoms and soothe the baby's distress. Contact your doctor if your baby has other symptoms, such as vomiting or diarrhea.

Conventional Medicine

A baby with colic who is fussy but has a fever, is extremely agitated, or has any other physical symptoms should be taken to a doctor for evaluation. Do not assume that it is an episode of colic.

Diet: Treatment of colic is primarily dietary. While breastfeeding is preferred, switching to a non-dairy formula such as a soy-based milk, goat's milk, or a whey hydrosylate milk may be useful. Less frequently, a lactase-treated milk (lactose free) and low-allergen milk can be tried. If the baby is breastfeeding, the mother should go on a low-allergen diet, which involves low gluten, low dairy, and cutting out processed foods. Avoiding foods that create gas in the mother (beans, broccoli, onions, spicy foods) is also essential.

Physical comforting: Feeding techniques that involve frequent, gentle burping are encouraged, as is rocking, cradling, and comforting the baby. Avoid overstimulating irritable babies when they are crying by reducing visual and auditory inputs. However, serene music and lullabies may be soothing and quieting. Massaging the baby may also be effective.

Herbal tea: Some herbal teas, such as peppermint tea, or tea with extract of chamomile, vervain, licorice, fennel, and balm mint have been shown to ease colic. These can be drunk by breastfeeding mothers, or a weak tea can be given directly to infants with a medicine dropper.

Infant drops: Simethicone infant drops are worth a try, but have had mixed reviews as to their effectiveness. If an infant over six months of age is colicky, dicyclomine is sometimes prescribed; however, it does have side effects such as sedation, blurred vision, dizziness, and dry mouth.

Traditional Chinese Medicine

Herbs: If the pain is not relieved after taking these remedies, consult a doctor immediately.
• **Formula one:** Mix 2 g of dried peppermint, or 3 g of fresh peppermint, with 3 g of fresh ginger. Boil these ingredients in 3 cups of water, and simmer for two to three minutes. Strain the tea, add 1–2 tbsp of honey, and stir well. Let the tea cool to a warm temperature and give your child 2–4 oz, using a dropper, every one to two hours.

• **Formula two:** Combine 4 g of Jin Yin Hua (honeysuckle flower), 3 g of Shen Gan Cao (raw licorice), and five pieces of Da Zhao (Chinese jujube). Place the ingredients in 3 cups of water and bring to a boil. Simmer for three to five minutes and strain. Give your child 3–5 fl oz of cooled tea every half an hour to one hour for a total of three to five times.

Acupressure: Press the Hegu points, located on the back of the hands between the thumb and first finger, with strong pressure. Press the Nei Guan point, in the center of the wrist on the palm side about 2 inches below the crease, with medium pressure. Press each point for one to three minutes at a time to reduce the pain.

Naturopathy

Diet: Allergies, particularly an intolerance to milk proteins from a cow's-milk-based formula, may cause colic in some infants. Infants who are sensitive to milk may be given a hypoallergenic formula containing extensively hydrolyzed proteins. If this does not work try a soy-based formula, or even goat's milk. If your child appears allergic to this as well, consult a pediatrician. If a baby is breastfed, certain foods in the mother's diet, such as cows' milk, may provoke an allergic reaction in the baby. Cow's milk proteins have been found at higher levels in milk from breastfeeding mothers with colicky infants than in milk from mothers with non-colicky infants.

Tip: FOODS FOR MOM TO AVOID

There are certain foods and drinks that have a reputation for aggravating colicky pains, and as a result, they are best avoided by mothers breastfeeding colicky babies. The most common culprits include any of the following: cucumbers, citrus fruit, raw peppers, cabbage, beans, raw onion, brussels sprouts, alcohol, coffee, and very spicy foods.

Tip: LAVENDER MASSAGE

Add a few drops of lavender oil to baby oil and massage a colicky baby's back and chest to release tense muscles and calm the spirit.

Supplements: Lactobacillus acidophilus and Bifidus provide the bowel with friendly intestinal bacteria (flora), which will ease digestion and may help resolve colic. A breastfeeding mother should take 1 tsp twice a day. Give a bottle-fed baby ⅛ tsp of acidophilus and ⅛ tsp of bifidus powder twice a day dissolved in his or her formula.

Herbs: Nursing mothers should drink 1 cup of chamomile tea twice a day. Give a bottle-fed infant 1 tbsp of tea three times a day mixed in formula or water. Fennel has been traditionally used to treat colic. Nursing mothers can drink 1 cup of fennel tea, on its own or mixed with chamomile, up to three times a day, or give a breastfeeding baby 1 tsp of the tea four times a day. Nursing mothers can also drink 1 cup of ginger tea twice a day to relieve colic in their infants.

Homeopathy

The remedies below can ease the distress and pain of a recent, acute bout of colic. Regular, severe colic is best dealt with by a practitioner.

Nux vomica: This is a possible remedy for colicky pains in breastfeeding babies whose mothers have been eating spicy food.

Lycopodium: If strong colic pain tends to come on in the late afternoon, often lasting until the early evening, try Lycopodium. Symptoms include loud, audible rumbling and gurgling sounds coming from the abdomen. Lycopodium is also appropriate for colic pain that arises in breastfed babies whose mothers have been eating an excessively high-fiber diet.

Mag phos: To relieve symptoms of colic that develop with teething pains, use Mag phos. Excessive amounts of gas are produced that can temporarily relieve discomfort. Symptoms also include an instinctive pressing of the knees up to the belly in order to try and gain relief. Warmth locally applied and gentle massage ease pain.

Chamomile: This is appropriate if the baby is extremely fussy, irritable, and inconsolable. Babies may arch their backs when crying, and may seem better after passing gas.

Herbalism

Colic is commonly described as excessive, inconsolable crying from an otherwise healthy baby. Some research has suggested that colic is related to excess gas; however, this is not the case with every child. The following herbs and doses can be clarified by your herbal medicine practitioner.

Chamomile: This plant's sweet, aromatic flowers soothe the stomach, relieve excess gas, and act as a mild sedative. The active constituent, apigenin, calms nerves and relieves anxiety, making chamomile good for soothing night terrors and anxiety in children.

Fennel seed: Recognized for its antispasmodic action, fennel is well known as a herbal remedy for colic. The essential oils, flavonoids, and plant sterols it contains reduce spasms in the digestive system and decrease the production of gas. There is the potential for allergy with this herb, although it is rare, but should be monitored for.

Tip: USE A HOT WATER BOTTLE

Place a warm hot water bottle wrapped in a towel on your lap and lay your baby across, stomach down. This will relax the muscle cramps and calm your baby.

Vomiting

Diagnosis

Vomiting is your body's way of ridding itself of an infection or toxins. In most cases it is caused by a viral gastrointestinal infection. Common triggers include overeating, eating rich foods, food poisoning, stomach bugs, motion sickness, a weak stomach, food allergies, and pregnancy (morning sickness). Most cases of vomiting can be safely treated at home. However, if there is blood in the vomit, accompanying severe stomach pain, indications of dehydration, or the vomiting is prolonged, consult a doctor.

DANGER: If the vomiting is severe and accompanied by a high fever, headache, and a stiff neck, this could indicate meningitis. Get medical help immediately. If there is a serious pain anywhere in the abdomen or groin, always seek immediate medical advice.

Symptoms

- Vomiting
- Dry and parched lips and mouth
- Stomachache
- Diarrhea
- Fever and sweating
- Headaches

Treatment Goal

It is important to stay hydrated and replace any fluids lost by the body. Sip water continuously until the cause of the vomiting is identified and resolved. Treatment aims to relieve symptoms until the cause can be eradicated.

Conventional Medicine

Stay hydrated: Rehydration should be attempted with a solution containing salts, some sugar, and electrolytes, such as Gatorade®. If fluids cannot be kept down, and signs of dehydration are present, such as dizziness, reduced urination, dry mouth and eyes, and dry skin, then this is a medical emergency that requires intravenous fluid rehydration. Consult your doctor.

Diet: Avoid solid foods and instead drink small amounts of cool liquid, but not acidic citric or sweetened juices. Progress to easily digested foods such as toast, crackers, rice, and broth soups. If these are tolerated, plain soft foods such as pasta can be eaten. Fatty foods and dairy products should be avoided.

Medication: If dietary changes do not help stop the vomiting, anti-sickness drugs may be needed. Most of them act on the central nervous system and so have sedating side effects. Compazine® and Phenergan® medications can be used rectally, intravenously, or orally. Reglan® (metoclopramide) is another common anti-vomiting drug. These drugs are not normally given to children or pregnant women. Morning sickness can be treated with vitamin B6 (pyridoxine).

Traditional Chinese Medicine

Herbs: For each formula, place the herbs in a glass or ceramic pot and add 3 cups of water. Bring to the boil and simmer for 30 minutes. Strain and drink 1 cup twice a day.
• To treat vomiting due to a stomach bug or cold: Combine 10 g of Huang Qin (baical skullcap root), 10 g of Jin Yin Hua (honeysuckle flower), 12 g of Zi Su Gen (perilla), 6 g of Bo He (field mint), 8 g of fresh ginger, and 4 g of dried ginger. For a summer cold, add 10 g of Huo Xiang (agastache), 10 g of Zhu Ru (bamboo shavings), and 10 g of Xiang Ru (aromatic madder). If it is a winter cold, add 10 g of Bai Zhi (angelica dahurica), and 10 g of Zi Su Ye (perilla leaf). Drink one hour before or after meals.
• To treat vomiting due to food poisoning: Mix 10 g of Huang Qin (baical skullcap root), 6 g of Huang Lian (coptis root), 6 g of Chen Pi (tangerine peel), 10 g of Mu Xiang (costus root), 10 g of Lian Qiao (forsythia root), 6 g of Sha Ren (cardamom), 15 g of Bian Dou (hyacinth bean), 8 g of Shen Qu (medicated leaven), and 8 g of Hou Po (magnolia bark).

• To treat vomiting due to chronic digestive deficiency: Mix 15 g of Fuling (poria), 12 g of Wu Wei Zi (schisandra fruit), 12 g of Tai Zi Shen (pseudostellaria), 12 g of Fa Ban Xia (pinellia rhizome), 6 g of Chen Pi (tangerine peel), 8 g of Sha Ren (cardamom), 10 g of Wu Zhu Yu (evodia fruit), 15 g of Bai Zhu (white atractylodes rhizome), and 15 g of Shan Yao (Chinese yam).

Acupressure: Use the tip of your thumb to apply strong pressure to the Nei Guan point, located in the center of the wrist on the palm side about 2 inches above the crease, for one to two minutes. Also press the Susanli point, on the lower leg, 1 inch to the outside of and 3 inches below the kneecap.

Naturopathy

Diet: Eat a nourishing diet composed primarily of whole grains, fresh fruits and vegetables, and some fish and lean chicken. Stay hydrated, as dehydration can cause serious problems. Drink herbal tea, broths, soups and water.

Supplements: A good multivitamin/multimineral has been shown to lower the incidence of vomiting in non-pregnant women. If pregnant, make sure you take a prenatal multivitamin. Follow the instructions on the label. Some prenatal vitamins can lead to feelings of nausea. Talk to your doctor about this. You may need to take them at a different time or with food, or switch brands. In studies, Vitamin B6 has shown to help with nausea. Take 30 mg twice a day. Activated charcoal absorbs toxins in the digestive tract if you have been exposed to micro-organisms in food or water. Take 500–1,000 mg throughout the day.

Herbs: Ginger is a useful herb for treating vomiting. However, do not treat pregnancy-related vomiting with ginger for longer than the first two months of pregnancy, and do not take more than 250 mg of ginger four times a day during pregnancy without first consulting your doctor. Ginger is available as a standardized extract in pill form (take 100–200 mg), a fresh powder (take ½–¾ tsp), and a fresh root (take a ¼–½ inch peeled slice). These doses can be taken every four hours or up to three times a day. You can also drink several cups of ginger tea or ginger ale a day, but be sure to buy products that include real ginger. Peppermint is another herb that can soothe the stomach. Mix a drop or two of peppermint oil into juice, or make mint tea. Pour boiling water through a strainer containing some dried peppermint or spearmint. Let the fluid sit for a few minutes, add some sugar or honey if desired, and drink. Do not take peppermint if you are pregnant or have acid reflux.

Homeopathy

The remedies listed below can bring relief to vomiting due to an obvious trigger, such as a stomach bug or overindulging in food and alcohol. Cases of vomiting that do not have any obvious cause should be assessed by a medical professional, as should vomiting accompanied by severe abdominal pain or blood in the vomit.

Veratrum album: Consider this remedy to treat violent bouts of vomiting. Vomiting is accompanied by drenching sweats and exhaustion to the point of collapse. Symptoms include an unquenchable thirst for long drinks of cold water and gnawing hunger, despite severe nausea.

Arsenicum album: Symptoms are similar to those described above, but there is no hunger and a thirst for small sips of fluids rather than long drinks. In addition, patients are likely to feel chilled to the bone, and are restless despite feeling prostrated.

Nux vomica: If vomiting results from drinking too much alcohol, try Nux vomica. Symptoms that respond well tend to be those of the classic hangover. Nausea and vomiting is combined with a throbbing headache that radiates from the back of the head to the front. There is also likely to be dizziness and the scalp may feel sensitive. Seek conventional medical advice about headaches that are linked to nausea or vomiting.

Herbalism

Mint: There are many different species of mint, that all have a long history of calming stomach troubles that lead to vomiting. The leaves are the part of the plant most often used, and, when dried, can be steeped in hot water to make a tea to decrease vomiting. Many of the medicinal properties from plants in the mint family come from a class of compounds called essential oils, such as menthol, carvone, and limonene. These compounds disappear quickly when heated, so keep mint tea covered when steeping.

Ginger root: Either capsules of dried ginger root, or an infusion of the chopped dried or fresh root can be used to calm the stomach and decrease vomiting. The effect of ginger is due to several medicinal compounds, including gingerol, shogaol, and zingerone. Ginger is also useful for vomiting that accompanies motion sickness and, in prudent amounts, nausea and vomiting associated with pregnancy.

Constipation

Diagnosis

Constipation is defined as infrequent or irregular bowel movements. Stools may be hard, small, and dry with a pebblelike consistency. Bowel movements may also cause difficulty or pain. Although most people have a bowel movement at least once a day, there is no standard on what is "normal." It is possible to move your bowels every day and still be constipated if the stools are hard and difficult to pass, and some healthy people regularly do not have a bowel movement for a few days at a time.

Many things can trigger constipation. These include a change in your diet, such as a lack of fiber or too much processed food, an intolerance to certain foods, dehydration, traveling or a change of routine, not getting enough exercise, and emotional stress. The best way to avoid constipation is to eat a balanced diet that is high in fiber, including plenty of fresh fruit and vegetables, and drink at least eight to ten glasses of water a day. Prunes and plum juice can also be beneficial.

Symptoms

- Going for a long time without having a bowel movement
- Hard stools that are difficult to pass
- Stomachache, often at mealtimes
- Bloated stomach
- Bad breath
- Abdominal discomfort
- Fever
- Lethargy
- Muscle aches
- Irritability

Treatment Goal

To relieve symptoms of constipation. Consult your doctor if this is an on-going problem.

Conventional Medicine

Identify the cause: Medical treatment of constipation involves multiple therapies, but it is also important to make sure that there are no coexisting diseases causing the constipation. Diseases such as hypothyroidism, diabetes, and depression, some neurological disorders, and connective tissue diseases are linked to constipation. Many medications can also cause constipation, including antihistamines, blood pressure medications, water pills, calcium, iron supplements, and narcotics. Review the medications you are taking.

Diet and exercise: General lifestyle measures to relieve constipation include exercising daily (for example, about 20 minutes of rapid walking a day), drinking at least 6 cups of water a day, and including plenty of fiber in your diet (ideally about 30 g a day). Take 2 tbsp of psyllium husks a day and eat at least 5 portions of fresh fruit and vegetables a day. If you use stimulant laxatives, decrease the amount you use.

Laxatives: Medications for constipation are grouped by category. Bulk laxatives, such as Metamucil®, which is psyllium, Citrucel®, and Fibercon® contain fiber. These are safe to use on a long-term basis. Stool softeners, such as mineral oil and docusate sodium (Colace™), are also less likely to interfere with the body's natural colonic activity. Osmotic laxatives, which include unabsorbed sugars such as sorbitol, polyethylene glycol, and lactose, and salts such as magnesium hydroxide (milk of magnesia), magnesium citrate, and sodium phosphate (fleet enema), are somewhat harsher and should only be used occasionally. Stimulant laxatives, such as aloe vera, senna, castor oil, and bisacodyl (Dulcolax™), are the harshest kind of laxatives. Aloe vera, a natural plant stimulant, can be used for occasional relief while implementing the dietary and lifestyle changes listed above. Rectal enemas and suppositories such as glycerin, tap water enema, and Fleets™ phosphate enema provide direct and immediate relief. A new medication called tegaserod (Zelnorm™) is known as a colonic serotonin receptor binder that speeds up bowel movements and improves consistency of the stool.

Traditional Chinese Medicine

Herbs:
• **To treat constipation due to excessive heat:** Symptoms include one bowel movement every few days, dry stools, yellow urine, abdominal pain, bloating, and bad breath. Combine 10 g Huang Qin (baical skullcap root), 5 g of Di Huang (Chinese foxglove), and 10 g of Huo Ma Ren (hemp seeds) in ceramic pot. Add 3 cups of water and boil for five minutes. Strain the liquid and drink the tea.

• To treat constipation due to yin deficiency: Symptoms may include dry skin, loss of memory, or night sweats. Place 15 g of Zhi Mu (anemarrhena rhizome), 15 g of Xuan Shen (ningpo figwort root), 12 g of Mai Men Dong (ophiopogon tuber), and 12 g of Dang Gui (Chinese angelica) in a ceramic pot. Add 3 cups of water and boil for five minutes. Drink the tea throughout the day. You can also take the patent Chinese medicine Ma Ren Chang Wan, which has Huo Ma Ren (hemp seeds) as its main ingredient. It helps smooth the intestine and promotes bowel movement.

Acupressure: Press the Guan Yuan point, located on the abdomen, about 3 inches below the navel. You can also press the Zhi Gou point on the outside of the forearm about 2 inches above the crease of the wrist between the two large bones in the forearm. Use the tip of your finger or thumb to press this point for one minute two or three times.

Diet: Honey soothes the bowel. Take 1 tbsp every morning, or add it to tea.

Naturopathy

Diet: Drink 10–12 glasses of water a day, sipping throughout the day. Drinking an inadequate amount of fluids is one of the biggest contributors to constipation. A whole food diet consisting of whole grains and fresh fruit and vegetables will provide enough fiber to keep your bowels moving. Other good foods high in fiber are beans, nuts, prunes, and figs. Flaxseeds are highly concentrated in fiber and contain essential fatty acids that are thought to coat your intestines, promoting smooth bowel movements. Do not cook with flaxseeds or subject them to heat; instead, sprinkle 2 tbsp on cereals or salads. Children should take 2 tsp of flaxseeds at a time. Consume fermented products regularly to supply your intestines with healthy flora that can assist in inducing gentle bowel movements. Kefir, unsweetened yogurt, and raw sauerkraut are all excellent choices. Fried foods and simple carbohydrates contribute to constipation. Avoid these foods as much as possible. Caffeine and alcohol are hard on the digestive system and are dehydrating as well. Avoid them as much as possible during episodes of constipation.

Supplements: Magnesium helps with acute constipation and improves gut motility. Take 250 mg of magnesium four times a day for four to six weeks, then cut down to twice a day. Take

> *Tip:* EXERCISE REGULARLY
>
> Exercise for at least 20 minutes four times a week to help with intestinal contraction. You can do any exercise you enjoy as long as you do it aerobically for 20 minutes without stopping.

a probiotic product daily that contains at least four billion active organisms to help digestion and elimination. Psyllium husks act as a bulk-forming laxative. Take 1 tsp or 5 g twice daily. Digestive enzymes assist with digestion, which will help with elimination. Take two pills with each meal.

Herbs: Cascara sagrada helps with acute constipation. Take 250 mg two to three times a day. Do not use this herb as a long-term solution as it can lead to dependence and gastric irritation. Taking 250 g of dandelion root

with each meal stimulates bile flow and improves constipation. Milk thistle improves liver function and bile flow. Take 200–250 mg of a standardized product to 80% silymarin with each meal. Aloe vera juice also improves bowel movements. Drink 1 cup twice daily or as directed on the label.

Homeopathy

Most of the homeopathic remedies listed below can help treat a recent episode of constipation. If constipation occurs regularly, it is best to seek a professional homeopathic assessment.

Bryonia: Use this remedy to treat constipation that results from dehydration. There is no urge to move your bowels, and when a stool is eventually passed, it is likely to be large, hard, and dry in texture, and therefore difficult to pass. This remedy is helpful for constipation that is associated with a throbbing headache.

Alumina: If constipation manifests itself as soft stools that are passed with difficulty, consider Alumina. Alternatively, stools that have a knotted or hard appearance may require a lot of straining to pass them. When this remedy is indicated there is a noticeable aggravation of the problem when eating a diet high in refined carbohydrates and potatoes.

Nux vomica: If there is a strong, constant urge to move your bowels, but nothing or very little is passed even after a lot of straining, use Nux vomica. The headaches associated with this condition closely resemble a hangover headache and often lodge at the back of the head. Common triggers that call for this remedy include too much stress and tension, or a diet that is high in junk foods.

Lycopodium: This can be helpful for treating an acute episode of constipation after traveling. Confirmatory symptoms include bloating and distention in the belly with noticeably loud rumbling and gurgling sounds. Constipation may alternate with diarrhea if there hasn't been a bowel movement for a few days.

Herbalism

Herbal medicines relieve constipation in two primary ways: as bulk-forming agents or stimulant laxatives.

Psyllium: The husks of psyllium seeds provide a safe source of fiber. Take 2 tsp, which contain about 7 g of fiber, two to three times daily for a total of about 10–30 g of fiber. Some people don't need as much as others and the amount of psyllium you should take depends on the severity of the constipation and your tolerance to the herb. Be sure to increase your water intake with any fiber product or it could make symptoms worse. Introduce psyllium slowly, with, for instance, 5 g of husks twice a day, and increase as necessary.

Stimulant laxatives: These increase the motion of the colon and cause changes in the colonic cells that lead to the accumulation of water, thereby improving constipation. The long-term use of stimulant laxatives, however, may cause normal bowel function to decrease as the nerve reflexes start to depend on the presence of the stimulant compounds in order to have a regular bowel movement. Stimulant laxatives should only be used in the short term

and with care. As the strength of the stimulant laxative goes up, so does the risk of side effects such as cramping, bloating, and diarrhea.

Aloe vera juice: This juice is made from the part of the aloe leaf that contains compounds called anthraquinone glycosides, which act as stimulant laxatives. You should take the minimum amount necessary to produce a soft stool, which is usually 40–170 mg of dehydrated juice in capsule form per day. As with other stimulant laxatives, the use of aloe vera juice for more than seven days in a row can lead to dependency. There are also studies that show that chronically consuming any plant with anthraquinone glycosides increases the risk of colon cancer.

Senna: This widely used stimulant laxative is usually taken in a cold or hot water tea. Tablets and extracts of senna are also available. Take the minimum amount of senna a day necessary to achieve a soft stool. Start with a tea made from 0.5 g (½ tsp) of the ground dried fruit and 1 cup of hot water, and drink once or twice a day. It may be necessary to increase the dosage to 1 g twice daily. Do not use long term.

Tip: AVOID THE REGULAR USE OF LAXATIVES

If you have an underlying tendency to constipation, avoid the temptation to rely on laxatives to manage the condition. If they are used as a long-term solution you may become dependent and it can be progressively more difficult to have a regular bowel movement without them.

Diarrhea

Diagnosis

Diarrhea occurs when the mucous membrane lining the intestinal walls becomes irritated and inflamed, causing stool content to pass through too quickly, absorbing a lot of liquid with it. It is usually accompanied by abdominal pains, nausea, and vomiting. Some blood may also be passed.

Diarrhea is often caused by a virus or bacteria passed from person to person. Diarrhea can be acute (short term), generally lasting around 24 hours. It can also be chronic (long term), which can last more than two weeks and is usually a sign of an intestinal disorder disease, such as irritable bowel syndrome. Those with chronic diarrhea, especially with blood mixed in, should seek medical help immediately. Diarrhea can also be a symptom of an intolerance to food, such as lactose and gluten intolerance. Children can get diarrhea from having too much fruit, fruit juice, or cold foods and drinks.

Symptoms

- Loose, watery stools/liquid feces
- Frequent bowel movements
- Loss of appetite
- Unpleasant-smelling stools
- Stomach cramps
- Bloating and flatulence
- Nausea and vomiting
- Fever
- Dehydration—symptoms include small amounts of dark urine, drowsiness, and thirst. Dehydration as a result of diarrhea is a particular risk for young children and the elderly

Treatment Goal

To establish the cause of the diarrhea and take measures to control symptoms and rehydrate the body.

Conventional Medicine

To treat diarrhea, conventional medicine focuses on rehydrating the body and getting nutrition levels back to normal. Wash your hands thoroughly and avoid preparing food while ill to prevent the spread of infection.

Rehydrate the body: To make a rehydration solution, mix 1 quart of clean, filtered water with 2 tbsp of sugar and ½ tsp each of baking soda and salt, to be sipped continuously throughout the day.

Diet: Soft complex carbohydrates, such as bananas, rice, potatoes, and toast, are recommended. Black tea is a natural antidiarrheal. Fruits and vegetables (except those mentioned above) should be excluded from the diet, as should sugary processed foods, dairy products, and fatty foods. Infants may continue to breastfeed, but breast milk should be supplemented with oral rehydration fluid as described above. Probiotics (beneficial bacteria that live in the gut) may be given as a supplement. Some botanical formulas containing mallow licorice and black walnut can be helpful in re-establishing a healthy gut during or immediately after an episode of diarrhea.

Medication: Do not give infants or small children over-the-counter or prescription antidiarrheal medications. Loperamide (Lomotil™), Kaopectate™, Imodium™, and bismuth subsalicylate (Pepto Bismol™) may be used in adults and children aged 12 and over as directed, but never for longer than three days.

Complications: There is cause for concern if diarrhea is accompanied by light headedness, a high fever, severe abdominal pain, blood and mucus in the stool, or if the diarrhea lasts for more than three days. In any of these cases, an examination of the abdomen and tests of the stool for bacteria, parasites, and blood are carried out. Intravenous rehydration is usually given. Extreme care should be taken when diarrhea affects the very young, as this group is particularly susceptible to dehydration.

Traditional Chinese Medicine

Herbs: For the below formulas, place the herbs in a glass or ceramic pot and add 3–4 cups of water. Bring to the boil and simmer for 30 minutes. Drink 1 cup twice a day.
• Acute diarrhea: Combine 12 g of Ge Geng (kudzu root), 6 g of Chen Pi (tangerine peel), 12 g of Cang Zhu (atractylodes rhizome), 10 g of Hou Po (magnolia bark), 5 g of Gan Cao (licorice root), and 5 g of fresh ginger.
• For diarrhea due to dampness and heat: Symptoms include yellow-brown stools, abdominal pain, a burning sensation in the anus, thirst, and small amounts of yellow urine. Mix 12 g of Bai Shao (white peony root), 5 g of Huang Lian (coptis root), 10 g of Huang Qin (scutellaria root), and 10 g of Bai Tou Weng (Chinese anemone root).
• To treat diarrhea due to emotional upset: Symptoms include pain in the stomach, sticky stools, anxiety or depression, poor appetite, and belching. Mix 10 g of Chai Hu (hare's ear root), 8 g of Bo He (field mint), 10 g of Mu Xiang (costus root), 12 g of Bai Shao (white peony root), 8 g of Zhi Ke (bitter orange), and 3 g of Gan Cao (licorice root).

Acupressure: Press the Hegu points on the back of the hands between the thumb and first finger, the Guan Yuan point, on the midline of the abdomen, about 3 inches below the navel, and Susanli point, 1 inch to the outside of and 3 inches below the kneecap, for one minute two to three times a day.

Diet: Foods those are easy to digest, such as gruel, buckwheat, noodles, and rice are recommended. Avoid foods that are too fibrous or greasy and raw and cold foods.

Naturopathy

Diet: It is critical to stay hydrated, so drink water throughout the day. In acute cases do not eat solid foods if you do not want to, but stay hydrated with water, soups, vegetable juices, sports drinks with electrolytes, and broths. Try a few tablespoons of carob powder in water. This has been shown to reduce the duration of diarrhea.

Supplements: Take a probiotic product containing at least 4 billion active organisms of Lactobacillus acidophilus and bifidus a day to help with digestion and fight infection. Saccahromyces has been shown to be effective in treating diarrhea caused by antibiotic use. Take 1,000–3,000 mg of L-glutamine, an amino acid that repairs the gut, three times a day. Lactase enzymes help to digest dairy sugars.

Take two with each meal that may contain dairy. Avoid magnesium and vitamin C during active episodes of diarrhea, as they can contribute to the condition.

Herbs: Ginger decreases intestinal inflammation. Take 500 mg in capsule form and/or 1–2 cups of ginger tea a day. Goldenseal kills many micro-organisms that may cause diarrhea and helps improve digestion. Marshmallow root is soothing to the digestive tract. Take 500 mg in capsule form three times a day. Drink 3 cups of slippery elm tea each day, or take 500 mg in capsule form every three days, for its soothing effect on the intestines. Red raspberry has traditionally been used to relieve symptoms of diarrhea. To make raspberry leaf tea, pour 1 cup of boiling water over 1–2 tsp of dried leaf. Let the herb steep for 10 minutes, then sweeten to taste. Raspberry leaf generally has a very pleasant taste. In capsule form take 5–10 g daily.

Homeopathy

The following advice can help to clear up a recent, mild bout of diarrhea that has been triggered by an obvious cause. Chronic diarrhea should be treated by a homeopathic practitioner.

Arsenicum album: If diarrhea is accompanied by a sense of being chilled to the bone and shivery, and if there is a profound sense of restlessness, exhaustion, and anxiety when feeling ill, use Arsenicum album. Burning pains in the digestive tract are temporarily soothed by taking small sips of warm drinks.

Podophyllum: If diarrhea is watery and produces little or no pain or cramps, consider Podophyllum. There is a feeling of profound weakness after emptying the bowels, and a very loud gurgling in the gut precedes an episode of diarrhea. Liquid stools are triggered by eating too much fruit or drinking an excessive amount of milk.

Veratrum album: If bouts of diarrhea lead to a state of exhaustion as a result of cramping pains and straining to clear the bowel, try Veratrum album. The skin takes on a pale appearance and is also likely to feel cold and clammy to the touch. There is also likely to be an unquenchable thirst for long drinks of cold water. Unusually, the appetite is unaffected during a bout of diarrhea.

Herbalism

Treatment depends on the cause of the diarrhea. For example, the most effective plants will differ according to whether the diarrhea is caused by a viral infection such as gastroenteritis, irritable bowel syndrome (IBS), inflammatory bowel disease, or a food intolerance or allergy. Nonetheless, there are some plants that can be helpful in calming the symptoms until the underlying cause is addressed. In cases of IBS, food intolerances or stress may need to be addressed. For calming, nervine herbs that may be useful, see p. 438.

Astringents: This class of plant contains compounds called tannins that, when they come into contact with tissue, either skin, or intestinal mucosa, cause drying and healing. In this way, plants with tannins can lessen the loss of water through the intestines. Tannins do not address the underlying cause of the diarrhea, and in cases of food poisoning or infection, when the diarrhea may actually help to rid the body of harmful substances, the overuse of astringents could worsen the problem. One common astringent is carob pod, which can ease the frequency and volume of diarrhea. Your herbal expert may advise adding a small amount of powder to food, to mask the taste and make it easier to take. Raspberry leaf can serve as an astringent and is best taken as an infusion.

Goldenseal: Your herbal medicine practitioner may advise using goldenseal in cases of diarrhea that is presumed to be from an infection in the intestines. The root is most commonly used in tincture form and the antibacterial effects are thought to be primarily due to the alkaloid compound, berberine, that it contains. Goldenseal is still a threatened plant in its natural habitat due to over harvesting, so any goldenseal product purchased should be from companies that cultivate it or obtain it from growers.

Nutmeg: This herb is used in small doses to help cases of diarrhea. It also has antimicrobial, anti-inflammatory, and analgesic properties that may all be useful in treating diarrhea. It is often used in tincture form by practitioners, but may also be taken in powdered form. It is not used in therapeutic doses in pregnancy.

Colitis

Diagnosis

Colitis is a type of inflammatory bowel disease where a superficial inflammation of the large intestine results in ulceration and bleeding. It is often mistaken for irritable bowel syndrome as the symptoms are similar. The exact cause of colitis is unknown but there is a hereditary link, which means it does tend to run in families

An endoscopy and barium enema X-ray examination is usually performed to determine the extent of the disease. Blood tests are also done. Once you have this condition the frequency and severity of flare-ups can be reduced. It is crucial to take preventive treatments, monitor symptoms, and consult your doctor if there is blood in your stools. Medication is usually sufficient to suppress the inflammation. In cases of chronic, ulcerative colitis, if the condition cannot be controlled by medical treatment, surgical removal of the large intestine is sometimes required.

DANGER: If at any time a high fever, bleeding from the rectum, vomiting, or jaundice develops, get immediate medical help.

Symptoms

- Bloody diarrhea
- Blood in stools
- Fever
- Stomach pain
- Symptoms can be present most of the time or infrequently

Treatment Goal

Symptoms can usually be relieved and controlled with medication, but surgery may eventually be necessary.

Conventional Medicine

Medical treatment of colitis depends on whether it is an acute (infectious) or chronic (ulcerative) condition.

To treat infectious colitis: An episode of acute colitis generally resolves itself in a matter of time. Antibiotics are sometimes prescribed to clear up the infection. Modifying your diet, as described below, is also recommended.

To treat ulcerative colitis: Treatment depends on the severity of the disease and the extent of the inflammation in the colon. General methods involve medication, surgery to remove the diseased colon, and modifying your diet to that described below. Stress reduction techniques have been shown to help keep colitis in a state of remission to a certain extent.

Diet: Foods that tend to cause inflammation of the colon include gluten (wheat, rye, and barley), dairy products, and soy. Rice is a better choice as a source of carbohydrates. Avoid alcohol and aspirin to decrease the risk of bleeding. Add 1 tbsp of loose psyllium husks to your diet on a daily basis for intestinal health. However, discontinue if you have diarrhea.

Supplements: Take a probiotic on a daily basis. Also take a multivitamin, as the body's ability to absorb certain nutrients may be impaired. Take 4 g of fish oil a day to decrease inflammation.

Medication: Anti-diarrhea drugs, sulfa drugs (sulfasalazine), medicated enemas, and steroid therapy are sometimes prescribed. In severe cases of chronic disease, immuno-suppressive drugs can be used.

Traditional Chinese Medicine

Herbs: Using any of the herbal combinations listed below, place the herbs in a ceramic pot and add 3 cups of water. Bring to the boil and then simmer for 30 minutes. Drink 1 cup twice a day.
• Formula one: 10 g of Bai Tou Weng (Chinese anemone root), 5 g Huang Lian (coptis root), 10 g of Huang Qin (baical skullcap root), and 12 g of Ma Zhi Xian (purslane).
• Formula two: 12 g of Di Yu (burnet-bloodwort root), 10 g of Huai Hua (pagoda tree flower), and 10 g of Bai Tou Weng (Chinese anemone root).

• Formula three (for severe diarrhea): 10 g of Wu Mei (mume fruit), 15 g of Zhu Ling (polyporus sclerotium), 12 g of Ze Xie (water plantain rhizome), 12 g of Fuling (poria), and 15 g of Qian Shi (euryale seed).

Acupressure: Using the tip of your finger or thumb, press the Hegu and Susanli points with strong pressure and the Guan Yuan with medium pressure for one to three minutes. Release and repeat. The Hegu points are located on the back of the hands between the thumb and first finger. The Susanli point is on the lower leg, 1 inch outside of and 3 inches below the kneecap. The Guan Yuan point is on the abdomen, about 2 inches below the navel.

Diet: Eat foods that are easy to digest such as rice porridge, carrots, zucchini, daikon radishes, and apple sauce. Avoid eating fatty and raw food.

Naturopathy

Diet: Eliminate the most common food allergens from your diet, including dairy, soy, citrus, peanuts, wheat, eggs, and tomatoes, for three weeks. Re-introduce each food one at a time every three days. Watch for any reactions, which may include gastrointestinal upset, mood changes, headaches, flushing, and worsening of symptoms. Carrageenan has been shown in animal studies to cause lesions in the intestinal tract. Carrageenan is used to stabilize proteins and is mostly found in chocolate milk and milk products. Although this has not been studied in humans, the foods that contain carrageenan should be avoided due to their allergenic properties and potential for intestinal irritation in patients with colitis. A rotation diet in which a different food is eaten every three to four days may be helpful in reducing symptoms. Raw vegetables may be difficult for some colitis patients to digest.

Supplements: Take a multivitamin/multimineral, following the directions on the label (a practitioner can recommend a good quality product). Take the following supplements: 200 mg of magnesium, 50 mg of zinc, 3 g of fish oils, 200 IU vitamin E, and 50,000 IU of vitamin A a day—pregnant women should not take more than 10,000 IU of vitamin A a day. Also, taking 1–2 enterocoated peppermint oil capsules after every meal can reduce spasms and bowel irritability.

Herbs: The following herbs can be used in tincture form at 30 drops three times a day to treat colitis: marshmallow root, for its soothing effect on the gastrointestinal (GI) tract; wild indigo, to treat GI infections; geranium, to reduce excess secretions in the GI tract; goldenseal, to inhibit the growth of bacteria in the GI tract; poke root, to heal ulcers in the intestines; comfrey, as an anti-inflammatory to promote tissue growth and wound healing; and fennel, to relieve spasm of the GI tract, distention, and flatulence. Do not take comfrey internally as it can damage the liver.

Homeopathy

Patients who suffer from this condition are likely to find themselves subject to recurrent episodes. As a chronic condition, colitis is best treated and managed by a professional homeopathic practitioner.

Herbalism

There are many types of colitis and some, such as ischemic colitis and ulcerative colitis, are potentially life threatening. The herbs mentioned below are suitable for treating the less severe forms.

Slippery elm powder: Demulcents or mucilaginous plants are commonly used to treat skin disorders as they coat and soothe the skin. In the same way, the compounds in these plants can repair the damaged intestinal mucosa of colitis. For example, slippery elm root powder provides a protective layer to the intestinal wall, preventing further damage and healing intestinal mucosa. Add slippery elm root powder to food throughout the day, or add 1 tsp to a cup of liquid to make a thick beverage, and drink several times a day.

Boswellia: Resin extracts of boswellia, studied in clinical trials, function as anti-inflammatories in ulcerative colitis. To treat ulcerative colitis, a common dose is 350–400 mg of boswellic acid three times daily, standardized to 30% or higher.

Tip: POSSIBLE TRIGGERS

Dietary strategies that may be helpful include reducing or eliminating dairy products. Also be aware that certain types of antibiotics can aggravate diarrhea. If you are prescribed antibiotics by your doctor, be sure to inform him or her that you suffer from colitis.

Marshmallow root: The mucilage content of this herb is very soothing and protective to the mucous membrane of the digestive tract. This is best prepared as a cold infusion, made by steeping 2 tsp of the root in a glass of water overnight.

Goldenseal: This herb is useful for short-term use as an antimicrobial, if it is needed to aid the clearing up any secondary infection. It is important to source cultivated sustainable sources since it is endangered in its natural habitat due to over harvesting. Garlic may also be used as an antimicrobial, and is much more readily available.

Calendula: Calendula's resins have vulnerary properties, and aid healing of the mucous membrane lining. Water extracts aren't very effective at extracting the resins, so 90% tinctures are best used in small doses, if tolerated well.

Chamomile: This herb is useful as an anti-inflammatory, antispasmodic, and calming nervine. Bisabolol (a volatile oil constituent) provides some of the anti-inflammatory and antispasmodic properties, while apigenin (a flavonoid) provides anxiolytic, or calming, properties, as well as anti-inflammatory actions. This herb can be taken as an infusion by steeping 2 tsp in boiling water for 10 minutes. It is best to keep the cup covered while infusing to prevent the volatile oils from escaping.

Irritable Bowel Syndrome

Diagnosis

When your body digests food, a series of muscular contractions moves the food through the gut, known as peristalsis. Irritable bowel syndrome (IBS) occurs when there is a loss of coordination between these muscular contractions. It is a common condition and can occur at any age, but usually starts during the teenage years. IBS often results from a combination of physical and psychological factors. For example, there is evidence that patients with irritable bowel syndrome have increased sensitivity to stimuli within the gut. As well as the intestinal symptoms, stress seems to be one of the main triggers. Many people find that the onset of their symptoms is often due to a major life event.

Symptoms

- Variable and erratic bowel habits, alternating between constipation and diarrhea
- Feeling full after small meals
- Abdominal bloating after meals
- Excessive gurgling noises in the stomach
- Generalized abdominal tenderness with bloating
- Right-sided abdominal pain
- Pain under the left ribs
- Heartburn

Treatment Goal

It is not possible to prevent IBS. Changes in diet, exercise, and stress management techniques can help reduce symptoms.

Conventional Medicine

Diet: Add 2 tbsp of loose psyllium husk to food a day—it can be sprinkled on cereal or salad. Introduce foods that are high in fiber into your diet. The fiber should be mixed with, or followed by, about 8 fl oz of water to prevent binding. In the long run this works well, although it may be a little uncomfortable initially. Avoid foods that irritate the gut such as gluten, sugar, and dairy products, although irritants do vary from person to person. Bifidus probiotics and Saccharomyces boullardi introduce and maintain beneficial bacteria in the gut. These are available from health food stores. Black tea is useful for easing episodes of diarrhea.

Reduce stress: Stress reduction is very important in IBS. It has been documented that IBS responds best to an integrated mind, body, diet, and medication treatment approach. With this in mind, meditation, T'ai chi, and yoga are beneficial.

Medication: The medication loperamide is used to treat diarrhea. For very severe unresponsive episodes of diarrhea, a medication called alosetron (Lotronex™) can be used. It can cause severe constipation and should be used carefully. Tegaserod (Zelnorm®) is used to treat chronic constipation that does not respond to dietary modification. The antispasmotic dicyclomine (Bentyl®) can be used to treat spasms and bloating pain, although lifestyle and diet modification are usually successful.

Traditional Chinese Medicine

Herbs: To make either of the decoctions below, mix the necessary herbs in a ceramic or glass pot. Add 3 cups of water, bring to a boil, and simmer for 30 minutes. Drink 1 cup twice daily.
• **To treat IBS with digestive function deficiency:** Symptoms include irregular bowel movements, diarrhea, and fatigue. Mix 12 g of Zhu Ling (polyporus sclerotium), 12 g of ginseng, 3 g of dried ginger, 8 g of Gui Zhi (cinnamon), 15 g of Fuling (poria), 15 g of Bai Zhu (white atractylodes rhizome), 6 g of Chen Pi (tangerine peel), and 12 g of Fa Ban Xia (pinellia rhizome).
• **To treat alternating diarrhea and constipation:** Symptoms include bloating after eating, accompanied with anxiety or depression. Combine 12 g of Chai Hu (hare's ear root), 6 g of Chen Pi (tangerine peel), 12 g of Bai Shao (white peony root), 10 g of Zhi Shi (immature fruit of bitter orange), 10 g of Xiang

Fu (nut grass rhizome), 6 g of Bo He (field mint), and 12 g of Bai Zhu (white atractylodes rhizome).

Acupressure: Self-massage the Susanli and the San Yin Jiao points, once or twice a day. The Susanli point is on the lower leg in a depression 4 inches below and 1 inch to the outside of the knee. The San Yin Jiao point is located in the center of the inside of the leg, about 3 inches above the anklebone. You can also massage the Pi Shu and Wei Shu points while lying on the stomach or in a sitting position. The Pi Shu point is located on the back 1½ inches lateral to the spine at the 11th vertebra. The Wei Shu point is 1½ inches lateral to the spine at the 12th vertebra.

Diet: Eat a balanced diet that includes plenty of neutral foods, such as corn, celery, potato, honey, sweet rice, and string beans. Avoid raw food and foods that are hard to digest, like cucumber, onions, and green pepper.

Naturopathy

Diet: It is important to follow a high-fiber diet rich in whole grains and fresh vegetables, fruits, and legumes. This will help reduce the irritation of the digestive system and keep your bowels moving. Replenish the healthy flora in your intestines by eating sauerkraut, kefir, and non-sweetened yogurt containing live probiotics. Identify any foods to which you are allergic or intolerant and eliminate them from your diet. Wheat, dairy, corn, soy, and citrus fruits are the most common allergens. Be conscious of how these foods make you feel—for example, lactose produces symptoms of IBS in those who are intolerant to it. Saturated fats, hydrogenated oils, and partially hydrogenated oils lead to acid reflux. Avoid foods that contain these substances, such as fried and greasy foods, heavy sauces, and red meats, as they are hard to digest and may aggravate symptoms. Avoid chilled drinks, as they inhibit digestion and may cause cramping. Also steer clear of the sweetener fructose, as research shows that IBS sufferers are sensitive to it.

Supplements: Digestive enzymes help your body digest food more efficiently, reducing irritation. The enzymes include lipases that digest fat, proteases that digest proteins, and amylases that digest starch. Take 2 capsules or tablets of a full spectrum enzyme product with each meal. Betaine hydrochloride supports stomach acid levels and helps with digestion. Take 1–2 capsules with each meal. Probiotics help digestion and prevents overgrowth of candida and other harmful microbes. Take a product containing four billion active organisms daily of lactobacillus acidophilus and bifidus.

Herbs: Abdominal pain, the most frequent and disabling symptom of IBS, improves when the intestinal smooth muscles are relaxed. Fennel seed is used to relieve spasms in the gastrointestinal tract, feelings of fullness, and flatulence. Take 1 tsp a day of tincture on an empty stomach. Also take 150 mg of gamma-oryzanol, a natural substance isolated from bran, three times a day for one month. Studies have shown that it protects the mucous lining of the gastrointestinal tract by regulating nervous system control and exerting antioxidant activity, all of which can help with IBS. Gentian root improves overall digestive function by stimulating the secretions of digestive juices; take 300 mg or 10 drops of tincture 15 minutes before meals. Drinking ginger root tea three times a day reduces bloating, gas, and diarrhea. You can also take 500 mg of ginger root in capsule form with each meal.

Homeopathy

This chronic condition is best treated by a homeopathic practitioner. The remedies listed below may be helpful, but long-term home prescribing and management of this condition is not encouraged. Homeopathic treatment for IBS can be given on its own or in conjunction with conventional medicine.

Arg nit: This remedy may be helpful if symptoms of IBS occur after ingesting too many sugary foods or drinks. Symptoms include passing gas and diarrhea that alternate with bouts of constipation, accompanied by severe bloating and swelling of the belly, which feels as though it's about to burst. High levels of anxiety and nervous tension will also aggravate digestive uneasiness.

Colocynthis: This remedy helps to relieve colicky pains that come on in waves after eating and drinking. These are eased temporarily by bending over, which is done instinctively as a way of applying pressure to the abdomen. Episodes of watery diarrhea are accompanied by excessive gas. Common triggers of IBS associated with this remedy include anger or emotional stress.

Lycopodium: If symptoms of IBS are associated with anticipation about an upcoming event, or eating too much hard-to-digest, high-fiber foods, such as beans, sprouts, and lentils, try Lycopodium. Common symptoms include alternating bouts of diarrhea and constipation, coupled with a very noisy and distended digestive tract. There is rumbling and gurgling in the abdomen, heartburn, and a tendency for acid to wash up into the throat when belching.

Herbalism

Peppermint: Peppermint is the most effective herb in treating IBS and the oil has been shown to decrease intestinal motion by acting on calcium channels in the cells. Menthol is the primary component of peppermint oil and produces many of the clinical effects. For IBS, it is best to use enteric-coated capsules so that the oil passes through to the intestines rather than being absorbed in the stomach, where it may contribute to heartburn. The daily dose is 0.6 ml of peppermint oil in enteric-coated tablets or capsules, often dosed as a 0.2 ml of peppermint oil in a capsule or tablet three times daily before food. Peppermint oil should not be used during pregnancy because it may cause the onset of menstruation, gallbladder disease (due to its activity in stimulating the production of bile), hiatus hernia, or acid reflux disease, because it relaxes the sphincter between the esophagus and stomach.

Tip: WARM COMPRESS

If you are experiencing abdominal cramping, lie down with a warm compress against your abdomen to relieve pain. Try using a hot water bottle.

Chamomile: This herb is useful as an anti-inflammatory , antispasmodic, and calming nervine. Bisabolol (a volatile oil constituent) provides some of the anti-inflammatory and antispasmodic properties, while apigenin (a flavonoid) provides anxiolytic, or calming, properties, as well as anti-inflammatory actions. Calming herbs can be very useful if stress and anxiety are playing a part in the IBS, as is often the case. This herb can be taken as an infusion by steeping 2 tsp in boiling water for 10 minutes. It is best to keep the cup covered while infusing to prevent the volatile oils from escaping.

Other herbs: Depending on an individual's symptoms of IBS, there are many other plants that can be helpful. Those that improve digestion, dispel gas, or generally calm the intestines are useful. Examples are teas, tinctures, or capsules of caraway, fennel, cardamom, and anise. A few pieces of fennel may be enough to soothe the symptoms of IBS. Intestinal bitters are calming and healing to the intestines, often because of the astringent tannins present in this class of plants, and are especially useful if diarrhea is the major symptom (see Diarrhea, p. 219). Anxiety may trigger IBS in some people; this can be addressed by using many different plants (see Anxiety, p. 448).

Gallstones

Diagnosis

Gallstones are small solid stones made up of cholesterol, salt, and calcium, that form in the gallbladder, a small organ positioned near the liver. Those with a family history of gallstones, who are overweight or have high cholesterol, or who have inflammatory stomach conditions, are more at risk. Women who have had several pregnancies or who are on a birth-control pill are also more susceptible. The symptoms of gallstones vary widely from mild discomfort to a severe pain that usually begins after eating. A poor diet, especially one high in fatty foods, is a contributory factor. In severe cases the patient can suffer from jaundice, nausea, and fever as the main bile duct can get blocked with migrating gallstones. If symptoms are acute, contact your doctor immediately for tests.

Symptoms

- Pains in the upper right side of the abdomen, or just below the ribs on the right side
- Pain in the right shoulder or between the shoulder blades
- Nausea and vomiting
- Loss of appetite
- Fever
- Frequency and severity of attacks is variable

Treatment Goal

To identify the cause of the gallstones and make any lifestyle changes necessary to prevent them from developing further. Treatment also aims to relieve symptoms and dissolve or remove any existing gallstones.

Conventional Medicine

The treatment of gallstones initially depends on an adequate diagnosis. Your doctor may take an ultrasound of the gallbladder to determine whether gallstones are present. If an infection of the gallbladder is suspected, a nuclear imaging study called a HIDA scan is done. The recurrence rate of gallstones is high after treatment unless, of course, the gallbladder is removed. Lifestyle modification, described below, is essential to preventing recurrence.

Diet: If you suffer from gallstones, it is necessary to make certain changes to your lifestyle. Substitute polyunsaturated fats in your diet with monounsaturated fats to prevent stones from developing. A slow and steady weight loss (about 2 lb a week is normal) in people who are overweight is appropriate, but rapid weight loss should be avoided as this can precipitate gallstones.

Surgery: Gallstones that are symptomatic are treated surgically by a cholecystectomy (removal of the gallbladder). The operation generally requires a short recovery period, particularly when performed through a laparascope. This involves inserting a scope into the abdomen and operating through it rather than cutting through the abdominal wall.

Dissolving the stones: Those who are too high risk for surgery, can take a medication that dissolves the gallstones. If there are five or less stones that are made of cholesterol rather than calcium, and that are less than ½ inch in size, ursodiol (Actigall™) is used. The stones can also be dissolved using a solvent called methyl tert-butyl ether (MTBE). The solvent is administered directly into the area of the stone through the skin with a long catheter, through which the solvent is infused before then catheter is drawn out. Finally, the stones can be shocked until they break up into very small pieces in a procedure called extracorporeal shock wave lithotripsy (ESWL).

Traditional Chinese Medicine

Herbs: The formulas below are designed to dispel gallstones. Using either of the herbal combinations, add 3 cups of water, bring to a boil, and simmer for 30 minutes. Strain the liquid and drink 1 cup two to three times a day. The clinical dosage may be heavier, but is reduced here for you to use safely. It is best to consult a professional TCM practitioner for a prescription of the Chinese herbal formulas.
• **To treat gallstones that have formed as a result of Qi stagnation:** Mix 10 g of Chai Hu (hare's ear root), 12 g of Yu Jin (turmeric tuber), 12 g of Xiang Fu (nut grass rhizome), 18 g of Jin Qian Cao (lysimachia), 10 g of Zhi Ke (bitter orange), and 12 g of Da Huang (rhubarb root and rhizome).
• **To treat gallstones that have formed as a result of dampness and heat:** Mix 10 g of Jin Yin Hua (honeysuckle flower), 10 g of Lian Qiao (forsythia fruit), 12 g of Yu Jin (turmeric tuber), 12 g of Yin Chen (artemisia), 10 g of Mu Xiang (costus root), 10 g of Huang Qin (baical skullcap root), and 10 g of Da Huang (rhubarb root and rhizome).

Acupressure: Gently press the Yang Ling Quan, Nei Guan, and Hegu points for one minute. Release and repeat to relieve the pain of a gallstone attack. The Yang Ling Quan point is on the outside of the leg by the knee in the depression just below the top of the fibula bone. The Nei Guan point is located in the center of the wrist on the palm side, about 2 inches below the crease. The Hegu points are located on the back of the hands between the thumb and first finger.

Diet: Chicory is good for the gallbladder.

 # Naturopathy

Diet: Studies show that vegetarians have a lower risk of getting gallstones than meat eaters. If you suffer from gallstones, try to reduce the amount of animal products in your diet and increase the amount of vegetables you eat. A fiber-rich diet, including whole grains, fresh fruit and vegetables, and oat bran eaten every day at regular intervals, reduces the likelihood of gallstones. Also eat beets, artichokes, and dandelion greens regularly to improve bile flow. Use good quality extra virgin olive oil in salads to improve bile flow, and limit your consumption of sugar and simple carbohydrates. Note: If you already have gallstones, raw vegetables such as lettuce and broccoli may make the symptoms worse.

Supplements: Take 1–2 capsules of lipase enzymes with food to improve the digestion of fat. Taking 1,000 mg of lecithin in the form of phophatidylcholine twice a day helps to increase the solubility of gallstones. Take a probiotic product containing at least four billion active organisms of Lactobacillus acidophilus and bifidus daily for help with digestion.

Herbs: Dandelion root improves bile flow; take 400 mg of the freeze-dried herb or 1 tsp of liquid extract twice a day. Take 100–175 mg of milk thistle two or three times a day to decrease cholesterol saturation and increase bile flow. Artichoke also improves bile flow. Take 1–2 ml of a tincture or 500 mg in capsule form with each meal. Take 150 mg of turmeric with each meal for its anti-inflammatory effects and its ability to relax the bile duct.

Homeopathy

The remedies below can be used to manage the discomfort of gallstones on a temporary basis. Once gallstones begin to move, conventional medical assessment is needed. After the immediate condition is resolved, preventative long-term homeopathic treatment can help to prevent recurrence. In cases that require the surgical removal of the gallbladder, homeopathy can provide pre- and postoperative support.

Chelidonium: Consider this remedy if pain is present underneath the right shoulder blade. Intense pain may lead to severe nausea and possibly vomiting. Alternatively, pains may seem to flit about in all directions, and feel more severe when bending forward, backward, or when coughing. Lying on the belly may give some relief.

Berberis: To ease crushing, stitching, and sharp pains around the right shoulder blade use Berberis. Pains are so severe that they render the patient prostrate and exhausted. Pain feels more intense when sitting or lying down, and motion of any kind aggravates it further. The pains are also changeable in nature.

China: If pains are triggering hyperexcitability, try China. Symptoms include weakness due to the loss of body fluids from profuse sweating. Intense pain, normally felt between the shoulder blades, can trigger episodes of vomiting. Movement intensifies pain and leads to palpitations and shortness of breath. There may also be a need to double over in an instinctive desire to apply pressure to the painful area.

Herbalism

The presence of gallstone is potentially life threatening and requires medical evaluation to avoid serious complications such as pancreatitis, cholangitis, and cholecystitis. Conventional medicine should be the first line of treatment, but herbal remedies can be useful as additional therapies, or during the period when definitive treatment is being sought. The two categories of herbs used to treat gallstones are choleretics and cholagogues.

To prevent gallstones: Choleretic plants cause the liver cells to make more bile, and cholagogue plants cause this bile to be released. By collectively increasing the flow of bile, these plants may help to clean out the bile duct system or gallbladder. Examples of choleretics are dandelion root and globe artichoke (Cynara). Examples of cholagogues are dandelion root, yellow dock root, liquorice, globe artichoke, and celandine. These plants work best when taken 20–30 minutes before meals, and if you are not constipated. To successfully increase bile flow, treatment must be followed by regular bowel movements so that the bile is eliminated from the body.

Stone root: Known for its antilithic properties, this herb is often used in helping to break up urinary- and gallstones, and gravel. It may be used as a preventative, but is often of great use when an aid is needed to help pass stones and gravel. This is most often taken as a root decoction, or tincture.

Antispasmodic herbs and analgesics may also be indicated. 🌿

Tip: MAINTAIN A GOOD DIET

To avoid recurring gallstones, do not eat foods that are high in saturated fats (including full-fat cheese, red meat, cream, and whole milk). Instead, opt for foods that are high in unrefined carbohydrates, and eat at least five portions of fresh fruit and vegetables each day. Choose fish as a source of protein rather than meat. If you crave meat from time to time, opt for chicken or turkey, but do not eat the skin, which contains a significant amount of fat. Certain foods, such as artichokes, asparagus, kelp, and barley water, are thought to be beneficial for those who are prone to gallstones and may be worth including in the diet. If you are in any doubt, consult a dietician.

Hemorrhoids

Diagnosis

Hemorrhoids, also know as piles, are small, blood-filled swellings caused by dilated varicose veins in the anal area. Some hemorrhoids can get better without medical treatment, particularly those caused by constipation. A doctor may recommend a change of diet that includes more roughage, especially green vegetables, fresh fruit, whole grain cereals, and bran. Drinking eight to ten glasses of water every day is also advisable. Mild cases can be treated using creams available directly from your local pharmacy. A few days' treatment is usually enough for the irritation to settle. To treat cases of hemorrhoids that protrude from the anus with swelling and pain, resting with a cooling pack applied to the anal area can be helpful. Severe cases need to be treated by a specialist. One possible treatment is rubber band ligation. The most serious cases require surgical removal, known as a hemorroidectomy.

Symptoms

- Itchiness in the anal area
- Pain and discomfort
- A lump may be felt in the anus
- Sensation that the bowel has not emptied completely
- Occasionally, anal bleeding after a bowel movement

Treatment Goal

To ease the pain and discomfort, and resolve the hemorrhoids.

Conventional Medicine

Stool softeners: Creating softer stools will ease the pain of bowel movements. Add loose psyllium husks to food to prevent the formation of hard stools, or use the over-the-counter stool softener docusate. Incorporating fiber into your diet and making sure you drink plenty of water also helps in this manner.

Topical treatment: Witch hazel can be used topically for its cooling and astringent properties. Over-the-counter topical local anesthetics, which may or may not be mixed with a corticosteroid, can relieve symptoms. These consist of benzocaine 20%, which is applied four times daily as needed for pain and itching, or of lidocaine 5%, which may be applied as required. These are for external use only. Keep in mind that although these are topical agents, they can be absorbed over time. Sitz baths involve sitting in warm water for about 15 minutes three times a day. This can be helpful at the first sign of symptoms.

Surgery: Surgical treatments may be needed if the remedies above are unsuccessful or inadequate. An external hemorrhoid excision can be performed to remove any external hemorrhoids. For internal hemorrhoids, rubber band ligation, which involves placing a small rubber band at the base of the hemorrhoid to cut off the blood supply so that it eventually shrinks and falls off, is performed. Infrared coagulation and bipolar electrocoagulation are other possible procedures. These are painless and can be done in a physician's office, but require special equipment that not all doctors have. For advanced hemorrhoids, direct current (DC) therapy is used, where an electric current is applied directly to the hemorrhoid to cut off its blood supply.

Tip: LIE ON YOUR SIDE IF PREGNANT

If you are pregnant, lying down on your left side and resting for about ½ an hour two or three times a day can help prevent hemorrhoids from occurring. It also helps to lie on your left side at night, if you're comfortable in that position, to relieve the pressure of the fetus on the veins serving the lower half of the body.

Traditional Chinese Medicine

Herbs: External patent herbs may be available from Chinese herbalists, for example, Hua Zhi Gao (a paste that shrinks hemorrhoids). You can also use these formulas.

• **Internal formula for hemorrhoids with constipation:** Mix 8 g of Da Huang (rhubarb root and rhizome), 8 g of Chai Hu (hare's ear root), 2 g of Sheng Ma (bugbane rhizome), 3 g of Gan Cao (licorice root), 8 g of Huang Qin (baical skullcap root), and 10 g of Dang Gui (Chinese angelica) with 2½ cups of water. Bring to a boil, simmer for 30 minutes, and strain. Drink ½ cup of this decoction three times a day for five to seven days. If you have diarrhea, do not use this formula.

• **Internal formula to reduce pain and swelling:** Add 15 g of Ku Shen (sophora root) to 3 cups of water. Bring to the boil and simmer for 30 minutes. Remove the herbs and boil two organic eggs, with shells, for five minutes.

Remove and peel the eggs and add 30 g of brown sugar to the herbal liquid. Drink the decoction and eat the eggs once a day for five days to complete one course of treatment. You can take two courses of treatment. If you do not see some improvement after one course, see your doctor.

• **External herbal formula:** Combine 15 g of Ma Zhi Xian (dried purslane), 10 g of Hua Jiao (fruit of Szechuan pepper), 12 g of Wu Bei Zi (gallnut of the Chinese sumac), 15 g of Fang Fen (ledebouriella root), 12 g of Ce Bai Ye (biota leaves), 10 g of Zhi Ke (bitter orange), and 15 g of Fuling (poria) in a ceramic pot. Add 6 cups of water, bring to a boil, and simmer for 30 minutes. Strain the herbs, let them cool to a warm temperature, and sit in the herbs. Let the anus soak in the herbs for 10–15 minutes twice a day, in the morning and evening, for five to seven days.

Naturopathy

Diet: An inadequate amount of fiber in the diet is one of the most common causes of hemorrhoids, and taking fiber has a consistent beneficial effect for relieving symptoms. Base your diet on whole foods like fresh vegetables, fruits, whole grains, beans, nuts, and seeds. Sprinkle ground flaxseeds, which contain high quantities of fiber and essential oils that help with bowel movements, on your cereal, homemade shakes, or salads. If you try to eat too much fiber at one time this may put too much pressure on your intestines, so eat

several light meals throughout the day rather than two or three large meals. Avoid trans-fatty acids and hydrogenated oils. They slow down the digestive system and contribute to inflammation. Drink 8–10 glasses of water throughout the day to keep hydrated and help stools pass more easily.

Supplements: Bioflavonoids are a type of plant compound that stabilizes and strengthens blood vessel walls and decreases inflammation. They have been found to reduce anal discomfort, pain, and discharge during an acute hemorrhoid attack. The major flavonoids found in citrus fruits—diosmin, hesperidin, and oxyrutins—appear to be beneficial. Take a bioflavonoid complex of 1,000 mg three times a day. Also take 500 mg of vitamin C three times a day to strengthen the rectal tissue.

Herbs: Witch hazel can be applied topically to act as an astringent, decrease the bleeding, and relieve the pain, itching, and swelling associated with hemorrhoids. Use a distilled liquid, ointment, or medicated pad as a compress, or apply a cream. You can also add 1 oz to a sitz bath. Butchers broom has anti-inflammatory and vein-constricting properties believed to improve the tone and integrity of veins and shrink swollen tissue. Take a standardized extract that provides 200–300 mg of ruscogenins a day. Horse chestnut is often recommended when there is poor circulation in the veins, or chronic venous insufficiency. It relieves symptoms such as swelling and inflammation and also strengthens blood vessel walls. Take 100 mg of standardized aescin daily. Horse chestnut can also be applied externally as a compress. Stoneroot, taken at 500 mg three times a day, reduces the swelling caused by hemorrhoids.

Hydrotherapy: Take two or three sitz baths each a day. Sit in a warm bath with your knees raised for 5–15 minutes. To increase circulation, alternate hot and cold sitz baths, sitting for one minute in warm water and for 30 seconds in cold.

Homeopathy

The remedies below can be helpful in easing the symptoms of a recently developed, mild to moderate episode of hemorrhoids. If you have an established problem with severe hemorrhoids, seek treatment from a homeopathic practitioner. This becomes a greater priority if you experience hemorrhoids in combination with other circulatory problems such as varicose veins.

Nux vomica: If hemorrhoids are linked to constipation, where although bowel movements occur each day (after lots of straining and urging) the bowel seldom feels cleared, use Nux vomica. Hemorrhoids bleed easily and are distressingly itchy, but are soothed by applying cool compresses.

Tip: DON'T STRAIN

Move your bowels only when you feel the urge and do not spend more than 15 minutes at a time sitting on the toilet. Straining may bring a lot of pressure into the pelvic area, which can lead to hemorrhoids.

Hamamelis: Use this remedy if hemorrhoids are tender and sore, with lots of prickling stinging pains. Hemorrhoids are likely to bleed quite profusely when very inflamed, and feel especially uncomfortable when touched or when you move suddenly.

Aloe: Use this remedy if hemorrhoids burn and itch, especially at night. There may also be pulsating, throbbing sensations in the rectum, especially after attempting to pass a stool.

Aesculus: To relieve acute hemorrhoids that occur due to long-term, underlying constipation and a sluggish bowel, use Aesculus. Pains in the affected area are characteristically sharp and lead to backache, with shooting pains traveling from the rectum up the back. Dryness in the bowel makes passing stools very painful, and there is a persistent feeling of discomfort.

Herbalism

The herbal approach to hemorrhoids includes preventing and treating constipation. Please see Constipation for further advice (p. 214).

Yarrow: Flowers of yarrow can be used as a poultice or salve to stop bleeding and act, like witch hazel, as an astringent. Both of these actions are important in controlling the swelling and bleeding associated with hemorrhoids. Yarrow's effectiveness is partly due to a compound, called achilleine, which stops bleeding.

Stone root: This astringent herb is either taken internally or incorporated into suppositories to treat hemorrhoids. Some herbalists use the whole plant, others use just the root. It contains numerous compounds, such as terpenoids and rosmaric acid, that account for its medicinal effects.

Multifaceted approach: There are many other herbs that are useful for treating hemorrhoids. It is important to treat constipation, and use a local, topical herb to help with swelling, bleeding, and pain. Many herbalists also address the health of the vascular system by using plants such as horse chestnut seed to tone the venous system and address any congestion. Open wounds associated with bleeding hemorrhoids can be treated with any of the vulnerary herbs, such as calendula. Also, mucilaginous herbs, such as slippery elm, can soften stools and coat the intestinal wall to make bowel movements more comfortable. Consult a herbal expert for a comprehensive treatment plan. 🌰

Tip: AVOID HEATED SEATS

Heated seats tend to raise the pressure in the veins of the rectum. When traveling by car on long journeys, avoid using heated seats if you are prone to hemorrhoids.

Urinary Tract Infection

Diagnosis

The urinary tract is composed of the kidneys, ureters, the bladder, and the urethra. A urinary tract infection (UTI) is defined as the presence of multiplying micro-organisms (bacteria) in the tract through which you pass urine from the kidneys via the bladder. UTI is much more common in women, because of the short length of the female urethra and its proximity to the anus. UTIs are rare in men under 60, but the incidence increases as both men and women get older, until they tend to be equally affected. To establish whether an infection is present, a clean midstream urine sample is taken and sent to the lab for examination. A level of 100,000 bacteria per milliliter of urine is regarded as a significant infection.

Symptoms

- Burning sensation when passing urine
- Frequent and compelling need to urinate
- Urine can be cloudy
- Urine can have an offensive odor
- Loin pain, with fever and chills (this indicates an upper infection of kidneys or ureters)

Treatment Goal

Treatment depends on why the infection has occurred. Most patients respond rapidly to antibiotics. A high intake of fluids is essential to help flush out the infection from the system. If UTIs keep occurring, it is essential to identify and treat the underlying cause.

Conventional Medicine

Antibiotics: Trimethoprim/sulfamethaxazole can be taken twice a day for three days. This antibiotic is generally well tolerated but can affect the skin and central nervous and gastrointestinal systems. If the bacteria causing the UTI is resistant to this antibiotic, ciprofloxacin (Cipro®) or levofloxacin (Levoquin®) can be used, as well as nitrofurantoin (Macrobid®). Symptoms should resolve in one or at the most two days after starting treatment. Phenazopyridine is sometimes prescribed along with an antibiotic to decrease the pain experienced on urination with a urinary tract infection. This medication turns the urine bright orange. It has been associated with infrequent but very severe allergic reactions.

Lifestyle modifications: Practice stress reduction techniques, avoid irritating soaps, and take showers rather than baths. Women should wipe front to back after urination.

Traditional Chinese Medicine

TCM can be an effective treatment for both acute and chronic UTIs.

Herbs: To prepare either of the formulas below, mix the herbs in a glass or ceramic pot and add 3 cups of water. Bring to a boil and simmer for 30 minutes. Strain and drink 1 cup twice a day.
• **Acute UTI:** Mix 12 g of Pu Gong Ying (dandelion), 12 g of Huang Bai (phellodendron), 12 g of Huang Qin (baical skullcap root), 12 g of Che Qian Cao (plantago), 10 g of Zhi Zi (cape jasmine fruit), 8 g of Gan Cao (licorice root), and 12 g of Bai Mao Gen (wooly grass rhizome). You can take this formula for seven days.
• **Chronic UTI:** Mix 12 g of Sheng Di Huang (Chinese foxglove root), 15 g of Fuling (poria), 15 g of Shan Yao (Chinese yam), 10 g of Huang Bai (phellodendron), 12 g of Zhi Mu (anemarrhena rhizome), 12 g of Han Lian Cao (eclipta), 12 g of Bai Zhu (white atractylodes rhizome), and 12 g of Huang Qin (baical skullcap root). You may take this formula for up to two months. If your stools loosen, stop treatment.

Acupressure: Use your thumbs to press the Zhong Ji and Guan Yuan points with gentle pressure for one minute. Breathing deeply, release the pressure for one inhalation and exhalation, and then reapply pressure. Repeat this six times once or twice a day. The Zhong Ji point is on the abdomen, about 4 inches below the navel. The Guan Yuan point is on the abdomen, about 3 inches below the navel.

Naturopathy

Diet: Eat natural diuretics such as watermelon, parsley, and celery, or make a juice out of these foods. Ginger and garlic, which can be added to vegetable broths, have powerful antimicrobial effects. Restrict your sugar intake while battling an infection, as it can feed bacteria. Spicy foods, caffeine, and alcohol can aggravate symptoms and should be avoided. Drink 9–12 cups of water a day, to increase your urinary output. Also drink 2–3 glasses of unsweetened cranberry juice a day to flush out the infection. If you are taking antibiotics, eat 1 cup of unsweetened yogurt two to three times a day to replenish some of the friendly bacteria in the gut that antibiotics can cause you to lose.

Supplements: Take 1,000 mg of vitamin C four times a day to help enhance immune function, inhibit E.coli bacteria, and acidify the urine to decrease bacterial growth. Probiotics prevent the overgrowth of harmful bacteria and replace healthy flora if you are taking antibiotics. Take a product that contains at least four billion organisms a day (two hours before or after taking antibiotics) for two months.

Tip: WEAR LOOSE CLOTHING

Avoid wearing clothing and underwear that hugs the body too tightly, such as tights, jeans, leggings, and underwear made from synthetic materials such as nylon. They do not allow for good ventilation around the genital area.

Herbs: Cranberry has been used for more than a century to prevent UTIs. Evidence suggests that it is the antioxidant flavonoids found in cranberry, called proanthocyanins, that prevent bacteria from sticking to the walls of the urinary tract. Take 400 mg of a standardized extract twice daily. Uva Ursi is an antimicrobial that fights E. coli. Take a standardized capsule that contains 250 mg of arbutin four times daily, make a tea by steeping 2 tsp of herb in 1 cup of hot water, or take 1–2 tsp of tincture in warm water. Uva ursi may turn urine green. Goldenseal has a long and well-documented history as a powerful antimicrobial agent. It can be taken as a tea made from 1 tsp of dried herb per cup of hot water, in capsule form at 1,000 mg, or as 1–2 tsp of tincture in warm water. Horsetail is an excellent diuretic and has a long history of use for urinary tract infections. Take 500 mg of the capsule or 2 ml of the tincture four times a day. Take 500 mg of D-mannose a day to prevent bacteria from sticking to the bladder wall. You can also try drinking an herbal tea consisting of buchu, horsetail, thyme leaf, and pipisissewa. To make a tea, steep 2 oz of the herbal mixture in 2 cups of boiling water in a glass or ceramic jar or teapot. Drink 2–5 cups a day for 7–10 days after all the symptoms have cleared. Pregnant women should omit yarrow from the mixture. Marshmallow root has soothing demulcent properties. Soak the herb in cold water for several hours, strain, and drink.

Homeopathy

The following remedies can be helpful in easing a recent, mild to moderate bladder infection. Remedies can be used alone or alongside conventional medicine. To be most effective, treatment should be combined with naturopathic measures such as increasing your fluid intake. If problems with UTIs are chronic, seek professional homeopathic support.

Cantharis: Take Cantharis at the first twinges of a UTI. When this remedy is helpful, severe burning pains when urinating develop rapidly. Symptoms feel more distressing when you are moving around, but you feel better when resting at night.

Arsenicum album: This remedy also treats burning pains, but is more suitable for pain that is most distressing at night and in the early hours of the morning. Burning sensations feel temporarily eased by contact with warmth. Symptoms include shivering and feeling chilly.

Pulsatilla: If discomfort and the urge to urinate are more distressing when lying down at night, try Pulsatilla. This remedy is especially helpful if a UTI results from being in chilly, damp surroundings, and if ignoring the urge to urinate brings on slight urinary incontinence. Although you may feel chilly, warmth in any form makes discomfort worse. Symptoms also include feeling weepy when ill, with a need for sympathy and attention.

Staphysagria: If symptoms develop after sexual intercourse, or after being catheterized for surgery, Staphysagria can help. There may be an inability to empty the bladder fully, and urine is likely to look concentrated and dark in color. There are also strong stinging sensations after passing water.

Herbalism

Cranberry: This fruit has been thought for some time to be of great benefit for those with UTIs. Many studies support its use as a preventive measure for people with frequent infections. However, data concerning its use to treat UTIs is either lacking or indeterminate. Cranberry's capacity to defend against UTIs is said to be from its ability to prevent bacteria from adhering to the bladder and urethra. To prevent, and possibly treat, UTIs it is best to drink 100% pure cranberry juice, which you can find at your local health food store. Most of the cranberry juice you find at the supermarket is highly diluted and contains a lot of added sugar. There is no certain recommended dosage for cranberry juice, though 3 fl oz has been shown to be beneficial for the prevention of UTIs while as much as 12–32 fl oz has been used to treat UTIs. The juice can be diluted in water as the pure form is often unpalatable.

Cranberry juice has few side effects. Mild stomach upset has been noted, along with the slim possibility of precipitating an attack of kidney stones in people who are already susceptible, but this only occurs in those taking excessive amounts of juice (greater than 32 fl oz per day).

Dandelion: This weed is often referred to as a "restoring" or "purifying" herb for the liver, gallbladder, intestines, and kidneys. Traditionally one of dandelion's purported benefits has been in the treatment of UTIs. There is some evidence that dandelion acts as a diuretic, increasing the flow of urine, which may explain its beneficial effects in the treatment of UTIs. Dandelion can be found in most health food stores in dried or tincture form. If using the dried herb, take 3–4 g as a tea two to three times a day. If using a tincture, take 5 ml diluted in water or juice three to four times daily. Dandelion is a member of the daisy/ragweed family, so should be used cautiously by those with allergies to plants in this family. Besides allergic reaction, other reported adverse effects are dermatitis and gallbladder irritation and obstruction. Do not use dandelion if there is a history of gallbladder problems.

Stinging nettle: Recent evidence shows promise that this plant can be used effectively to treat enlarged prostate and disorders of the kidneys, bladder, and urinary tract, as well as allergies. For UTIs, the suggested dosage is 1–2 g of the root as a tea two to three times daily. Many health food stores now sell stinging nettles as freeze-dried capsules, which can be a more convenient mode of delivery.

Corn silk: A very useful herb for the urinary system, corn silk has diuretic and antimicrobial properties. It soothes and protects mucous membranes, and cools irritation of the urinary system. The strands of corn silk can be made into a tea by infusing 2 tsp in a cup of boiling water for 10 minutes. Drink three times daily. Tinctures may also be used, if well tolerated during a urinary tract infection.

Cystitis

Diagnosis

Cystitis is a urinary infection that affects the bladder. The E. coli bacterium, which lives in the digestive tract, causes about 80% of all cases of cystitis. Women are particularly prone to this condition. This is thought to be due to the short length of their urethra (the tube that carries urine from the bladder out of the body) and its proximity to the anus. Women should wipe themselves after urinating from front to back, towards the anus, to avoid bringing bacteria from their intestinal tract into their urethra. Many women experience the condition when they first become sexually active or during periods of increased sexual activity. During intercourse, bacteria are pushed up into the urethra and to the bladder. Urinating before and after intercourse can be preventive, as this flushes out bacteria. Some women are particularly prone to this condition and suffer repeat attacks. Cystitis can be particularly troublesome during pregnancy, when the growing fetus puts pressure on the urinary tract.

Symptoms

- Painful burning sensation when urinating
- Frequent urge to pass urine
- Cloudy urine that smells unpleasant
- Occasionally, blood in urine
- Pain directly above the pubic bone

Treatment Goal

To get to the root cause of the cystitis and address it, while providing relief for the painful symptoms of the condition.

Conventional Medicine

Treatment of cystitis involves identifying the cause and avoiding risk factors wherever possible. Bubble baths, low estrogen, certain spermicides, altered vaginal flora, and toilet hygiene are some factors that contribute to urinary tract infections.

Drink plenty of fluids: Drinking enough water is important. Some natural herbs such as cranberry and uva ursa can be taken along with water as preventive measures.

Antibiotics: These are used to treat the infection. The antibiotic most frequently used to treat a urinary tract infection is trimethoprim/sulfamethaxazole (Bactrim™), taken twice a day for three days. It is the most cost-effective antibiotic, but does have some side effects such as gastrointestinal problems, depression, and anxiety. Some bacteria have become resistant to Bactrim™, in which case ciprofloxin, taken twice a day for two to five days, is used as an alternative. Nitrofurantoin (Macrobid™) is another common medication used for urinary tract infection. However, again, resistance is occurring and ciprofloxin may be a better choice. A recent study showed that a two- to four-day course of antibiotics is just as effective as longer duration treatments. The medication phenazopyridine (Pyridium™) is used for bladder pain and burning that occurs with a urinary tract infection. It is taken three times a day for two days. This medication causes the urine to turn a red-orange color and should not be used for more than a few days, or at all by children under 12 years old.

Traditional Chinese Medicine

Herbs:
• **Herbal decoction:** Combine 10 g of Che Qian Cao (plantago), 10 g of Jin Qian Cao (lysimachia), 10 g of Ze Lan (bugleweed), 12 g of Huang Bai (phellodendron), 12 g of Fuling (poria), 12 g of Zhu Ling (polyporus sclerotium), and 8 g of Shen Gan Cao (raw licorice) in a ceramic pot. Add 3 cups of water, bring to the boil, and simmer for 30 minutes before straining. Drink 1 cup twice a day.
• **Herbal decoction to treat yin deficiency and heat**: Mix 15 g of Zhi Mu (anemarrhena rhizome), 12 g of Shan Shen (mountain root), 12 g of Huang Bai (phellodendron), 12 g of Bai Mao Gen (wooly grass rhizome), 12 g of Cang Zhu (atractylodes rhizome), and 12 g of Jin Qian Cao (lysimachia). Use this mixture to make a decoction as described above.

Acupressure: Use the tip of your finger or thumb to press the San Yin Jiao, Zhong Ji, and Hegu points with medium pressure for one minute several times. The San Yin Jiao point is found on the inside of the leg, about 3 inches above the anklebone. The Hegu points are located on the back of the hands, between the thumb and first finger. The Zhong Ji point is on the abdomen, 4 inches below the navel.

Naturopathy

Diet: One of the best ways to treat cystitis is to increase the amount of times you urinate. Drink a glass of water every hour throughout the day. Cranberry juice has been used for more than a century to prevent and treat urinary tract infections. Evidence suggests that it is the antioxidant flavonoids called proanthocyanidins that prevent bacteria from adhering to the walls of the urinary tract. Cranberry juice should be unsweetened, especially if it is used by people with suppressed immune systems. Drink 4 fl oz three times throughout the day. Eat watermelons, celery, and parsley, which act as natural diuretics and will help flush out infection from the urinary system.

Supplements: Vitamin C enhances immune function, inhibits growth of E. coli (the bacteria most commonly responsible for cystitis), and makes urine more acidic so that bacteria cannot grow as easily. Vitamin A also enhances immune function. Take 25,000–50,000 IU of vitamin C and A daily. Pregnant women should not take more than 10,000 IU a day. Take a probiotic product that contains at least four billion active organisms daily to replace helpful bacteria in your gut. This is especially important if you are taking antibiotics, and the probiotics should be taken at least two hours after taking an antibiotic.

Herbs: Take 400–500 mg of cranberry in capsule form twice a day to help prevent bacteria from adhering to the bladder wall. D-mannose, taken at 500 mg four times a day, also prevents bacteria from attaching to the urinary tract and the bladder wall. Uva ursi contains arbutin, a chemical known to have antimicrobial activity against E. coli. Take 250 mg of uva ursi in capsule form or 5 ml of the tincture form four times a day. Horsetail is another herb traditionally used to treat urinary tract infections. Take 500 mg or 2 ml of the tincture four times a day. Juniper berry helps increase urination to rid the bladder of bacteria. You can make juniper tea by adding 1 cup of boiling water to 1 tbsp of juniper berries and allowing the berries to steep for 20 minutes. The usual dosage is to drink 1 cup twice a day. A formula that contains this herb along with the other herbs listed may be more effective.

Hydrotherapy: A hot sitz bath is a potent therapy for cystitis. Take it at least once a day and add apple cider vinegar or garlic oil for a stronger effect.

Homeopathy

The following remedies can help to ease the discomfort, and shorten the duration, of an acute episode of cystitis. Homeopathy can be used as a first line of defense until a medical evaluation is done, but should not be used as an alternative to conventional care. If cystitis becomes a chronic problem, consult a professional homeopath.

Cantharis: This is the first choice for treating classic symptoms of cystitis, such as burning sensations before, during, and after urinating. There is a constant, distressing urge to pass water, but only a very small amount of urine is passed at a time. Scalding and burning sensations flare up violently and quickly. Symptoms are characteristically soothed by contact with warmth and massage, while moving around and drinking coffee aggravates symptoms.

Arsenicum album: This is a strong candidate if burning pains are associated with a sense of being generally chilly, exhausted, and restless when feeling ill. Symptoms include burning sensations while urinating that are temporarily soothed by taking a warm bath or applying warm compresses to the affected area. Symptoms tend to feel worse at night, including shivering, nausea, and anxiety.

Staphysagria: This can help ease symptoms that set in after any medical procedures involving catheterization, or are triggered by sexual intercourse. Classic symptoms include an unpleasant sensation of being unable to completely empty the bladder. Urine passed appears dark and concentrated, and stinging, burning sensations occur after urinating.

Sarsaparilla: If passing urine is most painful as the bladder becomes more empty, try Sarsaparilla. There may also be a tendency for slight urinary incontinence at night, and symptoms are noticeably worse when premenstrual.

Herbalism

The following herbs can be taken in combination to treat an infectious condition, or may be used separately for their soothing and healing properties.

Uva ursi: An astringent and slightly sweet plant, uva ursi increases urination and renal circulation, while acting as a urinary antiseptic. The key constituent, arbutin, is converted to its active component, hydroquinone, in the alkaline environment that uva ursi creates. A tincture or dried leaf tea might be recommended by your herbal medicine practitioner. Limit use to one week or less, and no more than five times in a year, due to some concerns about the safety of long-term use of hydroquinone.

Tip: PREVENTING INFECTION

If you develop bladder infections easily, always pass water when you feel the need, however busy you may be. Not doing so can encourage an infection to develop.

Buchu: This herb has a sharp, spicy, and bitter taste. It is a urinary tract anti-inflammatory, diuretic, and slightly antiseptic. Diosphenol is one of the flavonoids that may contribute to diuretic and antimicrobial actions. A tincture or infusion may be taken.

Marshmallow root: This sweet, cooling, nutritious plant has polysaccharides and mucilage properties that soothe and ease pain and inflammation in the urinary tract. A cold infusion or a tincture may be used, but a water extract may be better tolerated during cystitis. Your herbal expert can advise on how much tea or tincture to take daily, and whether this treatment might prevent the absorption of other medications you may be taking.

Corn silk: Sweet and cooling, corn silk (the silky threads on a kernel of corn) soothes and coats the urinary tract, while also eliminating microbes and encouraging urination. Corn silk is used to treat inflammation of the bladder and kidneys. Your herbal medicine practitioner may recommend taking an infusion of the dried herb, or a tincture.

Kidney Stones

Diagnosis

Kidney stones generally start off as a minute crystal in the kidneys, usually caused by a high concentration of calcium in the urine. They can also be caused by dehydration, infection, and various kidney disorders.

Kidney stones vary greatly in size. If the stone is ¼ inch or smaller, the attack will usually stop after a few hours when the stone is passed in the urine. However, if the stone gets stuck, the process of passing it can take several days. Discharging a kidney stone from the bladder through the urethra is often painless, or at worst will cause a slight pain when urinating. There are many methods of removing stones.

A stone lodged in the ureter can be removed by a cystoscope (via the bladder). Those in the kidneys are accessed via a small cut in the back, from where the stone is either pulled out or broken up using shock waves.

Symptoms

- Sudden, intense pain of an intermittent nature
- Nausea and vomiting
- Blood in the urine
- Reduced urine flow and output
- Frequent urinary infections

Treatment Goal

To ease the pain of severe attacks and prevent recurrences of kidney stones. This may involve changes to your diet and drinking plenty of fluids.

Conventional Medicine

Treatment aims to control pain, identify any complications such as infection or obstruction, and reduce the recurrence of kidney stones. Generally, urgent medical attention is needed if fever and chills are present along with other symptoms of kidney stones. Also, if there is a history of kidney failure, if a sufferer is pregnant, or if the patient has a single kidney, seek immediate help.

Pain relief: Non-steroidal anti-inflammatory drugs (NSAIDs) are used to reduce pain. Intravenous NSAIDs such as ketorolac can be given for immediate relief. If this does not work, intravenous narcotic analgesics are given.

Remove the stone: It is thought that increasing fluids either orally or intravenously can help to push stones out, but some doctors feel this is dangerous as it may cause an obstruction. Extracorporeal shockwave lithotripsy, or ESWL, (in which sound waves are used to break up stones) is a common method of stone ablation. Percutaneous nephrolithotomy, a procedure done under sedation or anesthesia to remove stone fragments, is performed if stones are too big to be removed by ESWL, or if ESWL fails. The procedure does require a short hospital stay. Ureteroscopy is another procedure that can be performed to remove stones.

Modify your lifestyle: Depending on what kind of kidney stone develops (different stones are made up of different minerals), general lifestyle modifications can be taken to prevent recurrence. In general, drinking 2 liters of water a day helps to keep the dilution and flow of urine at a level that discourages stone development. A high fiber diet is also recommended. Avoid carbonated beverages that contain phosphates as these have been associated with the development of stones. Grapefruit juice should also be avoided as it has been linked to the formation of kidney stones in some studies. Avoiding calcium is generally thought to be unhelpful, and some doctors even advocate calcium supplementation as a preventive measure. Generally, avoiding a high-protein diet, particularly animal protein, is wise. It is recommended that you also avoid too much salt and fat in the diet, alcohol, and foods that are high in oxalate, such as beets, black tea, chocolate, figs, pepper, lamb, parsley, poppy seeds, spinach, soy, and Swiss chard. Oxalate combines with calcium to form a salt that causes kidney stones.

Supplements: Taking magnesium (as a salt of aspartate, which does not cause diarrhea) helps inhibit stone formation, as does taking 25–100 mg of vitamin B6 a day. There is some evidence that omega-3 fatty acids found in fish oil (taken at about 4 g a day) reduce oxalate stone formation. Since acidification of the urine is a problem in stone formation, a greens alkalinizing powder such as Xymogen® BioAlkalizer should be effective, although this has not been the subject of research.

Medication: Hydrochlorothiazide, chorthalidone, amiloride, cellulose sodium phosphate, allopurinol, potassium citrate, or calcium carbonate may be recommended for prevention.

Traditional Chinese Medicine

A combination of herbal medicine and acupuncture works best if the stone is smaller then ³⁄₈ inch in diameter and if the patient has normal kidney function. If the patient has kidney disease or kidney dysfunction, consult a doctor before treatment. If the stone is stuck in the wall of the kidney, or if the patient has a narrow urinary tract, other treatments, such as surgery, should be considered.

Herbs: To make a decoction, mix the herbs of one of the formulas below in a glass or ceramic pot. Add 3 cups of water, bring to the boil, and simmer for 30 minutes. Strain and drink 1 cup twice a day.

- **Formula one:** Mix 10 g of Jin Qian Cao (lysimachia), 12 g of Xia Ku Cao (common self-heal fruit-spike), 15 g of Hu Tao Ren (walnut), 10 g of Che Qian Zi (plantago seed), 12 g of Shi Wei (pyrrosia leaves), 12 g of Bian Xu (knotwood), and 12 g of Qu Mai (aerial parts and flower of Chinese pink dianthus).

- **Formula two:** Mix 10 g of Chen Xiang (aloeswood), 10 g of Mu Xiang (costus root), 12 g of Bin Long (betel nut), 12 g of Wang Bu Liu Xing (vaccaria seeds), 10 g of Tao Ren (peach kernel), 15 g of Niu Xi (achyranthes root), 12 g of Zao Jiao Ci (spine of Chinese honeylocust fruit), 12 g of Ru Xiang (frankincense), 12 g of Mo Yao (myrrh), and 12 g of Chuan Lian Zi (sichuan pagoda tree fruit).

- **Formula three:** Mix 10 g of Dan Shen (salvia root), 12 g of Huang Qi (milk-vetch root), 12 g of Hong Hua (safflower flower), 12 g of Gou Ji Zi (wolfberry), 10 g of Gui Zhi (cinnamon), 12 g of Jin Qian Cao (lysimachia), 12 g of Ze Xie (water plantain rhizome), and 15 g of Hua Shi (talcum).

Diet: Foods that are good for the kidneys are chives, duck, plums, star anise, tangerines, and egg yolks.

Naturopathy

Diet: Staying hydrated is important in the treatment and prevention of this condition. If you have kidney stones, make sure you drink plenty of water every day. A vegetarian diet may help prevent the formation of kidney stones in the first place, as research shows that vegetarians have a lower rate of developing condition. Follow a diet based on whole grains, fresh vegetables, and legumes. If you do eat meat, opt for lean cuts. Eat foods that are rich in magnesium such as barley, bran, corn, buckwheat, rye, oats, brown rice, potatoes, and bananas. Freshly squeezed lemon juice helps acidify the urine and eases the passage of calcium oxalate stones. Drink a 8 fl oz three times a day. Dilute it with a little water to minimize its tartness. Avoid naturally carbonated and mineral waters, as their calcium content can be high.

Supplements: Magnesium prevents the formation of calcium oxalate crystals. The citrate form may be most effective; take 400–500 mg of magnesium daily. Vitamin B6 is deficient in those with kidney stones, and also reduces calcium oxalate levels. Take 50 mg a day. Take 120 mg of IP-6 (inositol hexophosphate) a day as it also reduces calcium oxalate crystals in the urine. Vitamin A deficiency is considered a risk factor for kidney stone formation. Take 5,000 IU daily. Vitamin C supplementation should be kept below 2,000 mg a day. Vitamin C can potentially form oxalates, which make up kidney stones, in high amounts.

Herbs: Take 400 mg of a standardized cranberry extract twice a day; it has been shown to reduce urinary calcium in those with a history of kidney stones. Drinking aloe vera juice may also reduce urinary crystals. Uva ursi is traditionally used for urinary tract infections, and relieves pain and cleanses the urinary tract. Take 250–500 mg three times a day, but do not use this herb for more than two weeks. Drink 2–4 cups of juniper berry tea, a strong diuretic kidney cleanser, every day until the stones pass. Horsetail also has diuretic qualities. You can take 2 g a day of the capsule form or drink 2–3 cups of the tea a day.

Hydrotherapy: A hot sitz bath can help relieve pain. Drink lemon juice, tea, or water while sitting in the bath to speed up the elimination of stones.

> *Tip:* AVOID ANTACIDS
>
> Antacids that contain aluminum are known to contribute to kidney stone formation, especially if taken with milk.

Homeopathy

Since kidney stones tend to be a recurrent problem, they require professional medical treatment and homeopathic support. Treatment from a homeopath will aim to help at both preventive and acute levels (but not simultaneously) to relieve the situation. The long-term aim of homeopathic constitutional treatment (ideally in combination with dietary and nutritional guidance) is to discourage the body from producing kidney stones. Should an acute episode of pain occur, any of the remedies below can be used in a supplementary way to conventional pain relief. If removal of the stone or stones is needed by conventional means, your homeopath will also be able to prescribe to support a swift recovery.

Nux vomica: To ease spasmodic pain, especially that due to renal colic, which tends to be right-sided, radiating to the genitals and the leg, use Nux vomica. Pain and discomfort are more distressing and intense when lying on the back, and there are severe problems when trying to urinate.

Berberis: Use this remedy if there are smarting, burning pains that radiate in all directions and are sharp enough to make the patient hold their breath. There is a burning sensation in the urethra, especially between attempts to urinate. Jarring movement and getting up from a sitting position increase the pain.

Cantharis: This remedy has a reputation for easing pain and inflammation that affects the kidneys and bladder. It is useful when pains come on quickly and violently, causing unbearable cutting, burning sensations around the kidneys and bladder. Applying pressure to the glans of the penis temporarily eases the pains of renal colic. Trying to urinate increases distress, while massaging and applying warmth to the painful area feel soothing.

Herbalism

The herbal approach to kidney stones is to prevent the formation of stones in the first place, as well as treating symptoms during the passage of a kidney stone. A full examination of the person's digestion and function of the gastrointestinal tract is also necessary, as abnormalities in uric acid and oxalates (common components of kidney stones) should be addressed. Herbal diuretics can help to increase the flow of urine through the kidneys and help to prevent the formation of kidney stones. Some herbal diuretics such as juniper, parsley, and lovage rely on their volatile oils for this effect. However, these cause a loss of water by irritating the kidney tissue, which, over time, can be damaging to the kidney or aggravate pre-existing kidney disease. These herbs should be used carefully, under the guidance of a herbal expert.

Goldenrod: This herbal diuretic may help facilitate the elimination of kidney stones, probably due to its flavonoid and saponin compounds. Make a decoction by placing 3–5 g of the above-ground parts of the plant in 1 cup of boiling water. Let the herb steep for a few minutes, strain, and drink the liquid several times a day as necessary for acute urinary pain, or once or twice daily as a preventive measure.

Stone root: Known for its antilithic properties, this herb is often used in helping to break up urinary- and gallstones, and gravel. It may be used as a preventative, but is often of great use when an aid is needed to help pass stones and gravel. This is most often taken as a root decoction, or tincture.

Pain relief: An infusion or tincture of Hydrangea arborescens root can calm the urinary system and help with pain. A tincture of cramp bark can ease pain by acting as an antispasmodic on the urinary tract muscles. Couch grass rhizome is used in tincture form and is also calming, but it is more of a coating, or demulcent, herb for the urinary system, and has a mild diuretic effect.

5

Respiratory System
and
Circulation

Flu

Diagnosis

The influenza virus is a highly contagious respiratory infection. There are usually several outbreaks of different flu strains every winter. Once you have been infected by a particular strain of flu you become immune to it. Flu shots are designed to fight the flu bug that is prevalent in a particular year, so immunization is necessary on an annual basis. Influenza is spread through sneezing and coughing, when water droplets carrying the virus become airborne and are breathed in by others. It is also passed on through the spread of germs due to poor hand-washing hygiene. Symptoms, which include fever, chills, headache, aches and pains, and exhaustion, begin after an incubation period of one to four days and usually continue for about a week.

DANGER: Occasionally, pneumonia can develop from a bad attack of flu. Infants, the elderly, and people with heart or lung disease are more prone to complications.

Symptoms

- An elevated temperature (above 98.6°F)
- Fever and chills
- Sweating
- A flushed face
- Headache
- Loss of appetite
- Muscular aches and pains
- Weakness
- Feeling lethargic and tired
- Sore throat
- Cough
- Feeling under the weather and rundown

Treatment Goal

It is usually possible to treat flu at home. Stay in bed and get as much rest as possible. A bad attack of flu can last for up to two weeks. It is not unusual to feel extreme fatigue for a couple of weeks afterwards. Both conventional and complementary therapies aim to relieve symptoms and encourage recovery as quickly as possible.

Conventional Medicine

Flu shot: It is possible to protect against infection by getting the flu vaccine. However, the vaccine does not protect against every strain of flu. It is recommended for the elderly, debilitated, immune compromised (people who have illnesses that affect their immune systems), asthmatics, and chemotherapy patients. Good hand washing is probably the best preventive measure against spreading flu germs.

Herbs: Some herbs with natural viral suppression properties can be taken during the flu season. One that has had some success is larch (found in a Thorne product called Larix®). Elderberry extract can be used in the same way. These herbs can also be used at the onset of flu symptoms.

Tamiflu®: Upon exposure to flu, high-risk patients (the elderly, debilitated, immune compromised, asthmatics, and chemotherapy patients) are encouraged to take the drug Tamiflu® within the first 72 hours. It can sometimes lessen the severity and duration of symptoms if taken on the day of exposure.

Rest and fluids: Treating an active case of flu involves taking rest, plenty of fluids, and non-steroidal anti-inflammatory drugs for aches and pains are advisable.

When should I see a doctor? Complications include dehydration and electrolyte imbalance, pneumonia, and problems related to immobility. If a patient is unable to take oral fluids, is disoriented, has a fever of over 102°F (or 103°F in a child), and does not respond to conventional treatment, seek medical attention.

Traditional Chinese Medicine

Herbs: Combine 10 g of Jin Yin Hua (honeysuckle flower), 12 g of Lian Qiao (forsythia fruit), 12 g of Ban Lan Gen (isatis root), 10 g of Da Qin Ye (woad leaf), and 3 g of Gan Cao (licorice root) in a ceramic or glass pot. Add 3 cups of water, bring the mixture to a boil, and simmer for 30 minutes. Strain and drink 1 cup two to three times a day for three to five days.

Acupressure: The Feng Chi points are at the back of the head at the base of the skull, about 2 inches on either side of the center point. The Hegu point is located on the back of the hand in the depression between the thumb and the first finger. Press with medium pressure for one to two minutes. Repeat five times twice a day.

Diet: Eat light food with seasoning such as ginger, garlic, onions, olives, and daikon radishes. These foods are good for helping recovery.

Naturopathy

Diet: Eat light foods such as soups, steamed vegetables, and broths. Add ginger, garlic, and onions to your soup for their antimicrobial and anti-inflammatory effects. If you do not have an appetite, do not eat, but make sure you stay hydrated with water and herbal teas. Try to eat some berries and citrus fruit. These contain bioflavonoids and vitamin C, which help stimulate the immune system. Eliminate foods that weaken your immune system and cause mucus, including dairy products, and any foods to which you are allergic. Caffeine depletes zinc, an important mineral for healing, so avoid black tea, coffee, and chocolate.

Supplements: Vitamin C increases white blood cell activity and supports immune function. Vitamin A with beta-carotene has powerful immune-boosting and antioxidant effects. Take 15,000 IU of each vitamin a day. Pregnant women should not take more than 10,000 IU of vitamin A a day. Zinc gluconate lozenges act as immune stimulants. Dissolve a single lozenge in a glass of water and drink every two hours.

Herbs: Elderberry prevents the influenza virus from replicating. Adults should take 1 tbsp four times a day and children should take 1 tbsp twice a day. Lomatium dissectum has strong antiviral activity and is traditionally used by herbalists for flu. Take 500 mg in capsule form or 4 ml four times a day. A combination of echinacea and goldenseal can be taken at 500 mg or 2 ml to enhance immune function and dry up mucus. Take 500 mg of oregano oil four times daily or 300–450 mg of garlic twice a day for their powerful antiviral effects. Andrographis, taken at 400 mg three times a day, can be used to prevent flu.

Homeopathy

Any of the following homeopathic remedies can support the body through a bout of flu, reducing distress and discomfort, and shortening the duration of symptoms. A well-chosen homeopathic remedy may also reduce the possibility of complications setting in.

Baptisia: If a profound sense of exhaustion is combined with restlessness, try Baptisia. The muscles generally feel very sore and heavy. The throat is also sore and it is very difficult to swallow solids due to pain and inflammation.

Gelsemium: This remedy can ease classic flu symptoms that develop slowly over two or three days. Symptoms include an overwhelming sense of listlessness, droopiness, and heaviness, accompanied by aching muscles, and shivering. The eyes have a droopy, glassy look, the face is likely to be flushed, and lips may be cracked and dry. Sufferers tend to want to be left alone in peace and quiet to rest.

Eupatorium perfoliatum: Use this remedy to treat severe flu symptoms that manifest as aching deep in the bones and a bruised, tender sensation in the muscles. Symptoms include feeling chilly, weak, and restless, with aching in the arms, legs, back, and torso. This remedy can also help treat nausea and lethargy.

Mercurius: To ease the later stages of a bout of flu when the initial feverish stage has passed, use Mercurius.

Herbalism

Elderberry: The fruit of this plant can be used to treat flu. Studies have shown elderberry to reduce the duration of flu symptoms. To make a syrup, speak with a herbalist for the best preparation methods. Specific formulations of elderberry juice can be bought at your local health food store—raw elderberry juice can be quite toxic and is not recommended. Take the formulated juice orally at the onset of symptoms for three to five days. Diarrhea and vomiting have been reported with use of elderberry juice, although this side effect is greatly decreased with specific formulations.

Echinacea: This is a popular and effective immune modulator. It has been demonstrated that echinacea may work better if taken as soon as the symptoms of colds and flu develop. It is often used in respiratory infections, and helps to eliminate and reduce duration of symptoms. The roots are most commonly used, although research shows that the aerial parts are effective, too.

Astragalus: This herb is well known for its immune-stimulating effects and is often used for its antibacterial and antiviral properties. Astragalus root can be used as a decoction, or taken in capsule form. It may be incompatible with immunosuppressive drugs and advice should be sought from a herbal practitioner before using if on medication.

Fever and Chills

Diagnosis

A fever occurs when the core body temperature rises above the normal range (an oral reading of 98.6–100°F). A fever generally accompanies infectious ailments and acts as the body's mechanism for fighting infection. Occasionally, a fever can develop as a result of other conditions such as gastroenteritis, heatstroke, and dehydration, and more rarely as a result of more serious conditions such as meningitis.

As your core temperature rises, your extremities begin to feel cold and send out a signal to the muscles. The muscles begin to shake involuntarily, a condition known as chills. Chills in turn create body heat, which raises a fever. Your body effectively "cooks" the bacteria by generating high temperatures.

DANGER: If a fever is accompanied by lethargy, a rash of purple spots, or persists for more than 48 hours, call your doctor as a matter or urgency.

Symptoms

- Flushed face
- Hot forehead
- Alternating feeling of being burning hot then freezing cold
- Trembling sensation, or involuntary shaking
- General feeling of being unwell

Treatment Goal

To establish the cause of the fever and treat it accordingly. Treatment also aims to bring down the fever and alleviate any discomfort.

Conventional Medicine

The appropriate treatment of a fever is dependent on the causes, the most common of which tend to be dehydration, infection, and hyperthyroidism. It is important to treat the underlying problem rather than just the fever. In general, a fever of under 103°F in a child and under 102°F in an adult can usually be treated at home unless other symptoms are present. A very high fever can be a sign of a serious problem and requires professional medical help.

NSAIDs: To treat a fever associated with a viral infection, treatment usually involves non-steroidal anti-inflammatory drugs (NSAIDs).

Tip: DRINK WATER

Make it a priority to increase your fluid intake when you have a fever. Your thirst reflex does not always provide an accurate guide regarding the amount of liquid that your body requires, so drink a moderate amount of water even if you do not feel thirsty. Drink plain water, and avoid coffee, which has diuretic properties that encourage the body to eliminate rather than conserve fluid.

Ibuprofen is the primary choice for both children and adults. Adults can take up to 800 mg every six hours. Children above two years old can be given 7.5–10 mg per 2.2 lb of body weight every six hours, but no more than three times a day—this should not exceed the adult dosage. NSAIDs should not be taken by anyone with a peptic ulcer, as they may cause gastric irritation or bleeding. Acetaminophen is another treatment option, but do not take this drug if you have liver disease or if you drink alcohol regularly. Aspirin can also lower a fever, but again, the potential for gastric irritation is high in susceptible individuals. Aspirin should not be given to anyone under 16 years of age.

Keep cool: Drink cool beverages to relieve any symptoms of dehydration that may occur with a fever. Dehydration may be the cause of the fever, and rehydrating may resolve it. Cool baths are also effective, as are rubbing alcohol and witch hazel massages. Cooling blankets, which are available in First Aid Facilities, can be used if there is no response to the above methods. Intravenous rehydration can also be carried out.

Traditional Chinese Medicine

Herbs: The following decoction can be used to treat fever and chills that occur simultaneously. Combine 10 g of Gui Zhi (cinnamon), 12 g of Bai Shao (white peony root), 8 g of Huang Qin (baical skullcap root), 10 g of Chai Hu (hare's ear root), 8 g of Jing Jie (schizonepeta stem and bud), 3 pieces of Da Zhao (Chinese jujube), 5 g of Gan Cao (licorice root), and 5 g of fresh ginger root. Place the herbs in a ceramic pot and add 3 cups of water. Bring the mixture to a boil and simmer for 30 minutes. Strain and drink 1 cup two or three times a day. This decoction will help reduce the symptoms and speed up recovery.

Diet: Make a tea using a 1 oz of ginger chopped into small chips. Place the ginger in a bowl and add boiling water. Cover for 5–10 minutes, then add 1 oz of brown sugar, and stir well. Drink the tea while it is hot. You can also try eating a porridge made from 1/3 cup of rice and five to six Chinese jujubes. Place the ingredients in a pot and add 3 cups of water. Bring them to a boil and cook until the rice is soft. Add a chopped green onion. The porridge should have a creamy consistency.

Naturopathy

Diet: Eat a diet based on broths, soups, and teas. Avoid solid foods if there is no appetite for them. Add ginger, garlic, and onions to soups and broths to boost your immunity and help the respiratory tract heal. Avoid sugar, processed foods, dairy, and junk foods, which suppress your immune system. Stay hydrated by sipping on water or tea throughout the day. This will also expel toxins and keep the respiratory tract from drying out.

Supplements: Take 500 mg of vitamin C several times a day to support the immune system and help healing. If your stools become loose cut back the vitamin C by taking a dose every two hours. Also take 250–500 mg of bioflavonoids a day to stimulate the immune system.

Herbs: Take 900 mg of echinacea a day in capsule form, or 2–4 ml of tincture four times a day, to stimulate the immune system. Taking 5–10 ml of elderberry tincture three times a day is helpful in fighting viral infections, which may be causing the fever. Yarrow induces sweat to help break a fever. Take 300 mg in capsule form, 2 ml of tincture, or 1 cup of fresh tea four times a day. Taking 500 mg or 2 ml of ginger can also help to break a fever and reduce inflammation. You can also drink ginger tea throughout the day. Oregano oil, taken at 500 mg three times a day, has antiviral effects. Garlic, at a dosage of 300–500 mg three times a day, combats infection and supports the immune system.

Hydrotherapy: Sit on a chair and place your feet in a bucket of warm water for 15 minutes. Dry them and put on a pair of cotton socks that have been soaked in cold water and wrung out. Cover the cotton socks with a pair of wool socks and leave on overnight. This measure diverts blood flow to the feet and away from the upper body, thus reducing fever.

Tip: CHILD'S HERBAL TEA

Brew a fever-reducing herbal tea using equal parts of lemon balm leaf, chamomile flower, peppermint leaf, licorice root, and elderflower. These herbs promote perspiration, calm and relax the nervous system, and cool fever. Give a child over two years old ½ cup four times a day. A breastfeeding mother can drink 1 cup four times a day.

Homeopathy

For homeopathic home prescribing to be most effective, combine with additional holistic measures that can help bring down a fever.

Aconite: Use this remedy to treat a fever that develops after exposure to dry, cold winds. The patient feels fine on going to bed, but wakes from sleep feeling panicky and restless with an accompanying fever. Symptoms emerge dramatically and abruptly, and include a burning, hot head and chilled, shivery body.

Belladonna: This remedy is also appropriate for symptoms that develop violently and dramatically. Feeling irritable and having a short temper are key symptoms that call for Belladonna. Additional symptoms include hot, dry, bright red skin that radiates heat.

Arsenicum album: To treat a fever that peaks in the early hours of the morning and causes a significant amount of anxiety and restlessness, try Arsenicum album. Despite having a fever, there is a persistent sense of feeling chilled to the bone. A sufferer feels most comfortable if the body is kept warm, and the head is exposed to fresh air.

Pulsatilla: Consider this remedy to treat a fever that has been triggered by exposure to cold and wet conditions. Warm rooms make feverishness intolerable, while contact with fresh cool air feels soothing.

Herbalism

It is generally not advised to aim to lower a slightly raised temperature too soon, as this is the body responding to fight off an infection; but it is important to be aware of age-appropriate temperature ranges, and to watch out for other symptoms.

Tip: AVOID EATING

The exertion involved in digesting food can cause the body temperature to rise even further. Therefore, try to avoid eating when a high temperature is present.

Peppermint: This is a cooling herb, often used in treating a fever. It is often used alongside yarrow and elderflower for fever. For younger people, catnip is often a preferred choice over peppermint. Peppermint is very readily available, and can be obtained from health stores. Some also use the fresh leaves in herbal tea infusions.

Boneset: This popular herb is effective in reducing fever. Dosage recommendations are to infuse 2 tsp of dried herb in 1 cup of boiling water, and drink 1 cup every hour while fever is high. There is a chance of nausea and vomiting if too much is consumed.

Yarrow: This plant is a diaphoretic herb that combines well with peppermint and elderflower for fevers. It is often available in tincture and dried herb form. As a tea, 2 tsp per cup of boiling water can be used; drink a cup of this infusion three times a day. A lesser amount is often used of each herb if used in combination.

Asthma

Diagnosis

Asthma is an inflammatory condition that affects the airways. When the tubes (the bronchioles) that carry air to the lungs are irritated, they become swollen and obstruct the flow of air, filling up with sticky mucus in the process. This causes wheezing and breathing problems. Asthmatics tend to be sensitive to various types of irritants in the atmosphere that can trigger a contraction in the airways. Common irritants include pet fur, feathers, hair, dander, saliva, house dust mites, perfumes and other fragranced products, environmental pollutants, cigarette smoke, and cold and foggy atmospheres, plus exercise, stress, and anxiety. There is also a genetic predisposition to the condition.

DANGER: A severe asthma attack that makes breathing extremely difficult is a frightening experience. Other symptoms such as rapid heartbeat may also develop. If a severe asthma attack occurs, seek immediate medical help.

Symptoms

- Wheezing
- A dry, irritating, persistent cough
- Night-time cough
- Breathlessness
- Persistent coughs and colds
- Gasping when breathing in
- Pains and feelings of tightness in the chest
- Morning cough

Treatment Goal

Treatment aims to control symptoms. Asthma is a condition that requires conventional medication. Complementary therapies can help to ease symptoms as part of an integrated approach.

Conventional Medicine

Status asthmaticus is severe unremitting asthma that does not respond to treatment. It is a major medical emergency and immediate help must be sought from a hospital emergency room, where oxygen, breathing treatments, and intravenous medication can be administered.

Make lifestyle changes: It is important to identify and avoid any triggers of asthma attacks, and make lifestyle changes when necessary. Excluding dairy from the diet may be helpful. Keep the child's surroundings as clear of dust as possible and practice stress-reduction techniques such as deep breathing and meditation.

Medication: The type of medication used to treat asthma in children above five years old varies according to the severity of the condition.

A short-acting inhaler (belonging to a class of drugs called beta agonists) can be used as needed for immediate, short-term relief from a wheezing episode. This is usually sufficient for cases of asthma where attacks are infrequent. For mild but persistent asthma, a low-dose inhaler of corticosteroid is used. Other classes of medication can be used as well, such as cromolyn sodium, montelukast, ipratropium, and theophylline. For severe asthma, combinations of these medications are used. A steroid such as prednisolone may need to be taken for a short period of time.

Traditional Chinese Medicine

TCM treatment for acute and chronic cases of asthma includes strengthening the Qi of the lungs and spleen, tonifying the kidneys and lungs, and complementing conventional medication. Herbal decoctions and pills are not a replacement for inhalers or other medication, which must be used as recommended by your doctor. However, you can consult a doctor about the possibility of reducing your medication by utilizing herbal remedies.

Herbs: Place the herbs from any of the formulas in a ceramic pot. Add 3 cups of water, bring to a boil, and simmer for 30 minutes.
• To strengthen the lungs and spleen Qi: Symptoms include fatigue, frequent cough with white or clear phlegm, or loose stools and distention in the abdomen. Combine 10 g of ginseng, 12 g of Bai Zhu (white atractylodes rhizome), 15 g of Fuling (poria), 12 g of Huang Qi (milk-vetch root), 12 g of Wu Wei Zi

(schisandra fruit), 12 g of San Bai Pi (mulberry root bark), 6 g of Chen Pi (tangerine peel), 12 g of Fa Ban Xia (pinellia rhizome), and 5 g of Gan Cao (licorice root). Drink 1 cup twice a day for three to six months.

• To tonify the kidneys and lungs: Symptoms include shortness of breath at the slightest movement and difficulty inhaling. Combine 12 g of Wu Wei Zi (schisandra fruit), 15 g of Shan Yao (Chinese yam), 12 g of Tu Si Zi (Chinese dodder seed), 15 g of Fuling (poria),

12 g of Shu Di Huang (cooked Chinese foxglove), 12 g of Shan Zhu Yu (Asiatic cornelian cherry), and 8 g of Rui Gui Zhi (inner bark of Saigon cinnamon). Drink 1 cup three times a day for three months.

• Patent herbal pills: Ding Chuang Wan or Zhi Shu Ding Chuan Wan can be taken to complement conventional medication. Take as directed on the label or consult a TCM practitioner.

Naturopathy

Diet: Eat a simple diet that includes lightly steamed vegetables, fresh fruit, whole grains, lean poultry and fish (fish consumption in children has been shown to decrease the risk of developing asthma). Eliminate dairy products and foods made from white flour from your diet, as they cause mucus to form. Sprinkle ground flaxseeds on salads and cereals to obtain some of the omega-3 fatty acids that help reduce inflammation. Drink water regularly throughout the day to flush out mucus from your body.

Supplements: Take 4–8 g of fish oils a day for their anti-inflammatory components. Magnesium has been shown to relax the bronchial tubes and improve lung function. Take 250 mg three times a day, but reduce it if the stools become loose. Take 1,000 mg of Vitamin C two to four times a day for its anti-allergen benefits, but again cut back if stools loosen. Vitamin B12 reduces asthma symptoms in some people and can be taken at 1,500 mcg orally or 400 mcg sub-lingually (under the tongue). N-acetylcysteine (NAC) is been used with some success in those with respiratory conditions, including asthma. Take 500 mg two to three times a day.

Herbs: Take 500–1,000 mg of astragalus twice a day to strengthen the lungs and to prevent respiratory infections. Lycopene, taken at

> *Tip:* SIP A WARM DRINK
>
> When a mild episode of asthma has been triggered by exposure to cold winds, rest in a comfortably warm room and sip a hot drink to encourage the airways to relax.

10 mg three times a day, can help with exercise-induced asthma. Also take 1,000 mg of quercetin three times a day for its anti-inflammatory benefits. Other herbs act as antihistamines (histamines are substances released in the body that produce swelling and constrict bronchial passages) to open air passages and relieve wheezing. These herbs include anise, ginger, peppermint, and chamomile. Studies show that chamomile may slow allergic reactions, such as those that trigger asthma attacks, by increasing the production of cortisone in the adrenal glands, which reduces lung inflammation and makes breathing easier. Make a tea using some or all of these herbs to help with asthma.

Homeopathy

Asthma is unlikely to be adequately managed by home prescribing. The homeopathic remedies suggested below can help ease mild, acute asthma symptoms, but should not be used as long-term remedies. Treatment from a homeopathic practitioner can be very beneficial.

Kali carb: If asthma symptoms are aggravated by movement, or by exposure to very cold or hot conditions, try Kali carb. There is likely to be an unpleasant sour taste in the mouth, and a cold sensation in the chest during coughing episodes. Coughing spasms are frequent in an effort to raise mucus that seems determined to stay in the chest. Symptoms tend to be more severe around 2–4 a.m.

Aconite: This remedy is helpful if wheezy symptoms are brought on by exposure to very dry, cold winds. Sufferers may go to bed feeling fine, but wake from a short sleep feeling terrified and short of breath. Coughing spasms are likely to sound hoarse and dry, and there may be a hot sensation in the lungs, followed by a tingling sensation once the coughing spasm is over. Symptoms are also often brought on by shock or fright when feeling panicky, terror-stricken, and restless.

Arsenicum album: If symptoms tend to get worse around 12–2 a.m., Arsenicum album may be suitable. Symptoms include anxiety coupled with a sense of restlessness. Sufferers may feel chilled, but although warmth is desirable, the head and face feel better for contact with cool, fresh air. Bouts of coughing and wheezing may be triggered by smoky atmospheres, or strong perfume.

Herbalism

Ephedra: A herb that is prescribed by qualified herbal practitioners, which is very useful for those with asthma. It is a great bronchodilator, and helps to relieve bronchospasm by relaxing the airways. This herb is also particularly useful in those with asthma triggered by allergies, due to its antihistamine properties. Speak with your herbal practitioner before using. It shouldn't be used by those with cardiovascular problems, or an enlarged prostate, diabetes, glaucoma, or a number of other conditions.

Tip: STAY RELAXED

If you begin wheezing when lying down, sit up to allow the chest to naturally expand. However difficult, try to relax your chest as much as you can. The muscles in the chest instinctively tense and tighten in response to feelings of anxiety and panic, making it harder to breathe.

Licorice: This herb has many properties useful in helping with asthma. It has demulcent properties that help to soothe, coat, and protect the mucous membranes. It is antispasmodic, so helps to relax the airways. It is also a useful expectorant, which is beneficial if the asthma is triggered by allergies and mucous is forming. It also has anti-inflammatory properties. Licorice is not recommended for those with high blood pressure, but short-term use may be suitable. Speak with your qualified herbal practitioner if you have other health complaints, or use medication .

Boswellia: The breathing difficulties associated with asthma are due to overactive muscles that line our airways, the excessive production of mucus, and long-term inflammation of the airways. Current research shows that boswellia contains certain chemical compounds that protect against inflammation, making this herb very useful in the treatment of chronic asthma. It is important to note that the extracts used were of the resin, which is believed to contain the active components; they did not contain raw plant material. Boswellia should not be taken at the same time as certain prescription asthma medication, and your herbal expert will be able to advise you.

Croup

Diagnosis

Croup is a condition that inflames the airways, resulting in a barking cough and difficulty breathing. It generally affects children under five years old. As a child ages, the chances of developing croup decrease, and symptoms become less severe in those that have the complaint. Some children are prone to the condition, and it is thought that allergies may trigger recurrent bouts of croup. Croup tends to develop quickly and is usually caused by a viral infection in the upper airways. In most cases, it clears up on its own in a couple of days. However, the coughing and breathing problems that croup causes may last for some time longer. Very rarely, croup is a sign of a much more serious illness, such as diphtheria. The croup virus can be transferred through airborne water droplets by coughing and sneezing, or is passed on by physical contact. In serious cases, children may be admitted to hospital.

Symptoms

- Cold symptoms
- Characteristic deep, barking cough
- Hoarseness and noisy breathing
- Occasionally, voice loss
- Fever and raised temperature
- Symptoms are worse at night and after naps

Treatment Goal

Croup is a viral infection and cannot be treated with antibiotics. It can generally be treated at home through conventional or alternative therapies to relieve symptoms and prevent recurrence.

Conventional Medicine

The medical name for this viral illness is laryngotracheobronchitis. The treatment focuses on protecting the breathing passages.

Comfort the child: Most acute cases of croup can be managed at home through rest, hydration, and a light diet.

Steam inhalation: Immediate relief may be achieved with hot steam by, for example, standing close to a hot shower, with parental supervision, and inhaling deeply. Releasing cool mist into the room via a humidifier is also suggested.

When to see a doctor: If the condition does not improve within a few days, or if the child is obviously struggling to breath (i.e., you can see the muscles in between the ribs being used, or the muscles around the neck protruding with the tissue in between sinking in), take the child to the emergency room, where oxygen will be administered. Another danger sign is a breathing sound called stridor (like a wheezing, whistling noise), which is a sign of progressive closure of the airway, requiring emergency evaluation. Another treatment is epinephrine which can be released into the airways in a mist every 20 minutes to relax the muscles in the airways. Steroids (usually prednisone) are given intravenously or by mouth.

Traditional Chinese Medicine

Herbs: Combine 6 g of Huang Qin (scutellaria root), 8 g of Lian Qiao (forsythia fruit), 6 g of Jin Yin Hua (honeysuckle flower), 8 g of Zhi Zi (cape jasmine fruit), 6 g of Gan Cao (licorice root), 8 g of Xin Ren (apricot kernel), 3 g of Ma Huang (ephedra stem), and 5 g of Bo He (field mint) in a glass or ceramic pot. Add 3 cups of water, bring to a boil, and simmer for 30 minutes. Strain the liquid and give your child 1 cup twice a day.

Acupressure: Press the Tian Tu point, found along the central line of the throat at the depression in the collarbone. Also press the Fei Shu points on the back, which are 3–4 inches below the neck at the third thoracic vertebra, 1½ inches to either side of the spinal cord. The Ding Chuan points are on the center of the back at the base of the neck, ½ inch to either side. Seat the patient and use your fingertip to apply gentle pressure to these points for one to two minutes and repeat three times twice a day. See a doctor to monitor your child's condition.

Diet: Eat daikon radishes and food that is heat cleaning, such as watermelon, mung beans, purslane, peppermint, apples, wheat and wheat bran, mandarins, eggplant, spinach, button mushrooms, and cucumber.

Naturopathy

Diet: Encourage the child to drink plenty of fluids to thin the mucus and make it easier to cough. To ease coughing spasms, encourage the child to drink either warm soups and drinks or cold beverages, depending on what makes them feel better. Avoid dairy products as these can thicken and increase mucus.

Herbs: Prepare a tea using equal parts of marshmallow root (to soothe an irritated throat), mullein (to promote expectoration), osha root (to help clear the lungs), and licorice (for its antiviral and anti-inflammatory properties and to sweeten). Feed your child 3 tbsp three times a day, or mix it with juice.

Homeopathy

Any of the following homeopathic remedies can be used to relieve the symptoms of a mild, acute bout of croup. Should your child experience very severe and recurrent symptoms, this is a situation that will benefit from evaluation and treatment by an experienced homeopathic practitioner. They will aim to strengthen your child's system so that the episodes of croup become less frequent and less severe until they have phased themselves out.

Aconite: To treat croup symptoms that develop after your child has been out in dry, cold winds, or has had an upsetting or traumatic experience, use Aconite. The child may go to bed seeming fine, but wake abruptly from sleep in a state of panic, anxiety, and distress. There

is likely to be a dry, hoarse cough that triggers feelings of fear and tension, making breathing even more difficult.

Spongia: If coughs are harsh and rasping, and feel most distressful when talking or inhaling, or when feeling excited, consider using Spongia. Symptoms tend to come on just as the child is falling asleep.

Drosera: Try this remedy if croup symptoms develop or get more intense after midnight, and when a croupy cough comes on immediately after lying down. The child may be extremely hoarse, and coughing takes so much effort that the child must hold his or her sides and may retch or vomit. Stooping aggravates symptoms, while contact with fresh air may help.

Herbalism

There is no suitable herbal remedy for this condition.

Bronchitis

Diagnosis

Bronchitis is caused when a chest infection leads to the inflammation and swelling of the airways that connect to the lungs. It is a common disease among smokers and residents of polluted cities, and can be aggravated by cold, damp weather conditions, especially fog. Like many disorders, bronchitis can be acute (short term) or chronic (long term, when symptoms persist and recur at regular intervals). Acute bronchitis usually lasts around 10 days. Most often it accompanies or closely follows a cold or flu, and is contagious. Chronic bronchitis is more severe, and recovery is even harder for those with additional severe illnesses. Pulmonary hypertension and chronic respiratory failure are possible complications of chronic bronchitis.

DANGER: If you start coughing up mucus tinged with blood, see a doctor. It could indicate a more serious condition such as pneumonia, tuberculosis, or lung cancer.

Symptoms

- Flu symptoms in the upper respiratory tract
- A dry, hacking cough
- Pain and discomfort in the chest
- Chesty cough
- Copious phlegm
- Rapid breathing that is often accompanied by wheezing
- Fever
- Loss of appetite
- General lethargy
- Symptoms may be worse at night

Treatment Goal

To establish the cause of the bronchitis and treat it accordingly.

Conventional Medicine

To treat acute bronchitis: Treatment is dependent on several factors. In patients who do not smoke or have lung disease, bronchitis will usually resolve without medical therapy. Rest, fluids, and deep-breathing practices will help ease symptoms. High doses of vitamin C may also be helpful. Occasionally, coughing can interfere with sleep. In these cases, a non-sedating cough suppressant such as benzoate is effective. The cough should be allowed if it is tolerable as it helps to eliminate the virus. Inhalers such as albuterol are sometimes prescribed, but not generally in routine and uncomplicated cases.

To treat chronic bronchitis: When bronchitis occurs in smokers, or ex smokers with chronic lung disease, treatment involves taking antibiotics and using an inhaler. Ampicillin, cephalosporins, tetracylines, sulfonamides, and azithromycin are the antibiotics commonly used. These are prescribed, along with an inhaler that relaxes the lungs and eases breathing.

Preventive measures: To prevent bronchitis from recurring, identify and eliminate allergens from your diet and the immediate environment. Dairy is a food that is commonly associated with respiratory problems. If you are a smoker, attempt to stop.

Traditional Chinese Medicine

Herbs: For each formula, place the raw herbs in a glass or ceramic pot, add 3 cups of water, and bring the mixture to a boil. Simmer for 30 minutes, strain the liquid, and drink 1 cup twice a day.
• **To treat coughs with thick yellow or green mucus:** Mix 10 g of Huang Qin (baical skullcap root), 12 g of Xin Ren (apricot kernel), 6 g of Bo He (field mint), 15 g of Jie Geng (balloon flower root), 6 g of Chen Pi (tangerine peel), 12 g of Lian Qiao (forsythia fruit), and 6 g of Gan Cao (licorice root).
• **To treat coughs with clear mucus, and chronic bronchitis:** Combine 12 g of Shang Bai Pi (mulberry root bark), 10 g of Zi Su Ye (perilla leaf), 12 g of Jie Geng (balloon flower root), 15 g of Fuling (poria), 12 g of Bai Zhu (white

atractylodes rhizome), 10 g of ginseng, 10 g of Chai Hu (hare's ear root), and 6 g of Gan Cao (licorice root).

Acupressure: Press the Feng Chi and Da Zhui points for one minute at a time, using light to medium pressure. The Feng Chi points are at the back of the head at the base of the skull, 2 inches on either side of the center point. The Da Zhui point is on the spine in the depression below the seventh cervical vertebra (at the base of the neck).

Diet: Foods that promote lung health include carrots, button mushrooms, garlic, leeks, grapes, honey, pears, radishes, tangerines, and pumpkin. Foods that help dispel phlegm include apricots, fresh ginger, and lychee.

Naturopathy

Diet: Eat a simple diet of steamed vegetables, fresh fruit, whole grains, and lean poultry, and fish. Avoid mucus-forming foods such as dairy products. Instead eat chicken and vegetable soup with garlic, onions, and ginger to thin mucus, support the immune system, and for their anti-inflammatory effects. Sprinkle some ground flaxseeds on your food to obtain some of the omega-3 fatty acids that help ease inflammation. If you are taking antibiotics to resolve bronchitis, add kefir and sauerkraut to your diet to replenish the beneficial flora in your gut that may be lost. Drinking water at regular intervals throughout the day will also help to flush mucus from your body.

Supplements: N-acetylcysteine (NAC) thins phlegm and makes it easier to cough up mucus. Take 300–500 mg twice daily. Also take 1,000 mg of vitamin C two to four times a day for its anti-allergenic benefits and its ability to enhance the immune system. If loose stools develop, cut back the dose.

Herbs: Astragalus has been used to strengthen the lungs and to prevent respiratory infections. Taking 500–1,000 mg twice a day is an excellent treatment for acute and chronic bronchitis. Take an echinacea and goldenseal combination—500 mg in capsule form or 2 ml of tincture every day—to enhance immune function and dry up mucus. Mullein, taken at 500 mg in capsule form or 2 ml of tincture four times a day, promotes mucus discharge and soothes the respiratory system. Licorice can help to reduce coughing and also enhances the immune system. Take 500 mg in capsule form or 1 ml of tincture four times a day, but do not use licorice if you suffer from high blood pressure. It may also be helpful to take a formula that includes horehound, pleurisy root, plantain, marshmallow, and cherry bark, all of which have traditionally been used for bronchitis.

Aromatherapy: Add eucalyptus, peppermint, tea tree, and thyme essential oils to a bath or a steam inhalation to drain congestion.

Tip: STAY RESTED

Rest as much as possible during an acute attack of bronchitis, to provide the body with energy to fight the infection. Try to keep your body at a comfortable and stable temperature.

Homeopathy

Any of the following remedies may help ease symptoms and speed recovery from an acute attack of bronchitis. They can be used in a complementary way together with conventional treatment. A pattern of recurrent attacks of bronchitis that appear to be increasing in severity will be best dealt with by a homeopathic practitioner.

Ant tart: If bronchitis symptoms include rattling mucus in the chest, and coughing fits and shortness of breath that are eased when lying on the right side, try Ant tart. There is a need to sit upright to feel comfortable, and overheated rooms make discomfort more intense. Temporary relief is felt once mucus has been raised from the chest.

Ipecac: If coughing spasms are linked to an intense sensation of nausea, consider Ipecac. The effort of coughing causes the face to flush a purple-tinged color, and may result in retching and vomiting. Humidity and extreme temperature changes aggravate symptoms, while rest and exposure to cool air feels comforting.

Bryonia: This remedy can help to ease dry, irritating, tickly coughing spasms that come from the throat or top of the chest. Coughing leads to pain in the chest muscles, and is triggered or made worse by moving around. Eating and drinking can also trigger bouts of coughing.

Herbalism

Thyme: Thyme can be helpful in treating bronchitis. It can be taken as a tea, made from 1–2 g of dried herb and drunk two to three times a day. Thyme has been known to cause some mild gastrointestinal upset, and allergic reactions. Thyme is a useful antimicrobial, antispasmodic, and expectorant.

Chamomile: This herb contains two compounds, quercetin and apigenin, which may be anti-inflammatory and inhibit histamine release from mast cells, both of which could help to improve the symptoms of bronchitis. It is widely available in tea, tincture, pill, and capsule form.

Garlic: Garlic can be added to salads, soups, and other dishes to boost the immune system. Cooking garlic may destroy some of its medicinal qualities so try to eat it raw (chopped, pressed, or diced) whenever possible. Garlic is also widely available in pill or capsule form, which can be a more tolerable method of ingestion. Take 500 mg of capsule twice daily. When taken internally at high, therapeutic doses, garlic may interfere with certain anti-thrombotic drugs. 🌿

Cough

Diagnosis

Coughing is a reaction to an irritant, such as a respiratory infection, bacteria, or an allergen, that stimulates the production of mucus in the airways. As such, the coughing reflex is a vital part of the body's defense mechanisms. There are two types of cough: a dry, hard, tickly cough and a wet, rattling, productive cough that brings up phlegm. Most of the time a cough is nothing to worry about. A persistent night-time cough, however, can indicate a more serious problem, such as asthma, and it is important to seek medical advice if this is the case. Triggers and irritants include cold, damp weather conditions, especially fog, air pollution, and cigarette smoke.

DANGER: A cough that brings up blood or is accompanied by shortness of breath, or a long-term cough that refuses to resolve, requires medical attention.

Symptoms

- A dry, irritating cough
- A loose cough that rattles
- Coughing up phlegm that is green, white, or yellow, or foul smelling
- Chest pain
- Shortness of breath or wheezing
- Persistent night-time cough
- Fever and sweating
- Loss of appetite
- General lethargy

Treatment Goal

To alleviate symptoms while establishing the cause of the cough, and taking appropriate actions to resolve the underlying condition.

Conventional Medicine

Common causes of chronic cough are acid reflux (see p. 188), postnasal drip, and asthma (see p. 266). A chronic cough can also result as a side effect of a class of anti-hypertensive drugs called ACE inhibitors. A lung, bronchial, or sinus infection are the most common causes of a short-lived cough. Once the cause of the cough is determined, the underlying disease is treated.

Cough suppressants: A variety of medications, both narcotic and non-narcotic, exist to treat a cough that is a symptom of an acute upper respiratory tract infection, or to relieve cough symptoms while a diagnosis is being determined. Narcotic cough suppressants may be more effective but do have side effects. They are addictive, can cause constipation, and may interfere with natural sleeping patterns. Another prescription option is benzoanate, which numbs the cough reflex with minimal side effects. Dextromethorphan is a common over-the-counter preparation that can be effective.

Expectorants: Expectorants thin secretions so they can be coughed up more easily. They can be used in combination with cough suppressants for added relief.

Tip: WHEN TO TAKE COUGH SUPPRESSANTS

It is important to allow yourself to cough to expel the phlegm from your chest. This will allow the cough to resolve more quickly. Avoid taking cough suppressants until bedtime, when they can help you sleep undisturbed.

Traditional Chinese Medicine

Herbs: For either formula, place the raw herbs in a glass or ceramic pot and add 3 cups of water. Bring the mixture to a boil and simmer for 35 minutes. Strain and drink 1 cup twice a day.

• **Acute cough:** Mix 10 g of Huang Qin (baical skullcap root), 12 g of Xin Ren (apricot kernel), 6 g of Bo He (field mint), 15 g of Jie Geng (balloon flower root), 6 g of Chen Pi (tangerine peel), 12 g of Lian Qiao (forsythia fruit), and 6 g of Gan Cao (licorice root).

• **Chronic cough:** Combine 12 g of Sang Bai Pi (mulberry root bark), 10 g of Zi Su Ye (perilla leaf), 12 g of Jie Geng (balloon flower root), 15 g of Fuling (poria), 12 g of Bai Zhu (white atractylodes rhizome), 10 g of ginseng, 10 g of Chai Hu (hare's ear root), and 6 g of Gan Cao (licorice root).

Acupressure: While seated or lying on your stomach, have someone apply medium pressure to the Da Zhui and Fei Shu points for one to two minutes. The Da Zhui point is along the spine in the depression below the seventh cervical vertebra (at the base of neck). The Fei Shu points are also on the back, about 3–4 inches below the neck at the third thoracic vertebra, 1½ inches on either side of the spinal cord.

Diet: To treat a prolonged cough, boil 200 g of ginger juice and 200 g of honey in a pan. Dissolve 30 ml of this mixture in boiling water and drink it twice a day. A tea made from 6 g of licorice root, 30 g of honey, and 10 g of vinegar, boiled for 10 minutes, can also be soothing.

Naturopathy

Diet: Eat chicken soup made with onions, garlic, and ginger to help raise immunity, decrease inflammation, and dispel toxins. Hot barley soup also helps to reduce phlegm. Eliminate foods that increase mucus production such as dairy, sugar, junk food, and processed, refined foods. Drink a glass of water every hour to thin and dispel mucus.

Supplements: Take 500–1,000 mg of vitamin C three times a day to enhance the immune

system and for its anti-allergic benefit. N-acetylcysteine (NAC), taken at 300–500 mg twice a day can thin phlegm and make it easier to expectorate.

Herbs: Take 500 mg of licorice, or 1 ml in tincture form, to reduce coughing and enhance the immune system. However, do not use licorice if you suffer from high blood pressure. A combination of echinacea and goldenseal enhances immune function and dries up mucus. Take 500 mg in capsule form or 2 ml of tincture of this combination a day. Mullein, taken at 500 mg or 2 ml four times a day, promotes mucus discharge and soothes the respiratory system. Taking 500 mg of wild cherry bark, or 1 ml of tincture, three times a day can help reduce a wet cough. A herbal formula that includes horehound, pleurisy root, plantain, marshmallow, and cherry bark can also be helpful. Follow the instructions on the label.

Hydrotherapy: Let the hot water run in your shower for 20 minutes and then sit in the bathroom for 10–20 minutes. This will allow your body to expel toxins and thin mucus secretions. Add eucalyptus, peppermint, tea tree, and thyme oils to a bath or use them in a steam inhalation to ease congestion.

Homeopathy

The following remedies can help speed up recovery from an acute cough. For chronic coughs, it is best to seek the advice of a professional homeopathic practitioner.

Rumex: This remedy can be helpful in easing a cough that is set off by touching the throat. Bouts of coughing, choking, and retching are especially disturbing at night and trying to breathe deeply produces a raw, burning sensation in the chest. Any phlegm that is raised from the chest is likely to be thin and frothy.

Drosera: To ease bouts of coughing that begin as soon as you go to bed, and that begin with a maddening tickle or irritation, try Drosera. Coughing spasms may be severe enough to trigger a sweat or retching. Laughing and talking can aggravate the condition, or bring on a coughing spasm, while exposure to fresh air feels soothing.

Coccus cacti: If coughing spasms are triggered by exposure to hot, stuffy rooms, Coccus cacti can help. When this remedy is appropriate, sufferers swallow constantly in an effort to clear mucus from the throat. The mucus raised by a cough is likely to be stringy, clear, and rather sticky. Coughing spasms tend to be triggered by brushing the teeth or rinsing the mouth. Taking a stroll and sipping cool drinks give a temporary sense of relief.

Herbalism

A cough can be caused by a variety of underlying factors. Often, it is the body's attempt to clear the airways of an unwanted substance such as mucus that impedes the flow of air. Herbs that relieve congestion may improve a cough at the same time.

Licorice: A decoction of licorice root can be taken for a few days to alleviate coughs, especially a dry hacking cough that sometimes produces phlegm and that follows a postnasal drip. Licorice is a classic demulcent or mucilaginous herb, which coats the throat to stop the "tickle" from phlegm that triggers coughing. Boil 2 tbsp of chopped licorice root in 2–3 cups of water for 10 minutes and drink the decoction several times a day. As long as licorice is only consumed for a few days it is unlikely that the potential adverse effects this herb has on electrolytes and blood pressure will occur.

Eucalyptus oil: When this oil is inhaled it has a soothing and calming effect on the respiratory system, which can help alleviate a cough. Add a few drops of the oil to a vaporizer and breathe in, making sure your eyes are closed to protect against the irritating effects of the vapor. Do not swallow eucalyptus oil. Ingestion can cause severe side effects including depression of the central nervous system, nausea, and vomiting. Eucalyptus oil is not recommended for use in small children.

Lobelia: The flowers, as well as the rest of this plant, can be used to treat many respiratory conditions, from a simple cough to bronchitis.

Lobelia is thought to work by increasing airway diameter and promoting the secretion and expectoration of mucus. This herb is available on prescription from a qualified herbal medicine practitioner. Some adverse effects, such as nausea, dizziness, diarrhea, and tremors have been associated with lobelia. Do not take this herb if you have gastrointestinal problems, heart disorders, or are pregnant.

Thyme: This herb has been shown to be effective in treating coughs and congestion in studies. The recommended dose is 1 ml of tincture three times a day, but it can also be taken as a tea made from 1–2 g of dried herb two to three times a day. Thyme has been known to cause mild gastrointestinal upset and allergic reactions.

Elecampane: This herb that has been used for some time in traditional preparations as a decongestant. It has antibacterial effects and can serve as an expectorant and mucolytic (to break up mucus). Elecampane can be prepared as a cold infusion, using a small amount of dried shredded root. You can also take 1–2 ml of a tincture two to three times a day. Elecampane is generally considered safe with few reported side effects.

Pneumonia

Diagnosis

Pneumonia is an infection or inflammation of the lungs. It has a variety of causes, including infection by viruses, fungi, parasites, and bacteria. The streptococcus bacteria known as pneumococcus is the main cause of the most common type of pneumonia that occurs during the winter months. Although the majority of cases of pneumonia respond well to treatment, the infection can still be a very serious problem. The illness can range from mild to severe, and can even be life threatening in some cases.

The seriousness of the condition is often linked to the health of the patient at the time of infection. The elderly and less mobile, young children, diabetics, and those with heart disease and weakened immune systems are more prone to severe types of pneumonia. Occasionally, pneumonia develops after an infection of the throat, nose, ears, or sinuses and then spreads into the lungs. Those who are regularly exposed to cigarette smoke are more at risk as smoke injures the airways. Toxic fumes, industrial smoke, and other air pollutants may also damage lung function.

Symptoms

- Shivering fits, chills, fever, pains in the chest, and coughing
- Feeling ill, exhausted, and achy
- Coughing up yellow or brown phlegm, which is sometimes bloodstained
- Fast and shallow breathing
- Breathing and coughing is painful, with sharp pains in the chest
- Confusion (in the elderly)

Treatment Goal

It is important to determine the type of pneumonia you have in order to treat it in the best possible way. You should get plenty of rest and take plenty of fluids to help flush phlegm out of your system. If you are very unwell you may need to be hospitalized and given intravenous antibiotics.

Conventional Medicine

Treatment of pneumonia depends on whether the condition was caused by a virus or bacteria, and how the disease was caught. Generally, an x-ray is taken of the chest and lab tests are carried out to help determine whether pneumonia is present. Patients who are over 60, who smoke, who have cardiovascular conditions, pulmonary disease, immune suppression such as cancer, diabetes, HIV/AIDS, or who have had their spleen removed should receive the pneumococcal vaccine (Pneumovax®).

To treat bacterial pneumonia: A two-week course of antibiotics, usually Biaxin®, Levaquin®, or Zithromax®, to be taken orally, is prescribed to otherwise healthy patients. Smokers who suffer from pneumonia should give up cigarettes. Sicker patients are admitted to a hospital and given double the antibiotic treatment. Depending on the oxygen level in the blood, oxygen may also be administered. Hydration is also essential and intravenous hydration is sometimes needed.

To treat viral pneumonia: This type of condition requires bed rest and adequate hydration. Viral pneumonia related to flu can be vaccinated against. Amantadine and ribavirin are two medications that can be used to treat certain types of viral pneumonia, but treatment is generally supportive. Maintaining oxygen levels is the primary goal.

Traditional Chinese Medicine

Herbs: For each formula, combine the ingredients in a ceramic or glass pot and add 3 cups of water. Bring to a boil, simmer for 30 minutes, then strain. Drink 1 cup twice a day.
• **Acute pneumonia:** Mix 15 g of Yu Xing Cao (houttuynia), 12 g of Pu Gong Ying (dandelion), 10 g of Da Qin Ye (woad leaf), 12 g of Bai Jiang Cao (patrinia), and 15 g of Hu Zhang (bushy knotweed root and rhizome).
• **For loss of body fluid from perspiration:** In addition to the herbs above, mix 12 g of Zhu Ye (bamboo leaves), 12 g of Tian Hua Fen (trichosanthes root), and 12 g of Sang Bai Pi (mulberry root bark).
• **To treat patients with excess phlegm:** In addition to the herbs used in the first formula, mix 12 g of Gua Lou Ren (trichosanthes seed) and 12 g of Huang Qin (baical skullcap root).

Acupressure: Use the tip of your thumb to press the Hegu point, located on the back of the hand in the depression between the thumb and the first finger, with strong pressure for one to two minutes. Repeat on the opposite hand. While lying or sitting, have someone apply medium pressure using the tip of a finger to the Fei Shu points, found 3–4 inches below the back of the neck, 1½ inches on either side of the third thoracic vertebra. While seated, apply medium pressure to the Feng Long point, approximately halfway between the knee and the foot on the front of the lower leg, for one to two minutes.

Diet: Eat Daikon radishes and food that clears heat and phlegm, such as peppermint, wild chrysanthemum flowers, purslane, mung beans, red beans, bananas, and spinach.

> *Tip:* INTEGRATE THERAPIES
>
> Traditional Chinese medicine can be used in combination with conventional medicine to treat pneumonia.

Naturopathy

Diet: Eat small meals that consist of whole grains, fruits, fresh vegetables, and lean proteins frequently. Make sure you are drinking plenty of fluids to prevent dehydration and to thin secretions so that they are easier to cough up. Drink lots of soup, herbal tea, and water. Avoid dairy products, which can increase the production of mucus. Also avoid fats, refined sugars, and caffeine, all of which may depress your immune system.

Supplements: Take 15,000 IU of beta-carotene a day to protect the lungs from free radical damage (free radicals are elements that can be harmful to the cells of the body). Take 500 mg of N-acetylcysteine (NAC) two to three times a day; it is being used with some success for respiratory conditions. Vitamin C is an anti-inflammatory and helps stimulate the immune system. It can be beneficial to take 1,000 mg three to four times a day. Emulsified vitamin A, taken at 50,000 IU a day, can help repair immune function. Take 80 mg of zinc gluconate, which is needed for tissue repair and immune function, a day. Take 2–3 proteolytic enzyme capsules a day on an empty stomach to help reduce inflammation. Vitamin B complex, which can be taken at 100 mg three times a day, is important in the formation of red blood cells and antibodies. If your treatment requires an antibiotic, be sure to supplement probiotics such as acidophilus (3–10 billion units/daily) during the treatment and for at least two weeks afterward.

Homeopathy

The severity of this condition is dependent on the age and vitality of the patient. The suggestions below are appropriate for treating mild symptoms in those who are otherwise in good health. Patients should also seek a conventional medical opinion. Severe cases require prompt conventional medical assessment and treatment, but homeopathy can be helpful after the condition has cleared up. However, treatment is best given by an experienced homeopathic practitioner who will prescribe to strengthen the overall system.

Aconite: Consider this remedy if respiratory symptoms come on suddenly in response to exposure to dry, cold air. Coughing spasms sound harsh, and pains in the chest are shooting or burning, and feel much more distressing when not lying on the back. A high fever may also come on suddenly, where the head feels cool while the rest of the body is hot. Sufferers have a strong sense of anxiety and panic.

Phosphorus: If coughing bouts are much worse when first lying down, and there is yellow and possibly blood-streaked expectoration from the chest, try Phosphorus. The chest is likely to feel heavy and uncomfortable, with sharp pains in the left lung, or a narrow band of pain behind the breastbone. There is also a tendency to feel hot and bothered with a fever, and most symptoms feel worse in the early evening. Sufferers also tend to feel anxious and have a strong need for emotional reassurance.

Bryonia: If pain and distress intensifies with even the slightest movement, try Bryonia. When this remedy is helpful, patients tend to press a hand to the chest when coughing in an effort to keep the area as still as possible. Symptoms that respond well to Bryonia are generally brought on in response to over-exposure to dry, cold winds, but tend to develop slowly and insidiously. When feverish, thirst is marked, and there is a tendency to sweat profusely, especially in the early hours of the morning.

Existing Conditions
If you have any medical conditions or are taking any type of medicine it is imperative that you inform your practitioner, who will be able to advise you on safe use of conventional and complementary treatments.

Herbalism

If pneumonia is associated with fever, there are several herbs that may be helpful in reducing the fever (see p. 264).

Echinacea: This herb is an effective immune modulator and can help speed recovery. Echinacea works best when it is taken at the first sign of illness. A recommended dose is 250 mg in capsule form two to three times a day, or 20–40 drops of a tincture three times a day.

Garlic: Take garlic capsules as a general immune booster to treat pneumonia. Garlic has known antimicrobial and antiviral properties and aids fighting infection. An effective dosage is 1,000 mg three to four times a day. Or, you could simply take two crushed, or chopped, raw cloves of garlic each day for the duration of your illness. Garlic does have the potential to cause stomach irritation, so caution is advised when taking it.

Lobelia: This herb can be used to treat a range of respiratory conditions, including pneumonia. Lobelia is thought to act by many different mechanisms, including increasing airway diameter and promoting the secretion and expectoration of mucus. This herb is available from qualified herbal practitioners on prescription. Some adverse effects of lobelia have been reported such as nausea, dizziness, diarrhea, and tremors. Lobelia is a strong herb, so it is advised to consult a herbal medicine practitioner prior to taking it. Do not take it if you have gastrointestinal problems, heart disorders, or are pregnant.

Tip: USE A HUMIDIFIER

Using a mist humidifier will help soothe the respiratory tract and thin secretions to facilitate expectoration.

High Blood Pressure

Diagnosis

High blood pressure (hypertension) is a common condition that tends to run in families. There is no cure for high blood pressure and the cause is unknown, although certain lifestyle factors are thought to contribute to the condition.

The heart pumps to create the necessary pressure that allows blood to circulate. When the heart contracts, the highest pressure it produces is called the systolic pressure; when it relaxes, the lowest pressure it produces is the diastolic pressure. A normal blood pressure reading might be around 130/80—shorthand for a systolic pressure of 130 and a diastolic pressure of 80. Generally blood pressure is thought to be high when it is above 140/90. A permanently raised blood pressure may result in heart attack, stroke, or kidney failure.

Symptoms

- Most people with high blood pressure do not have symptoms and are unaware that they have the condition
- Those with severe high blood pressure or a rapid rise in pressure may experience headaches or blurred or impaired vision

Treatment Goal

There is no cure for high blood pressure but treatment exists to lower the pressure and manage the condition. Lifestyle factors should also be examined and changes introduced where necessary.

Conventional Medicine

Modify your lifestyle: Give up smoking and reduce the amount of alcohol you consume a day; men should drink no more that 30 ml a day and women no more than 15 ml. Follow a daily regime of about 20 minutes of moderate aerobic activity, such as a brisk walk. If other cardiac conditions are present, do not begin a vigorous exercise program without first having a medical assessment. Weight loss can also help to lower blood pressure. Cut out fatty foods, reduce the amount of salt you eat, and follow a Mediterranean diet of whole grains, white meat, fruit, vegetables, nuts, and olive oil. Supplements such as fish oil, arginine, hawthorn, and magnesium can be beneficial, and stress reduction is also important.

Medication: If an ideal blood pressure reading is not achieved by lifestyle modifications, or if readings are extremely high, then medication is prescribed. A mild diuretic such as hydrochlorothiazide or a beta blocker such as atenolol is usually the first choice. Sometimes a class of drugs known as "ACE inhibitors" are used, such as enalapril. The third common

group is calcium channel blockers, such as diltiazem. The choice of drug really depends on co-existing illnesses and symptoms. Blood pressure medications do have side effects and should be carefully used with close monitoring of blood pressure at the same time each day.

Severe cases: Extremely high blood pressure (over 160 systolic and 100 diastolic) should be treated immediately. Symptoms such as headache, impaired vision, and any changes in sensation, cognition, or muscle tone should be immediately evaluated. Pregnant women with high blood pressure should also be treated immediately.

Traditional Chinese Medicine

Herbs: For either formula, combine the herbs with 3 cups of water in a ceramic pot. Bring to a boil and simmer for 30 minutes. Strain and drink 1 cup twice a day.
• **For symptoms of dizziness, or occasional palpitations:** Mix 10 g of Tian Ma (gastrodia rhizome), 12 g of Gou Teng (stem and thorns of

gambir vine), 12 g of Chuan Niu Xi (Szechuan ox knee), 10 g of Du Zhong (eucommia bark), 12 g of Chuan Xiong (Szechuan lovage root), 12 g of Bai Shao (white peony root), 30 g of Long Gu (fossilized bone), and 30 g of Mu Li (oyster shell).

• **For symptoms of feeling overheated, sweating or night sweats, and lower back ache:** Combine 12 g of Shu Di Huang (cooked Chinese foxglove), 12 g of Shan Zhu Yu (Asiatic cornelian cherry), 15 g of Shan Yao (Chinese yam), 15 g of Fuling (poria), 12 g of Dan Pi (cortex of tree peony root), 12 g of Ze Xie (water plantain rhizome), 12 g of Zhi Mu (anemarrhena rhizome), 10 g of Huang Bai (phellodendron), 12 g of Gou Ji Zi (wolfberry), and 10 g of Ye Ju Hua (wild chrysanthemum flower).
• **When suffering insomnia, stress, and a light headache:** Combine 12 g of Dang Gui (Chinese angelica), 12 g of Bai Shao (white peony root), 12 g of Chuan Xiong (Szechuan lovage root), 12 g of Mu Gua (Chinese quince fruit), 12 g of Shuan Zhao Ren, and 12 g of Mai Men Dong (ophiopogon tuber).

Acupressure: Apply medium pressure to the Tai Yang point, situated in the depression at the temple. The Tai Chong point is located on the sole of the foot at the base of the large toe; press for one minute while in a sitting position and repeat two to three times during the day. The Susanli point is found on the lower leg 1 inch to the outside of and 3 inches below the kneecap. Press this point for one minute while in a sitting position and repeat.

Naturopathy

Diet: A whole food diet is key to lowering blood pressure. Your meals should be based on fresh vegetables, beans, nuts, and whole grains. High sodium and low potassium are common in people with hypertension. Eat foods that are high in potassium such as apples, bananas, asparagus, cabbage, tomatoes, kelp, and alfalfa, and restrict your salt intake by cutting out table salt, smoked meats, cheeses, and packaged foods. Add onions, garlic, and parsley to your food; they have been shown to bring down blood pressure. Celery, which can be blended with cucumber to make a juice, has also been shown to lower blood pressure. Avoid saturated fats, hydrogenated, and partially hydrogenated fats, which are found in margarine and refined vegetables oils, as they cause high blood pressure and place a burden on your heart. Dehydration can also contribute to hypertension, so make sure you drink at least eight glasses of water a day. Reduce the amount of caffeine you consume by cutting down on coffee, carbonated beverages, chocolate, and caffeinated tea.

Supplements: Try to obtain potassium from food, but if you are unable to, take 2,000 mg of a potassium supplement a day under the supervision of a doctor. Also take a combination of calcium (500 mg) and magnesium (250 mg) twice a day, which is commonly prescribed by naturopathic practitioners and other complementary therapists. Take 60–100 mg of coenzyme Q10 twice a day, as it has been shown to lower blood pressure and be supportive for overall heart function. Fish oil also helps lower blood pressure. Take 3–4 g a day, but be aware that you may have to take it for three months before you see any benefits. Taurine, taken at 6 g a day on an empty stomach, is an amino acid that has been shown in research to lower blood pressure.

Herbs: Take 250 mg of hawthorn a day; this herb dilates artery walls, decreases blood pressure, and serves as a heart tonic. Garlic has also been shown to lower blood pressure. Take 600 mg of an aged garlic extract twice a day. Passionflower, which can be taken at 250 mg in capsule form or 1 ml in tincture form, helps to decrease blood pressure associated with stress. Dandelion leaf, when taken at 300 mg or 2 ml three times a day, acts as a gentle, natural diuretic to lower blood pressure.

Homeopathy

High blood pressure is best treated by a combination of complementary and conventional therapies. If mild symptoms have recently developed, consult a homeopathic practitioner as a first resort to bring blood pressure down to a desirable level. In addition to advising on an appropriate homeopathic remedy, practitioners can assess the condition and provide guidance on making lifestyle changes that can help you manage high blood pressure. Some possible suggestions are listed below.

Stop smoking: If heart health and the circulatory system are compromised it is always advisable that you give up smoking. Complementary therapies, such as homeopathy, acupuncture, herbalism, or hypnotherapy, can be helpful in supporting your efforts.

Manage your stress: If you know high stress levels are contributing to high blood pressure readings, make a point of taking some time each day to relax. Tried and tested formal relaxation techniques include meditation, progressive muscular relaxation, visualization techniques, or a system of movement such as T'ai chi. Alternatively, you may benefit from attending a yoga class that will teach you how to breathe in order to feel relaxed and calm.

Diet: Avoid foods that have a reputation for raising blood pressure. These include caffeinated drinks (carbonated drinks as well as tea and coffee), saturated fats such as butter, cheese, cream, and red meat, salty snacks, and convenience "ready meals" and take-out dishes (particularly Chinese food).

Herbalism

Hawthorn: Hawthorn is a wonderful cardiovascular system tonic, and often used in cases of high blood pressure. This plant is rich in beneficial constituents of flavonoids and proanthocyanidins. The berries and tops are used, frequently in tea or tincture form. Infuse 1–2 tsp of hawthorn tops in a cup of boiling water and take three times daily as a tea. It is advisable to have blood pressure readings monitored when using herbs to help lower it.

Lime flowers: This herb has a gentle cardiotonic effect, and is often used in herbal blends for high blood pressure. It also has a gently relaxing effect, making it all the more useful for those who have stress as a contributing cause of high blood pressure. Lime flowers can be taken as a tea three times daily by infusing 1–2 tsp of the herb in boiling water for 10 minutes.

Flaxseed oil: This herb has been shown to be effective in reducing high blood pressure, probably due to the effects of the omega-3 fatty acids it contains. Although not as potent a source of omega-3s as cold-water fish (such as salmon or sardines), it is one of a few plants that contain this highly beneficial oil. Flaxseed oil is susceptible to oxidation and can become rancid when exposed to air for a long period of time; it should be refrigerated and used soon after opening. Your best option is to buy fresh flaxseed and store it in the refrigerator. Because the seeds are very durable, and will pass directly through the digestive system, it is best to freshly crush them before use. Use a mortar and pestle or coffee grinder to quickly crush the seeds. Sprinkle them on salads or cereals, or add them to a glass of water.

Garlic: Studies show that garlic can lower your blood pressure. It can be easily added to salads, soups, sandwiches, and marinades. Cooking garlic at a high temperature destroys some of its medicinal qualities so try to eat it raw whenever possible. Two cloves daily should be sufficient. Garlic is also widely available in pill or capsule form, and these do not have the potent odor that raw cloves do. Take 500 mg twice a day. When taken internally at high, therapeutic doses, garlic may interfere with certain anti-thrombotic drugs.

Overactive Thyroid

Diagnosis

The thyroid gland, located in the neck, produces hormones that regulate the rate of metabolism and are essential to the function of many systems in the body. An overactive thyroid is a condition involving the increased activity of the thyroid gland, whereby it produces more of the thyroid hormones than it should. This leads to an increase in the body's metabolic rate, which in turn causes the body's other functions to speed up. The thyroid gland can also become enlarged, resulting in the formation of a goiter, where the base of the neck becomes swollen.

If your doctor suspects an increase in your metabolic rate, he or she will examine the throat for an enlarged thyroid gland and carry out thyroid function tests.

Symptoms

- Nervousness, restlessness, and anxiety
- Trembling, shaking hands
- Rapid and pounding heartbeat
- Irritability due to the overstimulation of the nervous system
- Hot, sweaty hands and skin
- Weight loss despite increased appetite
- Severe general tiredness
- Insomnia
- Muscle pains and muscle tiredness
- Frequent bowel movements
- In women, irregular and light periods

Treatment Goal

To establish the presence of thyroid disease and take appropriate action.

Conventional Medicine

Treatment options for an overactive thyroid vary. Anti-thyroid medications are available, or surgery may be performed to remove all or part of the thyroid. If hyperthyroidism is associated with Grave's disease and bulging eyes, consult an ophthalmologist. As a general rule, eye protection should be worn at all times.

Modify your lifestyle: Avoid foods that contain iodine such as kelp, seaweed, spinach, and certain root vegetables. Since this condition increases your metabolism, it is important to also increase your calorie consumption and fluid intake, and avoid extreme physical exertion, particularly when symptoms are present.

Medication: Occasionally, Grave's disease (a certain type of hyperthyroidism) heals itself over a period of about six months to two years. Medication can be used to control the disease during this period and is then stopped when the condition resolves. The most common type of medication used is propylthiouracil, which inhibits the synthesis of thyroid in the gland and stops its conversion to an active form that increases metabolism. Another common medication is methimazole. Sometimes beta-blocker drugs are given to slow the heartbeat. This is symptomatic treatment only and does not help the thyroid disease itself.

Remove the thyroid: The most popular therapy to treat an overactive thyroid in the US is radioactive iodine (I131), which destroys the thyroid. Surgical removal of the thyroid (known as a thyroidectomy) may also be performed. In cases of what is called toxic nodular goiter, where small nodules in the gland produce too many thyroid hormones, removal is the only option.

Traditional Chinese Medicine

Herbs: For either formula, make a decoction by placing the herbs in a ceramic pot, adding 3 cups of water, and bringing to a boil. Simmer for 30 minutes then strain the liquid. Drink 1 cup twice a day.
• To treat symptoms of constipation, feeling overheated, and sweating profusely: Combine 12 g of Zhi Mu (anemarrhena rhizome), 15 g of Sheng Di Huang (Chinese foxglove root), 15 g of Xuan Shen (ningpo figwort root), 12 g of Xia Ku Cao (common self-heal fruit-spike), 12 g of Dan Pi (cortex of tree peony root), 12 g of Mai Men Dong (ophiopogon tuber), 10 g of Chai Hu (hare's ear root), and 10 g of Huang Bai (phellodendron).
• To treat symptoms of irritability, phlegm in the chest, and fatigue: Mix 12 g of Chai Hu (hare's ear root), 12 g of Bai Shao (white peony root), 10 g of Huang Qin (baical skullcap root), 12 g of Tai Zi Shen (pseudostellaria), 15 g of

Shan Yao (Chinese yam), 15 g of Fuling (poria), 15 g of Bai Zhu (white atractylodes rhizome), 3 g of Gan Cao (licorice root), and 12 g of Gua Lou (trichosanthes).

Acupressure: Use the tip of your thumb to apply strong pressure to the Hegu point, on the back of the hand between the thumb and the first finger, for one to two minutes. Repeat on the opposite hand. Use the tip of your finger to apply medium pressure to the Nei Guan point, in the center of the wrist on the palm side. In a sitting position, press the Tai Chong point, on the instep of the foot in the depression between the first and second toe, for one minute. Repeat two to three times a day.

Diet: Eat food that reduces heat and that is calming and cooling. Examples are apples, barley, button mushrooms, lettuce, mangoes, spinach, strawberries, persimmons, licorice, and aubergine.

Naturopathy

Diet: Eat brussels sprouts, cabbage, broccoli, cauliflower, kale, mustard greens, peaches, pears, soybeans, spinach, and turnips several times a day for their ability to suppress thyroid hormone production. Limit the amount of sea vegetables consumed because they contain iodine, which may over stimulate the thyroid gland. Also avoid stimulants such as coffee, carbonated drinks, caffeinated tea, and nicotine, which make symptoms worse. Brewer's yeast has high amounts of vitamin B and other important nutrients. Make a drink from the yeast or sprinkle it on your food.

Supplements: Those with an overactive thyroid need vitamin B complex to calm the nervous system. Take 50 mg three times a day. Vitamin C is also important to stabilize stressful conditions. Take 3,000–5,000 mg a day.

Herbs: Some studies have suggested that melissa helps to soothe the overactive thyroid gland, particularly if it is associated with Grave's disease. Take 2–4 ml of a tincture twice a day. You can also take 2–4 ml of motherwort tincture twice a day.

Homeopathy

This is a chronic condition and is best treated by an experienced practitioner who will try to rebalance the whole system. The remedies below give a small impression of some of the homeopathic remedies that may be considered to treat an overactive thyroid.

Phosphorus: If energy levels are leading to weight loss and veer from being high to low very quickly, Phosphorus may be used. Anxiety and restlessness is very marked, and there is a host of digestive disturbances and discomfort. These may manifest as indigestion, nausea, and burning in the stomach, and may be temporarily eased by cold drinks. Severe diarrhea may also be present. Sleep is likely to be disturbed, and sufferers tend to toss and turn before midnight, and wake feeling sleepy.

Thyroidinum: Symptoms include weight loss, breathlessness, frequent diarrhea with flatulence and cramping pains, and a marked inclination to be moody and irritable. Symptoms often slightly improve in the evening.

Calc phos: If patients tend to tremble, feel breathless, and experience mental and emotional restlessness, Calc phos may be used. Sleep is disturbed and patients may have night sweats and wake feeling unrefreshed. Colicky pains accompany diarrhea, as food moves quickly through the gut, and problems with malabsorption are common. Being under stress and pressure can aggravate symptoms, while rest can help.

Herbalism

Consult a herbal expert regarding the recommended dosages of the herbs below. A herbalist will determine the correct dose based on the patient's weight, age, and thyroid parameters.

Bugleweed: This unique plant possesses several medicinally active compounds believed to be helpful in treating an overactive thyroid and its associated symptoms. It can be taken as a tea or tincture. Bugleweed is a powerful herb, with largely unknown side effects, so consult a herbal expert before using it.

Motherwort: This herb does not treat the cause of an overactive thyroid, but is useful when palpitations are a symptom. It is considered a cardiotonic herb. Motherwort is also a relaxing nervine, which can help to calm and ease anxiety and agitation associated with an overactive thyroid. This can be taken as a herbal infusion (tea) three times daily, or as a tincture.

Underactive Thyroid

Diagnosis

An underactive thyroid results when the thyroid gland does not produce enough of the thyroid hormones. If the hormones are not produced in adequate amounts, the body's metabolism slows, leaving you feeling lethargic and rundown. Decreased metabolism can affect every organ of the body, including the brain, heart, skin, intestine, and muscles.

The main causes of an underactive thyroid are Hashimoto's thyroiditis (an autoimmune inflammation of the thyroid gland), an inherited problem with the thyroid gland, and complications arising from previous surgery to the thyroid gland. It can also be a side effect of certain medications, or can result from inadvertently taking large amounts of iodine, for example, in food supplements or, at times, shellfish such as shrimp.

An underactive thyroid is the most common disorder of the thyroid, and tends to affect women more than men. It is more prevalent among the elderly, but younger people are also susceptible.

Symptoms

- Increased sensitivity to cold
- Feelings of depression and lethargy
- No desire to exercise
- Weight gain
- Constipation
- Dry, rough, scaly skin
- Thin, dry hair
- Irregular periods
- Voice is deeper and more hoarse
- Loss of memory

Treatment Goal

A doctor will carry out tests to determine a diagnosis. Permanently decreased metabolism requires lifelong treatment with thyroid medication. Conventional and complementary therapies aim to rebalance hormone levels so that sufferers are able to lead completely normal lives.

Conventional Medicine

Hypothyroidism usually progresses slowly, but it can reach a dangerous level, especially if the thyroid has been removed. This condition is known as myxedema, and can cause a low temperature, low blood pressure, and a coma. Such cases are emergencies and must be treated at a hospital in intensive care.

Medication: Conventional medical treatment for an underactive thyroid is levothyroxine (T4), which is a synthetic form of thyroid, or some form of thyroid replacement. This may be given in combination with cytomel (T3). Natural thyroid replacements made by compounding pharmacists, who make up individual prescriptions other than those made by pharmaceutical companies, or Armour® thyroid (pig thyroid) are also available. The dosage varies from person to person, and is adjusted according to levels of thyroid stimulating hormone (TSH) in the blood. It generally takes six to eight weeks for the thyroid values to normalize after an adjustment is made. Because the change is gradual, patients are encouraged to be patient as they await improvement and testing.

Lifestyle modifications: A low calorie, high-fiber diet will help combat the effects of an underactive thyroid. Eliminate iodine-blocking foods such as pine nuts, almonds, and dark leafy greens from your diet. Exercise is also important.

Traditional Chinese Medicine

Herbs: According to traditional Chinese medicine, this condition is caused by a Qi deficiency. The following formula can help to tonify Qi. Combine 12 g of Huang Qi (milk-vetch root), 12 g of Tu Si Zi (Chinese dodder seed), 10 g of Ji Shen (jilin root), 12 g of Bai Zhu (white atractylodes rhizome), 12 g of Shu Di Huang (cooked Chinese foxglove), 12 g of Shan Zhu Yu (Asiatic cornelian cherry), 15 g of Fuling (poria), 15 g of Shan Yao (Chinese yam), and 12 g of Xian Lin Pi (aerial part of epimedium) in a ceramic pot. Add 3 cups of water, bring the liquid to a boil, and simmer for 30 minutes. Strain the liquid and drink 1 cup twice a day.

Acupressure: While sitting, use your fingertips to apply pressure to the Susanli point, on the lower leg, 1 inch to the outside and 3 inches below the kneecap. Press for one minute on each leg. Apply medium pressure with your fingertip to the Nei Guan point, located in the center of the wrist on the palm side, about 2 inches above the crease. The Tai Xi point is found in the depression midway between the inside anklebone and the Achilles tendon. With the tip of the finger, apply medium pressure to this point on both legs for one minute.

Diet: Eat foods that promote yang energy such as beef, beetroot, chicken livers, Chinese cabbage, carrots, figs, marjoram, peaches, shiitake mushrooms, sunflower seeds, longans, and cinnamon.

Naturopathy

Diet: Eat plenty of sea vegetables, such as kelp, nori, dulse, kombu, and wakame. These have high levels of iodine, which nourishes the thyroid gland. Essential fatty acids (EFAs) that are found in walnuts, flaxseeds, and oily fish, are also important for thyroid function. Avoid goitrogens, or foods that suppress thyroid function, such as brussels sprouts, cabbage, broccoli, cauliflower, kale, mustard greens, peaches, pears, soybeans, spinach, and turnips. Flourine and chloride inhibit the body's absorption of iodine; do not drink fluoride supplemented tap water and use fluoride-free toothpaste.

Supplements: Take 500 mg of L-tyrosine, an amino acid used to synthesize thyroid hormone, twice a day. Also take 3,000 g of fish oils a day to obtain the essential fatty acids (EFA) necessary for thyroid function.

Thyroid glandulars: Take a tablet of a thyroid glandular, an extract of an animal thyroid gland, three times a day to support thyroid function.

Homeopathy

This is a chronic condition and is best treated by an experienced practitioner who will try to rebalance the whole system. The remedies below give a small impression of some of the homeopathic remedies that may be considered to treat an underactive thyroid.

Calc carb: To treat classic symptoms associated with an underactive thyroid, including slow metabolism, easy weight gain, slow digestive processes leading to indigestion and constipation, clammy, sweaty skin, poor circulation, chapped, dry skin, and exhaustion,

Calc carb may be used. This remedy can be especially beneficial if an underactive thyroid gland is associated with menopausal symptoms.

Thyroidinum: This is a remedy that can be used to treat both under- or overactive thyroid glands. Symptoms include unexplained weight gain, sweating of the hands and feet, hair loss, feeling chilly, discomfort after eating, hot flushes, and sharp mood swings. In women, symptoms may improve following a period.

Herbalism

The primary treatment for an underactive thyroid is thyroid hormone replacement. Herbal remedies can be used to correct any underlying causes of the condition and ease symptoms.

Bladderwrack: This type of seaweed is used in treating hypothyroidism and goiter (the enlargement of the thyroid) due to iodine deficiency. It contains high levels of iodine, beta-carotene, potassium, zeazanthin, bromine, and mucilages, which heal and soothe the tissues. Infuse 1–2 tsp of the herb in 1 cup of boiling water to make a tea.

Guggul: This herb is effective in stimulating the thyroid to produce more thyroid hormone. Guggul has a high resin content, which is secreted by the plant when injured. Because resins are insoluble in water, making an alcohol extract is ideal. Take 20 drops of tincture three times a day.

Ashwagandha: This is an Ayurvedic herb, popularly used in treating those with an underactive thyroid. It is considered an adaptogen herb. This herb is also nourishing, and helps to alleviate underlying stress, gently picking up energy. It is often used in powdered form and put into capsules, or taken with water. In traditional Ayurvedic medicine, it is taken in warm milk.

Tip: AVOID TRIGGER FOODS

Certain foods have a reputation for possibly inhibiting thyroid gland function, and they should be avoided by those who have an underactive thyroid. Common culprits include cabbage, cauliflower, brussels sprouts, soy, and mustard greens. It may also be beneficial to steer clear of refined foods, white sugar, caffeine, alcohol, and large helpings of dairy products.

Anemia

Diagnosis

Anemia is a deficiency of red blood cells or hemoglobin that results in a reduced ability to carry and transfer oxygen to the body's tissues. Sufferers usually experience unusual levels of tiredness, although mild anemia may not produce any symptoms. Anemia can be divided into two types: that triggered by the decreased production of red blood cells and that caused by an increased loss of red blood cells. Red blood cells are manufactured in the bone marrow and have a life expectancy of approximately four months. To produce red blood cells, the body needs, among other things, iron, vitamin B12, and folic acid (one of the B group of vitamins). If one or more of these ingredients is lacking, anemia will develop.

Iron deficiency anemia is the most common type of anemia, often triggered by heavy blood loss, the body's inability to absorb iron from the diet, or a diet that lacks iron-rich foods. Vitamin B12 deficiency anemia is frequently caused either by the inability of the small bowel to absorb vitamin B12, or by a lack of food in the diet containing vitamin B12. Anemia can also be caused by a lack of folic acid. Folic acid is not stored in large amounts in the body and a continuous supply of the vitamin is needed.

Symptoms

- Unusual tiredness
- Difficulty in breathing/shortness of breath
- Dizziness/light-headedness
- Headaches
- Paleness

Treatment Goal

Anemia is usually detected through a routine blood test. It is not a disease in itself, but can be a warning of serious disease. It is vital to get accurate diagnosis and treat the condition before complications develop.

Conventional Medicine

The treatment of anemia is dependent on the cause and type of condition.

To treat iron deficiency anemia: Diagnostic tests are carried out to first determine that there is no hidden blood loss, for example, due to a heavy period, an ulcer, or other occult gastrointestinal bleeding. If blood loss is detected, medication is prescribed to treat the cause and prevent further loss. Iron pills are also prescribed, usually in the form of ferrous sulfate, in the amount of 60 mg of elemental iron three times a day. Copper is used in conjunction with iron to make red blood cells, so a mineral supplement containing copper at 100% of the recommended daily allowance is needed along with the iron. Iron pills can upset the stomach, but taking the iron with meals

and starting at a lower dose than recommended and gradually increasing it can alleviate discomfort. Foods that are high in iron, such as leafy green vegetables and red meat, should be included in your diet.

To treat anemia caused by a B12 or folate deficiency: B12 and folic acids levels can be obtained by a blood test. A Schilling urine test is also used to determine if the body is unable to absorb vitamin B12 adequately. Treatment involves B12 and folate injections every two to four weeks. Sub-lingual B12 (given under the tongue) can sometimes be effective.

Traditional Chinese Medicine

Herbs: Hemoglobin levels are expressed as the amount of hemoglobin in grams (g) per deciliter (dl) of whole blood. A Western medicine doctor can determine your hemoglobin count. If your hemoglobin is under normal range (12–16 g/dl for women and 14–18 g/dl for men), but above 8 g/dl, try the following formula. Mix 15 g of Shu Di Huang (cooked Chinese foxglove), 12 g of Dan Shen (salvia root), 15 g of Bai Zhu (white atractylodes rhizome), 15 g of Fuling (poria), 12 g of Huang Qi (milk-vetch root), 12 g of Dang Gui (Chinese angelica), and 5 pieces of Da Zhao (Chinese jujube) in a ceramic pot. Add 3 cups of water,

bring to a boil, and simmer for 30 minutes. Drink 1 cup twice a day. This decoction may cause loose bowel movements. Reduce the dose if this occurs and consult your doctor. If your hemoglobin levels are lower than 8 g/dl, consult your doctor about taking iron pills or other medication along with this formula.

Acupressure: Guan Yuan and Xue Hai, and San Yin Jiao are suggested pressure points for anemia. Apply gentle pressure with your fingertips to the Guan Yuan acupressure point, found about 3 inches below the navel. In a sitting position, also apply pressure on the Xue

Hai and San Yin Jiao points. With the knees flexed, rest your palms on the top of the thighs, with your fingers on your knees. Point your thumbs toward the floor to find the Xue Hai point, located on the inside of the upper thigh. The San Yin Jiao point is on the inside of the leg about 3 inches above the center of the anklebone.

Naturopathy

The treatment of anemia is dependent on the correct identification of its cause. The following recommendations are given with this in mind.

Diet: Plan your meals around foods that contain iron, such as liver, leeks, cashews, cherries, figs, organic grass-fed beef, and green leafy vegetables—except for spinach. Spinach contains oxalic acid, which inhibits iron absorption. For this reason also avoid rhubarb, tomatoes, chocolate, coffee, carbonated drinks, and black tea. Brewer's yeast is a good source of iron as well as other essential nutrients. Add 1 tbsp to cereals, juices, or salads daily.

Supplements: Take 50–100 mg of iron a day if you are iron deficient. Choose a product that includes citrate, gluconate, glycinate, or fumurate rather than iron sulfate (ferrous sulfate), which is not absorbed as well and can cause constipation. Take 500 mg of vitamin C with each pill to help your body absorb the iron. Do not take iron supplements if you do not have iron deficiency anemia. Vitamin B12 helps with all types of anemia, but if you are diagnosed with B12 deficiency anemia then you should take 1,000 mcg of B12 a day, which is higher than the recommended daily amount, or have B12 injections. For folic acid deficiency anemia, take 800–1,200 mcg a day, which is higher than the recommended daily amount. Also take 2,000 mg of spirulina a day, which has been shown to stimulate the production of red blood cells from bone marrow.

Herbs: Take 300 mg of gentian root, or 20 drops of tincture, before each meal to increase the gastric juices that help with iron absorption. You can also take 20 drops of yellow dock tincture with each meal, as it contains high levels or iron and helps with its absorption. Dandelion root, taken as 3,000–5,000 mg a day, has high levels of iron and detoxifies the liver. Pau d'Arco has blood-building qualities and can be taken at 100 mg three times a day. Take 300 mg of nettle leaves a day for their rich nutrient content.

Tip: TAKE VITAMIN C

Vitamin C appears to increase the absorption of iron. Eat foods rich in vitamin C, such as red, orange, and dark green fruit and vegetables, with every meal.

Homeopathy

The remedies suggested below can provide complementary support for iron deficiency anemia that has been thoroughly investigated and diagnosed by your doctor, and that is caused by an obvious reason, such as heavy periods. Other forms of anemia that fall into a chronic category will require professional medical assessment and case management.

Ferrum phos: This remedy is suitable for iron deficiency anemia with symptoms of a pale complexion and a tendency to blush easily and rapidly. There may also be, in women, palpitations with a rapid pulse rate and a heady feeling during a period.

Calc phos: If symptoms of iron deficiency anemia develop after an illness, consider using Calc phos. Symptoms may be especially noticeable in children who have poor muscle tone, weak digestion, and a history of cold hands and feet indicating poor circulation.

Herbalism

Anemia can be caused by a variety of nutritional, genetic, and environmental factors. While some forms of anemia may benefit from herbal therapy, most are not responsive. Below is a short list of herbs that have traditionally been used to treat anemia.

Siberian ginseng: One of the symptoms of anemia is fatigue, and Siberian ginseng has been shown to increase energy. Although this can be used to treat fatigue, it does not cure the underlying anemia. Siberian ginseng is different to panax ginseng, and is recommended over panax, which can be a little too stimulating for those who are particularly depleted.

Stinging nettle: The leaf of this plant is beneficial in treating iron-deficiency anemia owing to its high concentration of iron. Drink a tea made from 1–2 g of nettle two to three times daily. Many health food stores now sell stinging nettles in standardized extracts and freeze-dried capsules. You can also add stinging nettles to stews in place of spinach, to take advantage of their rich iron content.

Herbs containing vitamin C: Iron deficiency anemia may respond to vitamin C supplementation. You can take 250–500 mg in vitamin C tablets or incorporate any of a number of herbs high in vitamin C in to your meals.

6

Aches
and
Pains

Arthritis

Diagnosis

Arthritis is a painful condition of the joints. There are several different types of the disease—many are inflammatory while others are more degenerative in nature. It is uncertain what exactly triggers arthritis. It may be partly hereditary and it occurs three times more often in women than in men. People of all ages can develop arthritis—even children can be affected.

Osteoarthritis (also known as degenerative joint disease) is the most common form of arthritis. It is very painful and occurs when the joint cartilage begins to deteriorate and slowly wears away. People become affected by this type of arthritis in middle age. Factors that may contribute to the development of this disease include a genetic predisposition, being overweight, and previous damage to the joints through injury.

Rheumatoid arthritis affects the tissue connecting bones and joints, and is one of the most debilitating forms of arthritis. Pain in the joints almost always begins in the hands, especially in the knuckles, and often occurs in both hands simultaneously. The most obvious areas of damage are to the joints, but it can affect the whole body and in particular the fingers, wrists, elbows, and knees. It can occur at any age but usually starts in early middle age.

Symptoms

Osteoarthritis
- Pain and stiffness in joints, particularly the knees and hips
- Tender joints

Rheumatoid arthritis
- Joints swell and become red, stiff, and sore
- Morning stiffness
- Fatigue and flu-like aches and pains
- Fever
- Loss of appetite

Treatment Goal

There is no standard treatment for arthritis. Conventional and alternative therapies aim to slow the progressive deterioration as much as possible. Lifestyle changes, such as exercise, can also slow deterioration and relieve pain and stiffness.

Conventional Medicine

Exercise: Lifestyle modifications can be used to augment medication, or even replace it. Daily exercise, particularly aerobic aquatic exercise, is beneficial. Strength building of the muscles also seems to help ease the pain of arthritis, particularly quadriceps work, which is beneficial in the reduction of knee pain. Heat therapy and ultrasound therapy may also be helpful.

Diet: Adopt an anti-inflammatory diet. This involves reducing the amount of dairy, gluten, sugar, and processed foods you eat. Using anti-inflammatory herbs such as ginger, curcumin, and turmeric can also be beneficial. Begin a weight-loss program if necessary as this can help to ease symptoms.

Supplements: Take 4–7 g of fish oil (EPA and DHA in combination) a day. Although recent studies suggest that glucosamine and chondroiten are not as worthwhile as once thought, some case reports indicate otherwise. Some may find that they are beneficial while others do not. Capsaicin cream can be helpful when applied topically, but sometimes causes irritation. Vitamin D3 (cholecalciferol) has surfaced as an important vitamin in osteoarthritis. Doses much higher than the recommended daily allowance are used, so consult a doctor regarding an appropriate dosage.

Medication: Ibuprofen and other non-steroidal anti-inflammatory drugs (NSAIDs) are effective but are generally not recommended for long-term use as gastric bleeding is a side effect. Tylenol® is the medication of choice as it causes the least gastric side effects. Other mediations such as tramadol, propoxyphene, and codeine may be used for pain relief, but have sedating and constipating side effects and can be addictive; however, they do not cause gastric side effects. Cox 2 inhibitors such as celecoxib have less gastric risk but have known risks of increasing cardiovascular problems such as heart attacks. Joint injections with steroids are an effective short-term therapy. If all else fails, surgery, such as joint replacement surgery or osteotomy, which realigns the bones to reduce wear and pain, can be performed.

Traditional Chinese Medicine

Herbs: Chinese herbal remedies can be combined with acupressure to treat this condition.
• **Internal formula:** Combine 10 g of Qiang Huo (notopterygium root), 10 g of Du Huo (pubescent angelica root), 12 g of Sang Ji Sheng (mulberry mistletoe stem), 15 g of Niu Xi (achyranthes root), 15 g of Ji Xue Teng (millettia root), 10 g of Huang Bai (phellodendron), and 12 g of Cang Zhu (atractylodes rhizome) in a

ceramic pot and add 3 cups of water. Bring to a boil and simmer for 30 minutes. Strain and drink 1 cup twice a day.
• **External formula:** Combine 10 g of Chuan Wu (Szechuan aconite), 10 g of Cao Wu (wild aconite), 12 g of Gui Zhi (cinnamon), 12 g of Tao Ren (peach kernel), 10 g of Hong Hua (safflower flower), and 15 g of Niu Xi (achyranthes root) in a glass or ceramic pot. Add 3 cups of water, bring to a boil, and simmer for 30 minutes. Soak a towel in the warm liquid and apply to the affected joints, or soak the joints in the warm liquid for 20–30 minutes, once a day. Repeat for five to seven days.

Acupressure: Press the Ba Feng and Ba Xie points, and massage the Yang Ling Quan and Qu Chi points. The Ba Feng point is located on the instep of the foot between the bases of the big and second toes. The four Ba Xie points are located on the back of the hand at the base between each of the fingers. The Yang Ling Quan point is on the outside of the leg in the depression about 2 inches below the knee. The Qu Chi points are about 3 inches to the side of the nostrils in the depression just below the cheekbone.

Diet: Traditional Chinese medicine views dampness as one of the major causes of arthritis. Green onion, purslane, taro, honey, lychee, squash, and bitter melon are good for reducing dampness and can be combined with herbal remedies to treat arthritis.

Naturopathy

Diet: Dehydration has been linked to arthritis, so drink an 8 oz glass of water every couple of hours to keep your joints lubricated and your body hydrated. Eat foods that are high in essential fatty acids such as salmon, mackerel, and flaxseeds. These have anti-inflammatory properties and the fiber in flaxseeds will help keep your intestines clean. Eat plenty of onions, asparagus, cabbage, and garlic as these foods contain high levels of sulfur, which helps repair cartilage. Avoid non-organic, non-grass-fed meats, fried foods, sugar, dairy, refined carbohydrates, alcohol, and caffeine. Vegetables in the nightshade family, such as tomatoes, eggplant, potatoes, and peppers, contain a substance called solanine that triggers inflammation. Eliminate these foods for three to four weeks and see if you notice any improvement.

Supplements: A high-quality multivitamin will provide the proper nourishment to prevent joint damage. Follow the instructions on the container. Glucosamine sulfate, which is usually combined with chondroitin sulfate, reduces joint pain and rebuilds cartilage. Take 1,500 mg daily of glucosamine with 1,200 mg of chondroitin. Take 4,000–8,000 mg of methylsulfonylmethane (MSM) a day; it has natural anti-inflammatory benefits and contains sulfur, an important component of cartilage. Take 4–6 g of fish oil a day to reduce inflammation and lubricate joints, but allow two to three months for the full effects to become noticeable. Niacinamide has been clinically reported to help arthritic patients. It can be taken at 500 mg three times a day, and higher dosages should be supervised by a doctor. Take 250 mg of methionine, a sulfur-containing amino acid (sulfur is important for cartilage structure) that has been shown to have benefits in arthritic patients, four times a day. Take 1–3 g of vitamin C a day; it is beneficial in collagen synthesis repair—a major component of bone. Also take 1–2 capsules of protease enzyme on an empty stomach to reduce inflammation.

Herbs: Take 500 mg of bromelain three times a day for its anti-inflammatory effects. Cayenne cream, which depletes the nerves of a neurotransmitter that transmits pain messages to the brain, can be applied to the affected area two to four times a day. White willow relieves pain in the joints. Products should be standardized to contain 240 mg of salicin or 5 ml in tincture form; take this three times a day. Take 1,000 mg of yucca root, which has been traditionally used for arthritic pain, twice a day. Take 1–2 g of ginger, or 2 ml of tincture, three times a day for its anti-inflammatory benefits and pain relief.

Hydrotherapy: Soak in a hot bath with Epsom salts or mineral salts for at least 20 minutes. The minerals will replenish the body's mineral stores and provide relief.

Homeopathy

The tips given below may be helpful for relieving the occasional twinge of mild osteoarthritis. Long-term and severe problems that arise as a result of an established case of rheumatoid or osteoarthritis are best treated by an experienced homeopathic practitioner.

Ledum: Consider using this remedy to ease pain in the joints that is relieved by applying cool compresses, or bathing in cool water. Pain tends to move from the feet upward, and the affected joints may feel cool to the touch and slightly numb with pain.

Bryonia: If joints look red and swollen, and get worse as the day goes on but feel less painful while resting, try Bryonia. This is an remedy appropriate if joint pains are related to a low-grade state of toxicity in the system, causing constipation and headaches. Jarring movements make the pain more intense, while keeping the affected joint firm and supported relieves the discomfort.

Apis: If joints look rosy-pink and puffy, and localized pains are prickling or stinging, try Apis. Acute episodes of pain are likely to flare up quickly, and trigger a restless state of mind. Bathing in warm water intensifies the pain, while contact with cool air and cool compresses temporarily soothes.

Tip: STICK TO AN ANTI-INFLAMMATORY DIET

Certain foods have a reputation for aggravating inflammation, pain, and stiffness in joints and should be eliminated from the diet, or used in strict moderation. These items include red meat, products made from refined white sugar and flour, citrus fruit, tomatoes, peppers, eggplant, tea, coffee, and alcohol. Also avoid "instant," convenience foods that call for water to be added. These are often a rich source of chemical additives in the form of preservatives and flavorings.

Herbalism

Osteoarthritis treatments that include eliminating food allergies or intolerances, supplementing deficient vitamins, minerals, and amino acids, stretching and strengthening joints and associated muscles, and herbal approaches tend to be the most successful.

Counter-irritants: One interesting approach to decreasing inflammation and pain in a joint is to use a herbal "counter-irritant," which is thought to increase circulation and move toxins from the joint space. Mustard powder, a powerful counter-irritant, is combined with cornstarch and a small amount of warm water to create a "slurry" or paste that is applied to the affected joint. Smear the mustard paste on a sheet of gauze and cover with a hot pack. Leave the paste on for 15–20 minutes, checking to avoid blistering. Cayenne may also be applied topically for the same effect.

Devil's claw: This bitter root is used as medicine as an anti-inflammatory, to relieve arthritic pain and improve joint mobility. Clinical studies have shown devil's claw to be the most effective when taken in higher doses of powdered herb or as a powdered extract. You will not be advised to use this herb if you are diagnosed with peptic ulcers or acute gallbladder disease.

Anti-inflammatory herbs: Three herbs that are used as gentle, long-term, natural anti-inflammatories are turmeric, ginger, and Indian frankincense. A tincture or a capsule might be recommended. Black pepper or long pepper are recommended for use alongside turmeric, to aid bioavailabilty.

Rheumatoid Arthritis

Diagnosis

Rheumatoid arthritis is an aggressive inflammatory condition that affects the fingers, thumbs, wrists, knees, and feet. The tissue that surrounds the joint, called synovial fluid, allows for smooth movement between the bones. Rheumatoid arthritis develops when this fluid becomes damaged, causing inflammation, pain, and swelling of the joints. This inflammation can eventually destroy the joint, eating away at the cartilage and bone. It may involve many areas of the body, making you feel generally unwell, and in some severe cases it can affect the whole body and have crippling results.

No one knows what triggers the inflammation, but it is thought to be an autoimmune disease, in which the immune system creates antibodies that fight against the body's tissues. It is unclear why this occurs, but it is a common illness and tends to run in families. It can develop at any age, but usually starts in middle age. The severity of attacks is extremely variable and ranges from a single episode to severe disability.

Symptoms

- Acutely painful, hot, swollen joints
- Inflammatory skin nodules
- Puffy joints
- Fatigue, weakness, fever, and flu-like aches and pains
- Pains typically located in fingers, wrists, elbows, knees, and ankles
- Pain can be continual or variable
- Morning stiffness
- Occasionally, eye problems

Treatment Goal

To help to slow the rate of joint damage and minimize pain and inflammation.

Conventional Medicine

Medication to treat pain: Drugs used to treat rheumatoid arthritis are pain relievers such as acetaminophen and non-steroidal anti-inflammatory drugs (NSAIDs). NSAIDs have the added benefit of reducing inflammation as well as pain. Corticosteroids are given orally to treat severe or aggressive disease. Local infections of the joint can be used when there is swelling and loss of motion.

Medication to control the disease: Other classes of drugs are used to modify and control the disease. These drugs include methotrexate, sulfasalazine, leflunomide, hydroxycholoroquine, azathioprine, etanercept, and infliximab. Adalimumab is a newly approved rheumatoid arthritis disease-modifying drug that is given subcutaneously (under the skin). These drugs are strong and have side effects that are significant, but they are generally effective. They should not be used if pregnancy is a possibility, or if liver disease is present.

Physical therapy: Hydrotherapy (also called balneotherapy) is effective for soothing pain and is one of the oldest treatments for rheumatoid arthritis. It is often used in conjunction with other treatments. Thermotherapy is the application of heat or cold to sore joints, which can ease pain. Exercise is also usually recommended by a physiotherapist. A light daily routine to improve joint mobility, muscle strength, aerobic capacity, and function is ideal.

Diet and supplements: If you are overweight and suffer from rheumatoid arthritis, weight loss is important. Follow an anti-inflammatory program that excludes dairy and processed foods, avoids excess gluten and sugar, and includes the herbs ginger, curcumin, and turmeric. Doses of 600 mg of curcumin three times a day on an empty stomach are also effective. Fish oil is a natural anti-inflammatory and may be helpful at doses of 4 g daily. Selenium and vitamin E should also be supplemented at 400 IU a day and 400 mcg a day respectively.

Traditional Chinese Medicine

Herbs: Combine 12 g of Chuan Xiong (Szechuan lovage root), 12 g of Tao Ren (peach kernel), 12 g of Qiang Huo (notopterygium root), 12 g of Du Huo (pubescent angelica root), 12 g of Dan Gui (Chinese angelica root), 15 g of Niu Xi (achyranthes root), 12 g of Du Zhong (eucommia bark), 15 g of Bai Zhu (white atractylodes rhizome), and 15 g of Chi Xiao Dou (adzuki bean). Make a decoction by placing the herbs in a ceramic or glass pot and adding 3 cups of water. Bring to the boil, simmer for 30 minutes, and drink 1 cup twice a day. You may take this formula for five to seven days to relieve symptoms. Consult a TCM practitioner for longer-term use.

Acupressure: The Yang Ling Quan can be pressed once a day as a complementary therapy to herbal remedies. The Yang Ling Quan point is on the outside of the lower leg, parallel to the knee in the depression on the head of the fibula. You can also press the painful area with gentle pressure. However, if you have severe inflammation of the joints, first consult a doctor.

Diet: Eat food that is neutral and good for clearing dampness and heat. For example: apricot, beetroot, Chinese cabbage, carrots, corn, duck, and grapes. Avoid food that is overly warm, such as asparagus, brown sugar, butter, chives, ginger, and red or green peppers. Also, avoid food that is too cold in its properties, such as bamboo shoots, bananas, clams, grapefruit, and muskmelon.

Naturopathy

Diet: An anti-inflammatory diet is essential for the relief of pain. Deep-water fish, such as salmon, sea bass, tuna, trout, and mackerel, are rich sources of omega-3 fatty acids and have anti-inflammatory properties. Eliminate the top food allergens from your diet such as wheat, dairy, corn, and soy, as they increase inflammation in the joints. Vegetables from the nightshade family, including tomatoes, aubergine, potatoes, and peppers, also increase inflammation and should be avoided. Blueberries, cherries, and hawthorn berries are rich sources of flavonoids, particularly proanthocyanidins. These flavonoids exhibit membrane and collagen stabilizing, antioxidant, and anti-inflammatory actions as well as many other actions that are beneficial in the treatment of rheumatoid arthritis. Low levels of vitamin E have been found in the joint fluid of rheumatoid arthritis patients. The antioxidant properties of vitamin E are thought to protect joint cells from free radical damage. Food sources high in Vitamin E include broccoli, almonds, avocados, mangoes, peanuts, sunflower seeds, and Brazil nuts.

Supplements: A good-quality multivitamin/ multimineral will provide the proper nourishment to prevent joint destruction. Follow the dosage instructions on the label. Glucosamine sulfate reduces knee pain and rebuilds cartilage. Usually it is combined with chondroitin sulfate. Take 1,500 mg daily of glucosamine with 1,200 mg of chondroitin. Methylsulfonylmethane (MSM) has natural anti-inflammatory benefits and contains the mineral sulfur, an important component of cartilage. Take 4,000–8,000 mg daily. Take 500 mg of niacinamide, which has been reported to help arthritic patients, three times a day. Higher dosages should be supervised by a doctor. Take 250 mg of sulfur four times a day as it is important for cartilage structure. Vitamin C is beneficial in collagen synthesis repair, a major component of bone. Take 1–3 g a day. Protease enzyme breaks down protein molecules that promote inflammation. Take 2–3 capsules between meals.

Herbs: Take 500 mg of bromelain three times a day for its natural anti-inflammatory effects. Cayenne cream can deplete the nerves of a neurotransmitter that transmits pain messages to the brain. Try applying the cream to the affected area two to four times a day. Devil's claw helps with arthritic pain in the joints. Take 1,500–2,500 mg three times a day, but do not take it if you have a history of gallstones, heartburn, or ulcers. Take a white willow product standardized to contain 240 mg of salicin to relieve pain, or take 5 ml of a tincture three times a day. Take 1,000 mg of yucca root, which has been traditionally used for arthritic pain, twice a day. Ginger has anti-inflammatory benefits and relieves pain. Take 1–2 g or 1–2 ml of tincture three times a day, but do not take more than 1 g of ginger a day if you are pregnant. Celery seeds help clear uric acid from the joints of gout and arthritis sufferers. Boil 1 tsp of seeds in 1 cup of water for 15 minutes, strain, and sip. Dandelion dispels uric acid. Take 3 capsules daily, or 1 tbsp of juice or 1 cup tea twice daily for four to six weeks to reduce the frequency and intensity of pain, and to strengthen the connective tissue. Parsley juice is effective in combating and flushing out uric acid from the tissue, which eases painful limbs and joints. Take 1 tsp of parsley juice three times daily for six weeks. Wait three weeks before repeating.

Homeopathy

This is a chronic condition. Homeopathic treatment can provide a complementary route for reducing pain, inflammation, and stiffness. However, treatment should be given by an experienced homeopathic practitioner to see the best results. Some self-help strategies are suggested below, but it must be emphasized that these are stop-gap measures only, and should not be relied upon in the long term.

Bryonia: This remedy can be helpful for reducing heat, swelling, and stiffness in joints that respond obviously well to rest and are aggravated by movement. Joint pains can be accompanied by a generally "toxic" feeling with associated symptoms of frontal headache and constipation. Applying pressure and support to the tender joints gives some relief, while light touch feels uncomfortable.

Apis: If the affected area is rosy-pink, puffy, and swollen, and acutely sensitive to contact with heat, try Apis. Contact with cool air or cool compresses gives relief from stinging pains and discomfort.

Tip: SWIM

Try to keep the joints as mobile as possible. Swimming is an ideal form or exercise, as the buoyancy of the water provides gentle support for any affected joints.

Ledum: This is a potentially helpful acute remedy to relieve pain in a joint that has been subject to a steroid injection. Symptoms include a numb, cool sensation in the affected area that is relieved by applying a cool compress, or bathing in cool water.

Rhus tox: This is one of the leading remedies for rheumatism and arthritis. It is appropriate if stiffness in the joints is relieved by moving around, applying hot compresses, or soaking in warm water. The body feels restless, and symptoms may come on after overexertion or getting cold or wet.

Herbalism

Turmeric: This powerful anti-inflammatory agent is possibly as effective as anti-inflammatory medications such as ibuprofen or acetaminophen in controlling some of the symptoms of rheumatoid arthritis. The downside is that turmeric is very poorly absorbed. Newer research suggests that taking turmeric alongside long pepper or black pepper greatly aids absorption, making it a much more effective remedy. One of its isolated phytochemicals, curcumin, is often used for conditions such as rheumatoid arthritis in doses of 400–600 mg three times daily, though many practitioners prefer to use whole turmeric for the added effect of other compounds. Powdered turmeric root is often dosed at 0.5–1 g two or three times daily, and it may take several weeks for symptoms to improve. It is probably easiest to simply incorporate this amount of turmeric regularly into your cooking. It is also possible to purchase turmeric extract standardized to its curcuminoid content; the dose will depend on the exact product purchased. Some people experience a stomach upset with turmeric and with long-term medicinal use of turmeric care should be taken with any medications or supplements that thin the blood.

Green tea: The daily consumption of green tea can help to decrease inflammation and pain in rheumatoid arthritis, primarily through the actions of its compounds, called polyphenols, which are similar to the compounds in red wine and dark chocolate. Three to four cups of green tea a day can help with symptoms; decaffeinated tea should work just as well. You can also take green tea extracts standardized to the polyphenol percentage. These standardized extracts should be taken as directed on the label.

White willow bark: This herb naturally contains salicylates. These are aspririn-like phytochemicals (natural plant chemicals) that have an anti-inflammatory and pain-relieving effect on muscles and joints. Theoretically, people with salicylate sensitivity may react to this herb. The dried bark of this plant may be used to make a decoction, by bringing 1¼ cups of water containing 2 tsp of the bark to a boil in a saucepan and simmering for 10 minutes. This may be drunk three times daily. A tincture may also be used. 🐝

Osteoporosis

Diagnosis

Osteoporosis or brittle bone disease is a condition characterized by loss of bone density, where the amount of bone tissue in the body is below what is considered normal for a person of a particular sex and age. As a result, the bones become weak and take on the texture of honeycomb. Fractures can occur in areas where there is a greater percentage of weakened bone, such as the wrists, the hip joint, and in the vertebrae of the lower spine.

Osteoporosis is a widespread problem. Various factors are known to trigger osteoporosis, and many of them are unavoidable. Contributory factors include getting older, a family history of osteoporosis, being female, going through menopause/estrogen loss, and being underweight. Lifestyle factors play a role, such as lack of exercise, a poor diet that is lacking in calcium, smoking, and regularly drinking alcohol. Other triggers include the use of steroid drugs, an overactive thyroid gland, chronic liver or kidney disease, and vitamin D deficiency.

Symptoms

- A fractured or broken bone can be the first indication of problems
- Bending forward into a hunched position
- Shortening of the spine due to fractured vertebrae

Treatment Goal

If you think you may have osteoporosis or are at risk of it, have your bone density measured. Treatment aims to prevent further deterioration and protect against complications such as fractures and broken bones.

Conventional Medicine

Prevention is the most important goal. Risk factors such as poor nutrition should be identified and corrected wherever possible.

Exercise: Engage in physical activity on a daily basis. Performing weight bearing exercises, which work your bones and muscles, is especially important.

Vitamins and supplements: Increase your intake of vitamin D3 (cholecalciferol) to about 400–1,000 IU daily. Also take 45 mg of vitamin K2 and 1,800 mg of calcium hydroxyapetite a day. In postmenopausal women, minimal amounts of natural estrogen and natural progesterone may be helpful. However, estrogen should be avoided if breast cancer has been diagnosed in the past or if a strong family history exists.

Medication: The medications alendronate, raloxifend, and risedronate are approved for the treatment of osteoporosis for the prevention of bone loss. A bone density test should show that bone loss has stopped after one year of beginning medication.

Traditional Chinese Medicine

Herbs: For either formula, make a decoction be combining the ingredients in a ceramic or glass pot. Add 4 cups of water, bring to a boil, and simmer for 30 minutes. Strain and drink 1 cup twice a day. Take the formulas for one to three months.
• **Formula one:** This combination will benefit bones by nourishing the blood and improving circulation. Mix 10 g of Shan Zhu Yu (Asiatic cornelian cherry), 12 g of Dang Gui (Chinese angelica), 15 g of Di Huang (Chinese foxglove), 15 g of Dan Shen (salvia root), 12 g of Gou Ji Zi (wolfberry), 12 g of Ji Shen (jilin root), and 15 g of Ji Xue Teng (milletia root).
• **Formula two:** These herbs tonify kidney energy, which is important for bone health. Mix 30 g of Long Gu (fossilized bone), 30 g of Mu Li (oyster shell), 12 g of Sang Ji Sheng (mulberry mistletoe stem), 12 g of Niu Xi (achyranthes root), 15 g of Shu Di Huang (cooked Chinese foxglove), 12 g of Shan Zhu Yu (Asiatic cornelian cherry), 15 g of Shan Yao (Chinese yam), 15 g of Fuling (poria), and 12 g of Ze Xie (water plantain rhizome).

Acupressure: Press the Xuan Zhong point, found on the outside of the lower leg, about 3 inches above the anklebone. Take a seat and apply pressure to the Xuan Zhong point on each leg. Apply pressure for one to two minutes and repeat a couple of times a day.

Diet: Eat foods that strengthen the kidneys, such as black sesame seeds, string beans, sword beans, wheat, kidney, plums, mutton, chives, dill seed, tangerines, walnut, pork, clove, and fennel. Also eat foods that are rich in vitamin B, tonify the blood, and strengthen bones.

Naturopathy

Diet: Eat plenty of sea vegetables, green leafy vegetables (except spinach), soybeans, nuts, molasses, and unsweetened cultured yogurt. These foods contain high levels of calcium and other nutrients important in the absorption of calcium. Spinach, which contains oxalic acid, a substance that interferes with the absorption of calcium, should be avoided. Vitamin K is known for coagulation and bone formation, and can be found in high amounts in green vegetables such as collard greens, kale, and romaine lettuce. Processed sugars contribute to osteoporosis and should be cut out of your diet wherever possible. Moderate your levels of caffeine and alcohol consumption, as they contribute to bone loss. Unlike the popular belief, milk and milk products are not the best sources of calcium. This is largely due to intolerances to lactose and casein, which can lead to problems with absorption. Unsweetened yogurt is the exception.

Supplements: Calcium has been shown to be effective in helping to build bone mass. For optimum nutrition, the recommended calcium intake is between 1,000–1,500 mg per day, depending on your age, dietary intake, and other health conditions. Use the forms that most easily absorbed by the body, such as calcium citrate, malate, chelate, or hydroxyappatite. Vitamin D has also been shown to be effective in building bone mass by improving intestinal calcium absorption and reducing excretion of calcium in the urine. Your daily intake should be approximately 400 IU a day for prevention and 800–1,200 IU per day if you already have osteoporosis. Vitamin K reduces bone loss and low levels have been associated with fractures. Take 2–10 g a day—a smaller amount for prevention and a higher amount if you have osteoporosis. Do not take vitamin K if you are on anticoagulant medications. Ipriflavone has been shown to help bone strength when combined with calcium and vitamin D. Take 600 mg a day with food. Take 250–350 mg of magnesium twice a day as it is required for proper calcium metabolism. Fish oils can also improve calcium absorption and deposition into bones when taken at 4 g a day. Boron is a mineral that activates vitamin D and supports estrogen levels of effective calcium metabolism. Take 3–5 mg daily. Vitamin C, among its many other healthy functions, synthesizes collagen, an important component of bone. Take 340 mg a day of strontium, which has been shown to increase bone density when taken with calcium. Finally, take 2–3 capsules of betaine hydrochloric acid with each meal to improve stomach acid, which aids in the absorption of calcium.

Homeopathy

Due to its chronic nature, osteoporosis requires professional medical management. Homeopathic treatment can play a positive role in helping patients who suffer from poor bone density, but for the most successful outcome this support needs to come from an experienced practitioner. The practical suggestions below can help to discourage the condition from escalating.

Diet: If you suspect that your bone density is at risk, avoid foods that have a reputation for aggravating osteoporosis, such as alcohol, coffee, salt, and preserved meats. Instead, eat plenty of oily fish (especially sardines and salmon), green leafy vegetables, small amounts of dairy foods, and soy products.

Lose weight sensibly: Avoid crash diets that may be nutritionally challenging. Extreme fluctuations of weight can leave you more vulnerable to problems with bone density. This is especially the case if your periods stop as a result of drastic weight loss over a significant period of time.

Exercise: Regular weight-bearing exercise has been shown to play an important role in guarding against osteoporosis, especially when performed up to three or four times a week. Try regular walking, weight training, running, cycling, swimming, and dancing.

Herbalism

Red clover: There is evidence that red clover could be useful for osteoporosis. Its benefits are probably due to compounds called isoflavones (sometimes referred to as phytoestrogens) that have hormonal activity. There is also evidence that diets containing high levels of phytoestrogenic isoflavones are associated with low incidence of osteoporosis. Red clover can be ingested as a tea (made from 1–2 g and taken one to three times daily) or ½ dropper of an alcohol or glycerin tincture can be taken three times a day. However, the most effective preparation of red clover appears to be capsules of a semi-purified leaf extract where the standardization to the percentage of isoflavones is listed specifically

on the bottle. Some caution should be taken if you are also on medications that can thin the blood, and some people can react to red clover by developing a skin rash.

Horsetail: The presence of minerals like silica, potassium, and manganese has prompted people to consider the use of horsetail extract for osteoporosis treatment and prevention. There is some animal research to suggest the importance of silica in bone growth, and clinical trials suggest that horsetail may slightly increase bone density. In theory, horsetail may cause vitamin B1 (thiamine) to become depleted.

Muscle Cramps

Diagnosis

A muscle cramp is the result of an involuntarily contracted muscle that does not relax. Any of the body's muscles can cramp, but it is particularly common in the legs and feet, and the calf muscle tends to be the most affected. When a muscle involuntarily contracts, it is called a spasm, which becomes a cramp when the spasm is sustained. It is a common condition, and most people experience it at one time or another. Cramps generally arise after exercise, or due to an imbalance of body fluids, hormones, or salts (the "electrolytes" calcium, magnesium, and potassium), or because of dehydration. Poor circulation can also trigger cramps, as can some medications. Although not dangerous in themselves, in some cases cramps may be a symptom of an underlying condition.

Most muscle cramps can be stopped if the muscle is stretched. A cold pack can also be used to relax tense muscles. Following a cramp, a warm towel or heating pad can also alleviate pain or tenderness.

Symptoms

- Muscle spasm, leading to a rigid sensation
- Pain in the affected area

Treatment Goal

To ease the pain and discomfort of cramps and to prevent them from occurring. It is also important to get a correct diagnosis for the cause of the cramps to determine whether there is an underlying condition. The most common and usually the most effective treatment is daily stretching of the affected muscles.

Conventional Medicine

Muscle cramping is not a medical disease in itself but a symptom of another condition. The first step in conventional medicine is to make an accurate diagnosis and rule out a serious disease.

Castor oil: A castor oil pack is sometimes helpful in easing muscle cramps. Apply castor oil to a washcloth, warm it in the microwave, and place it on the affected area for 15 minutes. This can reduce the pain of muscle cramping and may help stop the cramping itself.

Diet and supplements: Deficient amounts of electrolytes in the body, particularly magnesium, calcium, and potassium, can lead to cramps. These deficiencies can usually be corrected by modifying your diet to include foods that are high in these nutrients, but magnesium supplements may also be needed. Keeping the body hydrated is also essential in the prevention of muscle cramping.

Muscle relaxants: These may be used if a doctor has determined that cramping is due to an injury and is short term. Muscle relaxants may also be necessary if the cramping is due to a neuromuscular condition. Plants such as valerian may also provide some relief for chronic cramping.

Traditional Chinese Medicine

Herbs: Combine 10 g of Yan Hu Suo (corydalis rhizome), 12 g of Bai Zhu (white atractylodes rhizome), 15 g of Fuling (poria), 10 g of Mu Xiang (costus root), 8 g of Zhi Ke (bitter orange), 5 g of Gan Cao (licorice root), and 3 g of Sha Ren (cardamom) in a glass or ceramic pot. Add 3 cups of water, bring to a boil, and simmer for 30 minutes. Strain the liquid and drink 1 cup twice a day.

Acupressure: Pressing the Qi Hai and Zhong Wan points is recommended for easing cramps. Lie down and use your fingertip to press the Qi Hai point, located in the center of the lower abdomen, about 1 inch below the navel, as you inhale. Also use your fingertip to press the Zhong Wan points, found just to the left and right of centerline of the upper abdomen, about 3 inches above the navel. Do not press these points too hard.

Diet: Licorice, spearmint, and peppermint tea are very helpful in treating cramps. You can also try crushing 30 g of lychee seeds and boiling them in water with 6 g of fresh ginger or dried orange peel. Drink 1 cup of tea once a day to help relieve pain.

Naturopathy

Diet: Follow a high-nutrient diet based on whole foods such as fresh vegetables, fruit, and grains. This sort of nutritional regime decreases inflammation and strengthens the liver. If you eat animal protein make sure it is antibiotic and hormone free. Eat cold-water fish such as salmon, mackerel, and herring, along with flaxseeds and walnuts, as they are a good source of essential fatty acids, which help in reducing inflammation. You can also sprinkle 1 tbsp of high-fiber ground flaxseeds on your cereal. Add some wheat germ and/or brewer's yeast to two of your meals a day. Avoid hydrogenated oils, and trans-fatty acids. These foods promote inflammation and worsen symptoms. Avoid alcohol as it dehydrates and throws out blood sugar levels, all of which aggravate cramping symptoms.

Supplements: Take 250 mg of magnesium twice a day as it is a natural muscle relaxant. Calcium works synergistically with magnesium to promote muscle and nerve relaxation and can be taken at 500 mg twice a day. Potassium deficiency can lead to muscle cramping, so protect against this by taking up to 300 mg a day. If taking blood pressure medication, potassium should be taken under medical supervision. B vitamins become depleted when undergoing stressful events, which causes muscle cramping in some people. You can take a 50 mg complex every day.

Massage: Have a massage that involves deep kneading to help relax muscles and improve circulation. Use a combination of rosemary, rose, and germanium oil in an essential oil solution and add these to a base oil, such as almond or apricot oil. Gently massage the oil into the affected area to improve circulation.

Homeopathy

The following remedies can be useful in shortening the duration and easing the severity of a recent bout of cramps. More established conditions are best treated by a practitioner.

Arnica: This is the main homeopathic remedy to consider to ease cramps that have come on after overexertion, especially in anyone who is unused to exercise and has overdone it as a result.

Nux vomica: If cramps (especially those that come on at night) are associated with high stress levels, poor, disturbed sleep, a hangover, or nausea, consider this remedy. Symptoms include a general sense of muscle tension and spasm, and a short temper and irritability in response to stress and mental and physical tension.

Veratrum album: If cramps in the calves set in during or after a bout of vomiting and diarrhea caused by dehydration, try Veratrum album. This remedy is especially helpful if massaging the affected area brings relief, and walking makes symptoms worse.

Herbalism

Herbal medicines can be used to ease cramps by improving circulation, restoring nutrients, and relieving muscle tension.

Anti-spasmodic tincture: Cramp bark is astringent and drying, and excellent at relieving cramping muscles due to tension and overuse. Khella, part of the parsley family, is used to treat mild forms of angina. These anti-spasmodic and pro-circulatory benefits extend to spasming muscles throughout the body. Black cohosh is a bitter herb used for the treatment of muscle cramps as well as menstrual cramps. Black cohosh also acts as a mild sedative, an anti-inflammatory, a circulatory stimulant, and a digestive stimulant. Greater celandine, a bitter and cooling herb, aids digestion and acts as an anti-inflammatory and anti-spasmodic. Celandine is especially indicated for relief of headaches due to shoulder and neck muscle spasm but this herb

is restricted to practitioner use. Chamomile is a wonderful herb for the relief of nervous tension and irritability. Chamomile gently sedates while inhibiting inflammation and spasm in muscles.

Valerian: The root of this herb is an effective anti-spasmodic, which helps to relieve muscle cramps. This is partly due to its valerenic acid and volatile oil content. Valerian can be taken in various forms, including tincture, capsule, and root infusion/decoction. All forms are readily available at herbal medicine stores, and some health food shops. If using the tincture, 3–5 ml can be taken three times daily. Valerian does have sedative properties, so caution is advised. However, some individuals may be more stimulated by it.

Chronic Fatigue Syndrome

Diagnosis

Chronic fatigue syndrome (CFS) is a condition characterized by profound and severe muscle fatigue. An overwhelming feeling of exhaustion tends to come on suddenly following any form of physical exertion, and is accompanied by problems with memory and concentration. Many people who feel "tired all the time" consult a doctor regarding CFS, but only a small percentage of these actually have the condition. Illnesses that mimic CFS include anemia, celiac disease, liver disease, lupus, low thyroid function, and multiple sclerosis. Although the basic underlying cause remains uncertain, research suggests that CFS is triggered by a combination of factors, including a genetic susceptibility and repeated infections, particularly of a flu virus.

Symptoms

- Muscle pain
- Aching joints
- Ongoing flu-like feelings
- Severe headaches
- Waking up still feeling tired
- Sore throat and enlarged glands
- Sensitivity to heat and cold
- Alcohol intolerance
- Low blood pressure
- Sensitivity to bright light and loud noise
- Depression

Treatment Goal

The most helpful method of managing this condition involves "pacing," where levels of physical and mental activity are carefully balanced to reflect the stage and severity of the illness. Treatment looks at making lifestyle adjustments, as well as ways of easing symptoms, to reduce the chances of long-term ill health and improve the quality of life.

Conventional Medicine

Medication: There are several medications that may be used to treat CFS, including antidepressants, non-steroidal anti-inflammatory drugs (NSAIDs) for pain, and triazolopyridine antidepressants such as trazodone for sleep.

Lifestyle changes: A low to moderate amount of daily exercise such as graded aerobic exercise is recommended. Performing T'ai chi daily has been shown to be helpful and craniosacral chiropractic techniques (which involve massaging the skull), therapeutic touch, massage, and yoga may also be beneficial. Stress reduction techniques such as meditation are also highly recommended. Support groups and behavioral therapy are often helpful as well.

Diet and supplements: Evaluating and optimizing the adrenal and nutritional status of the body should be part of treatment. Eat whole grains, fruits, vegetables, and lean meats, and avoid processed foods to optimize energy. Supplements such as coenzyme Q10 (CoQ10) may be considered, as they also increase energy in the cells. Adequate B vitamins are also essential.

Traditional Chinese Medicine

Herbs: For either formula, make a decoction by placing the ingredients in a ceramic or glass pot and adding 4 cups of water. Bring to a boil and simmer for 30 minutes. Strain the liquid and drink 1 cup two or three times a day.
• To treat fatigue due to Qi deficiency: Symptoms include tiredness, lethargy, poor appetite, and loose stools. Combine 12 g of Dan Shen (salvia root), 12 g of Bai Zhu (white atractylodes rhizome), 15 g of Fuling (poria), 15 g of Shan Yao (Chinese yam), 15 g of Huang Jing (Siberian Solomon seal rhizome), 6 g of Chen Pi (tangerine peel), and 3 g of Gan Cao (licorice root).
• To treat fatigue due to blood deficiency: Symptoms include tiredness, a poor memory, light-headedness, insomnia, or feeling overly sleepy. Combine 12 g of Shu Di Huang (cooked Chinese foxglove), 12 g of Shan Zhu Yu (Asiatic cornelian cherry), 15 g of Shan Yao (Chinese yam), 15 g of Dan Shen (salvia root), 15 g of Niu Xi (achyranthes root), and 12 g of Dang Gui (Chinese angelica).

> **Tip:** TRY TO EXERCISE
>
> Exercise helps CFS patients get stronger in some cases. However, most fatigue patients do not have the energy to exercise, are not motivated, or feel more tired after exercising. In any case, it is important to know what exercises are adequate and suitable for you. You may try walking or gentle movement like T'ai chi. However, if you feel tired, do not push yourself.

Acupressure: The Susanli point is on the lower leg in the depression 4 inches below and 1 inch to the outside of the knee. Press this point using the tip of the finger for about one minute and repeat. The Bai Hui point is on the top of the head at the midpoint of the line running up and over the head from ear to ear. The Guan Yuan point is in the middle of the abdomen, about 2 inches below the navel. Press with medium pressure.

Diet: Eat food that tonifies blood and Qi and food that nourishes the spleen and lungs. Such foods include black soybean, peach, chestnut, sweet basil, coriander, beef, polished rice, potato, string bean, sweet potato, carrot, grape, and leek.

Naturopathy

Diet: Try following a detoxification and cleansing diet for one to three weeks. This involves avoiding all foods and chemicals that may make symptoms worse, and instead eat a diet of dense nutrients. Eat plenty of sea vegetables and gluten-free grains such as brown rice, millet, and quinoa, and fresh vegetables. Seeds, nuts, and fresh fish are also beneficial. Wheat, dairy, corn, gluten-containing products, sugar, and fermented foods are some of the most common allergens.

After three weeks re-introduce the foods into the diet one at a time to identify any triggers. For CFS patients with candidiasis, all types of sugar, including milk products and fruit, should be avoided, as should caffeine, alcohol, and refined carbohydrates such as white flour and white rice. Caffeine depresses the adrenal glands, which secrete the hormones needed for energy. Also avoid refined sugar, which may cause hypoglycemia and induce fatigue.

Supplements: Probiotics can greatly improve digestion and reestablish a healthy balance in the intestines. A typical dose is one to two capsules two to three times per day, taken on an empty stomach. Make sure there are at least 4 billion healthy organisms in the formula. Digestive enzymes can supply your body with additional enzymes to digest fats, proteins, and carbohydrates. Products differ greatly—some contain lactase to digest milk, others contain hydrochloric acid to assist the stomach, and still others contain ox bile to help with the emulsification and digestion of fats. A typical dosage is one to two capsules with meals. Vitamin C helps the immune system, is required for healthy adrenal gland function, and helps with liver detoxification; take 3 g throughout the day. Magnesium is involved in more than 300 enzyme reactions in the body and is essential for energy production, muscle function, nerve conduction, and bone health. People with chronic fatigue syndrome often have a deficiency in magnesium and should take 250 mg three times a day. CoQ10 is necessary for energy production and cell function. It also helps with the repair and maintenance of tissues. A typical dose is 60–100 mg daily. Nicotinamide Adenine Dinucleotide (NADH) is a naturally occurring chemical that plays a significant role in cellular energy production. Take 10 mg a day on an empty stomach. Also take 500 mg of L-Carnitine three times a day; it is used by the body to convert fatty acids into energy.

Herbs: Those with CFS often have adrenal fatigue or weakness. Licorice can tonify the adrenal glands are as it works to increase levels of cortisol in the body. Take 1,000 mg two to three times daily, and take the de-glycyrrhizinated form if you suffer from high blood pressure. Ginkgo biloba improves circulation and improves memory. You can take 60–120 mg twice a day of a standardized product containing flavone glycosides and 6% terpene lactones.

Homeopathy

This condition demands attention and treatment from an experienced homeopath due to its chronic and complex nature, and its potentially severe symptoms. If the patient's energy levels are severely depleted, choosing the appropriate strength remedy and dosage can be difficult, and is best left in the hands of a trained practitioner. The advice below offers some guidelines on how best to support homeopathic remedies with lifestyle changes

Pace yourself: One of the most important things to bear in mind is not to overdo things on days when you do feel better, as this can trigger a relapse. Instead pace yourself, and stop after achieving about 50% of what you would ideally like to do. As frustrating as this may be, it will give you the best chance of building on your recovery.

Gentle exercise: Once your physical strength has shown signs of steadily building and increasing, it can be helpful to engage in some gentle yoga to encourage energy levels to improve, while also having a potentially beneficial effect on the immune system. Consult an experienced practitioner who will be able to tailor his or her advice to your individual situation.

Herbalism

Herbal medicines are used to treat CFS to support the adrenals, thereby reducing fatigue, and to modulate the immune system to bring it back into a normal state.

Licorice: One theory used to explain fatigue associated with CFS is that adrenal depletion from excessive daily stress leads to lower levels of cortisol, the body's natural anti-inflammatory. A compound in licorice called glycyrrhetinic acid prolongs the life of natural cortisol by inhibiting its breakdown. Licorice is also high in flavonoids, which are potent antioxidants that protect and strengthen tissues, making the body more resistant to infection. Take 2–4 ml of 1:1 tincture of licorice per day. Licorice used in the long term may cause high blood pressure, so make sure your blood pressure is monitored regularly.

Astragalus root: This herb has been used in Chinese medicine for centuries. It is considered to be a potent herb that tonifies the Qi (life energy) and is nutritive to the life force and body, hence its use in treating fatigue. Current research has shown astragalus to be effective for long-term use in the prevention of infection by supporting the immune system. Active constituents called saponins stimulate immune cells, including NK cells, which are depleted in CFS. Astragalus also demonstrates adaptogenic, diuretic, hypotensive, and antioxidant properties. Boil 10–30 g of dried root in water and drink the decoction daily. Astragalus is safe to use long term, but should not be used during acute infections.

Sprains

Diagnosis

A sprain occurs when you stretch or tear a ligament, a strong band of tissue that connects one bone to another to support your joints. The ankle and wrist are particularly vulnerable to sprains and are the most commonly affected parts of the body. Sprains generally result from a sports injury or a fall. They cause pain, swelling, and bruising in the affected joint, and the skin around the injury often turns blue. This occurs when the small blood vessels and fibers in the flesh burst, causing blood to enter the surrounding tissue. When this happens the injured area must be kept still or the bleeding may become worse. If you suffer a sprain, rest the affected joint for one or two days, but it is then important to start moving again to reduce the amount of scarring formed in the damaged area. When the pain and swelling have subsided, start exercising the injured part of the body gently. As with any activity, warm up slowly and begin with stretching exercises.

Symptoms

- Pain and tenderness
- Swelling
- Redness or bruising
- Loss of mobility in affected area

Treatment Goal

Consult a doctor to confirm that you do have a sprain. Conventional and complementary therapies can help to reduce the pain and discomfort and speed up recovery from an injury.

Conventional Medicine

Use the RICE therapy: The mainstay of treatment for a sprain is rest, ice, compression, and elevation (RICE). Elevate the affected joint whenever possible, and apply ice to the injury for 20 minutes three times a day. An Ace wrap (an elastic bandage) can be wrapped around the injury to provide support and compression. Most sprains heal completely with conservative treatment.

Splints and crutches: In the past mild sprains were sometimes put into a cast and immobilized, but this is now associated with injuries that require longer healing times. Plaster splinting is now reserved for more severe sprains, and usually remains on for three weeks. Crutches are used until a few steps can be taken without pain.

Medication: The pain caused by a sprain can be managed by using non-steroidal anti-inflammatory drugs (NSAIDs), such as ibuprofen and acetaminophen. If this does not take care of the pain, opioid analgesics (such as hydrocodone and oxycodone) can be used. Once swelling has subsided and you can begin to put weight on the affected joint, begin to exercise gently. Motion exercises and muscle strengthening are both important, and can be supervised by a physiotherapist if necessary.

Surgery: Severe sprains that do not respond to conservative management are treated with surgical repair.

Traditional Chinese Medicine

Herbs: Apply Wan Hua oil to the sprained area twice a day. It helps reduce pain and promotes local circulation. You can find this at a Chinese medicine pharmacy. You can also take Du Huo Ji Shen Wan or Yuan Hu Suo Zhi Tong pills in combination with acupressure and external herbal medicine.

Acupressure: Lie on your stomach and have someone press the Cheng Shan and Cheng Jin points on the back of your legs for one minute, then release and repeat. When the leg is stretched with the toes pointing out, the Cheng Shan point is in the depression between the muscles on the back of the leg. The Cheng Jin point can be found about 4 inches below the bend in the back of the leg.

Diet: As general practice, eat a well-balanced diet that includes plenty of fruits, vegetables, and grains. Drink plenty of water as part of your daily routine. Have fresh food, but avoid shrimp, beef, lamb, and chili peppers since they may interfere with your herbal treatment and increase heat in your body.

Naturopathy

Diet: Follow an anti-inflammatory diet to help with the healing process. Cold-water fish, such as salmon, sea bass, tuna, trout, and mackerel, contain high amounts of omega-3 essential fatty acids, which have been shown to fight inflammation. Pineapple contains bromelain, a powerful enzyme that has been shown to have anti-inflammatory effects on muscle and tissue. Bromelain also breaks down fibrin, a blood-clotting protein that can impede circulation and prevent tissues from draining properly. It also blocks the production of certain compounds that cause swelling and pain. Apples and onions are high in quercetin, a flavonoid that can help reduce inflammation in the joints and muscles. Include anti-inflammatory spices such as turmeric and ginger in your meals, and drink at least eight glasses of water a day, to flush out waste material and metabolites from the system, which increase inflammation and inhibit the healing process. Whole grains, fresh fruit, and vegetables should be a staple in your diet to providing the muscles with all the nourishment they need to assist in the healing process.

Supplements: Proteolytic enzymes destroy free radicals, which inhibit healing, and proteins involved in the inflammatory process. Take three tablets or capsules between meals. Vitamin C is required for the formation of connective tissue and to combat free radicals. Essential fatty acids such as flaxseed and fish oil reduce inflammation and promote tissue healing. Take 5 g of fish oils a day or 1–2 tbsp of flaxseed oil. Take 1,500 mg of glucosamine sulfate a day to provide the raw material for the body to manufacture ligaments and tendons. Take 50,000 IU of beta-carotene per day to make collagen, which can help repair connective tissue. Take 15–30 mg of zinc a day to help you heal faster, along with 2 mg of copper to avoid copper deficiency.

Herbs: Ginger has anti-inflammatory properties that help with pain, and is available in many different forms. You can take ginger as a standardized extract in pill form, 100–200 mg every four hours up to three times a day; as a fresh powder, ½–¾ tsp every four hours up to three times a day; or raw, ¼–½-inch (peeled) slice of ginger every four hours up to three times a day. Ginger tea is available in prepackaged bags or can be prepared by steeping ½ tsp of grated ginger root in 8 oz of very hot water for 5–10 minutes. A cup of tea, when steeped for this amount of time, can contain about 250 mg of ginger. Do not take more than 1 g of ginger a day if you are pregnant. Take 500 mg of bromelain three times a day for its natural anti-inflammatory effects. Turmeric makes the effect of bromelain stronger, has anti-inflammatory properties, and is a strong antioxidant. Take 250–500 mg of turmeric three times a day between meals. Boswellia also has strong anti-inflammatory properties. Take 1,500 mg three times a day, but make sure it is a product that contains 60–65% boswellic acids. White willow bark is a natural pain reliever. Take 30–60 mg a day of an extract standardized to salicin.

> *Tip:* USE CASTOR OIL
>
> To relieve pain and swelling, apply castor oil directly to the skin and cover it with a clean, soft cloth and plastic wrap. Place a heated towel over the pack and leave it on for 30–60 minutes. For the best results, repeat for three consecutive days.

Homeopathy

The remedies below can play a complementary role in speeding up recovery from a mild to moderate sprain, provided the necessary first aid measures have been taken. To treat a severe sprain that requires a plaster cast and even surgery, consult an experienced homeopathic practitioner.

Arnica: As well as helping the body deal with shock following an injury, Arnica will help ease pain and encourage the reabsorption of blood from engorged tissues.

Bryonia: If Arnica has been initially helpful in reducing pain and swelling, but has ceased to improve the situation any further, try Bryonia. Use it when pain is aggravated by movement of any kind, and there is an obvious improvement when keeping the affected limb firmly supported and rested.

Rhus tox: This remedy can help to relieve the pain and stiffness of a sprain that has passed the initial stage of trauma. Unlike the symptoms that respond well to Bryonia, pain and stiffness is made worse by resting, and is eased by gentle movement for a limited period of time. It can also be used to follow Arnica appropriately.

Ledum: If a sprain is stiff, painful, and hot, but not red in appearance, try using Ledum. Pain and discomfort is soothed and relieved by cool applications, and aggravated by becoming warm, especially in bed at night.

Ruta: This remedy can follow either Bryonia or Rhus tox to support the final stage of recovery from an established sprain. It is appropriate if stiffness and pain lodges in one area, as though a nail were sticking into the affected joint. Ruta can treat sprains that affect the wrists, knees, or ankles.

Herbalism

Compresses: Apply ice to acute sprains for three to five minutes as often as can be tolerated within the first 24–48 hours after the injury. On the third day, begin contrasting hot compresses (apply for three minutes) with ice packs (apply for 30 seconds). Arnica, which has anti-inflammatory action, can be applied in a gel or lotion form with the ice to assist tissue healing and decrease swelling and pain. The arnica should be continued for several days, even when you make the transition to ice alternating with heat.

Essential oils: Prior to applying ice or heat, massage a few drops of essential oil of wintergreen or peppermint, commonly available in small vials from stores that sell herbal medicines, into the sprain. These oils penetrate the skin and have anti-inflammatory action; in particular, the peppermint oil deadens the pain sensation transmitted by nerves, providing comfort as the sprain heals. Any oil or plant product applied topically has the potential to cause skin irritation in some people. If redness, itchiness, or blistering occurs, cease using the oils and check with a medical herbalist or your doctor for guidance. Dilute in base oil before applying to the skin to reduce incidence of irritation.

Comfrey: A poultice may be made by crushing the fresh root and applying it topically; holding it in place with a cloth. Alternatively, a compress may be made by decocting the dried root for 10 minutes and soaking a cloth in the strained liquid when cool enough. This can be applied to the affected area, and held in place with a waterproof barrier. Comfrey root helps to reduce the inflammation, but should not be used on broken skin or internally. Creams containing comfrey may also be obtained from a herbal store or practitioner.

Pain relief: Some herbs with pain-relieving properties include meadowsweet, turmeric, and cayenne. Combine equal parts of these herbs, except cayenne, which should only make up 2–5% of the blend. Infuse 1 tbsp of this mixture per cup of water and drink every three to four hours as needed for pain relief. 🌿

Tip: USE ARNICA CREAM

Apply arnica cream to the affected area as soon as possible after the injury has been sustained to ease bruising and swelling. However, do not use this cream if the surface of the skin has been broken, since it may cause inflammation at the edges of the wound or be absorbed systematically.

Tendonitis

Diagnosis

Tendonitis is the painful inflammation of a tendon, a sinew-like tissue that joins muscles to bones. When a tendon becomes inflamed, the action of pulling the muscle is irritating, causing pain and making movement difficult. The most common cause of tendonitis is the overuse of a particular muscle. This can occur through exercise, particularly when a new exercise program is begun or the level of exercise is increased. The risk of tendonitis also increases with age. The symptoms of tendonitis usually subside after a few days, but they can last for up to six weeks in more severe cases. The areas of the body that are prone to tendonitis include the Achilles tendon, shoulders, and wrists.

Symptoms

- Restricted movement in the affected area
- Tenderness and pain
- Swelling
- Weakness

Treatment Goal

Pain management is the primary goal. Once the pain has eased, treatment involves increasing the range of motion and building strength in the tendons to protect against further injuries.

Conventional Medicine

Rest and ice: Initial treatment is to immobilize the affected area and rest it from the trigger activity. However, a shoulder should not be immobilized as it may become "frozen." A sling, heel pads, or splints may be used at the discretion of the doctor to keep the area stable. Applying ice to the affected site for 15–20 minutes is often helpful.

Exercise: Once the initial pain has subsided, begin an exercise program to restore the range of motion and strengthen the tendons. Hydrotherapy, or water aerobics, is a good form of exercise to restore muscle function, as the buoyancy of the water supports the body. Physical therapy is recommended to strengthen tendons and prevent recurrence.

Medication: Non-steroidal anti-inflammatory drugs (NSAIDs) can be used to relieve pain as needed. Steroids are sometimes injected into the joint associated with the tendonitis.

Ultrasound therapy: High-power focal ultrasound therapy, also known as shock-wave therapy (a non-invasive treatment in which high-energy shock waves are passed through the skin to the affected area), can have positive effects if small calcium deposits have developed in the tendon. Therapeutic ultrasound without focal pulses can be used to treat pain and swelling with or without calcifications.

Traditional Chinese Medicine

Herbs: Consult a doctor of Chinese medicine for a particular herbal medicine that can reduce the pain and inflammation. The herbs recommended will depend on the particular condition. In some cases, you may only need acupuncture treatment.

Acupressure: Consult your doctor before performing acupressure to treat your condition. Treatment may not be suitable for your condition.

Diet: No specific foods are recommended for tendonitis; however, maintain a well-balanced diet to promote good health. Eat fresh food and drink adequate amounts of water daily. Avoid shrimp, beef, lamb, and chili peppers. They may interfere with your herbal treatment and increase heat in the body.

Naturopathy

Inflammation is the cause of pain and discomfort in cases of tendonitis. See Sprains (p. 331) for guidelines on an anti-inflammatory diet as well as supplements and herbs that can help ease the pain of tendonitis by reducing inflammation. Below are some suggestions of other types of therapies that can relieve the pain.

Prolotherapy: With this treatment, a solution of simple compounds (usually dextrose or calcium carbonate) is injected at the point of the injury. This triggers an inflammation response that increases the blood supply and delivers the nutrients necessary to promote the growth of new cells and repair damaged connective tissue. Consult a naturopathic practitioner who practices prolotherapy regarding treatment.

Massage and hydrotherapy: Massage may be helpful in relieving pain and improving range of motion. Find a qualified massage therapist who has experience with tendonitis. Apply ice to the area for the first 48 hours and then try contrast hydrotherapy, alternating hot and cold applications. Soak the affected part for three minutes in hot water, then 30 seconds in cold water.

Ultrasonography (phonophoresis): This type of therapy involves using high-frequency sound to heat an area and increase the blood supply. This treatment can be offered by a chiropractor or sports injury clinic.

TENS: Transcutaneous electrical nerve stimulation (TENS) electricity can be used to control pain. This treatment can be offered by a chiropractor or at any sports injury clinic.

Homeopathy

The following remedies can be helpful in providing complementary support to ease the pain and distress of a recent mild to moderate episode of tendon inflammation. However, more severe examples of this problem, such as those involving the Achilles tendon, will require professional homeopathic assessment and treatment.

Ruta: Consider using this remedy if the affected area feels broken, achy, sore, and bruised internally. Inflamed tendons in the ankle joint are tender enough to cause temporary lameness. This may lead to a feeling of general weakness in the legs, with a tendency for the knees to give way when going up and down stairs.

Bryonia: If inflammation and pain are obviously aggravated by even the slightest movement, and clearly eased by keeping the affected area as still and rested as possible, use Bryonia.

Rhus tox: This remedy can be helpful if the affected area feels hot and inflamed, and if tearing pains are noticeably troublesome when trying to rest. Symptoms temporarily improve with gentle movement, and by taking a warm bath or shower.

Herbalism

As with many musculoskeletal problems such as shin splints and repetitive strain injuries, arnica and rue are good topical treatments to combat the inflammation, leading to pain relief and healing of the damaged tissues.

Arnica and rue: Start by icing the site for three to five minutes, then apply a poultice of arnica flowers with about 1 tsp of rue oil added, or as advised by your herbal medicine practitioner. This herbal blend should only be used topically, and can be applied several times per day. In between applications and at night, a castor oil pack would be useful (see below).

Castor oil: This oil can be massaged into the inflamed area. Alternatively, to make a pack, soak a washcloth and apply it to the site, covering it with plastic wrap and an elastic bandage to hold it in place. Allow 30–60 minutes to let the castor oil soak into the tissues. You can also apply the oil before going to bed and leave it on overnight. The castor oil acts to calm the pain, redness, swelling, and inflammation associated with the tendonitis.

Comfrey: Comfrey can be used topically to relieve pain and fight the inflammation associated with tendonitis. Comfrey is cooling and moisturizing and acts as a mild analgesic and potent anti-inflammatory. You might be advised to use a poultice of fresh or moistened roots and leaves by mashing them into a paste (add water if needed). Place the poultice on the affected tendon when you are not using the other treatments described above. Ointments or oils with comfrey can also be used. Do not use comfrey on broken skin. It is also not advised to use comfrey root internally.

Wintergreen oil: Wintergreen essential oil has anti-inflammatory properties and may be used topically by diluting a few drops in base oil or cream, and massaging into the affected area. Wintergreen contains salicylates, which may cause sensitivity in some. It is also used for rheumatic joints, muscle pain, and neuralgia.

Headache

Diagnosis

Headaches involve mild to severe pain in one or more parts of the head, and can also cause problems in the neck. A headache can occur for a variety of reasons—and sometimes for no reason at all. They can be triggered by being overtired, feeling stressed, watching too much TV, or sitting in front of a computer for a long period of time. Eating the wrong types of foods can often cause problems, as can missing a meal altogether. Some common medical conditions associated with headaches include colds, flu, sinusitis and catarrh, earache, toothache, dehydration, and sunstroke. While painful, the majority of headaches do not indicate a serious disorder. A tension headache, the most common type of headache, results from the contraction of the head and neck muscles.

DANGER: If any of the following symptoms occur, contact your doctor immediately: a sudden, severe headache accompanied by nausea and vomiting; persistent and recurring headaches accompanied by problems with memory; a high fever with neck stiffness; loss of feeling in the arms and legs; and/or convulsion.

Symptoms

- Head pain can range from a mild ache to a deep throbbing
- Throbbing and pulsating pain may be worse on one side of the head
- Feeling of tightness and constriction in the head
- Pain may be accompanied by other symptoms such as nausea and visual disturbances
- Sensitivity to loud noises and bright lights
- Irritability and tiredness

Treatment Goal

It may be possible to identify a pattern of when headaches occur and thereby pinpoint a trigger. Treatment aims to relieve acute symptoms, rule out any serious complications, and identify and avoid triggers.

Conventional Medicine

To treat headaches it is necessary to identify the type of headache experienced. Headaches can be vascular in nature, such as migraines, tension headaches, or cluster headaches, or due to an infection, trauma medication, high blood pressure, or a tumor. Depression and anxiety can also be associated with headaches. A severe headache that comes on suddenly should be evaluated by a doctor.

Keep a diary: A headache diary should be kept so that triggers can be tracked. Once a cause can be isolated, make any necessary modifications to your lifestyle or diet to avoid further episodes.

Preventive measures: Magnesium supplements in the form of magnesium aspartate can be helpful in preventing headaches. Coenzyme Q10, 300 mg per day,

can improve headaches, as can riboflavin, 150 mg per day. Beta-blocker drugs are also used as a preventive measure. Relaxation and stress-reduction techniques are also worthwhile and have been shown to help prevent headaches.

Medication: The medication usually used to treat tension headaches (the most common type) is acetaminophen or non-steroidal anti-inflammatory drugs. Caffeine is sometimes added to these preparations to enhance the body's ability to absorb the drugs.

Traditional Chinese Medicine

Herbs: For each formula, place the herbs in a ceramic or glass pot. Add 3 cups of water, bring to a boil, and simmer for 30 minutes. Strain the liquid and drink 1 cup twice a day. Consult a TCM practitioner for diagnosis and advice on herbal remedies before using the formulas below.
• **To treat headaches caused by blood stagnation:** Symptoms include nausea, sharp spasms of pain, and irritation from bright lights and sounds. Mix 10 g of Chuan Xiong (Szechuan lovage root), 12 g of Chi Shao (red

peony root), 10 g of Dang Gui (Chinese angelica), 12 g of Yan Hu Suo (corydalis rhizome), and 12 g of Niu Xi (achyranthes root).
• **To treat sinus headaches:** Symptoms include pain and pressure in the sinuses. Mix 10 g of Bai Zhi (angelica dahurica), 12 g of Fang Fen (ledebouriella root), 10 g of Chai Hu (hare's ear root), 12 g of Bai Shao (white peony root), 3 g of Gan Cao (licorice root), and 12 g of Niu Bang Zi (great burdock fruit seed).
• **To treat headaches due to Qi and blood deficiency:** Symptoms include a dull pain,

tiredness, and dizziness. Mix 12 g of Huang Jing (Siberian Solomon seal rhizome), 12 g of Huang Qi (milk-vetch root), 12 g of Tai Zi Shen (pseudostellaria), 12 g of Dan Shen (salvia root), and six pieces of Da Zhao (Chinese jujube).

Acupressure: Press the Tai Yang, Feng Chi, and Shu Gu points. The Feng Chi points are at the back of the head and at the base of the skull, 2 inches from either side of the center point. The Tai Yang point is at the temple, in the depression between the lateral end of the eyebrow and eyelid. Press these points and hold for one minute. The Shu Gu point is on the outside edge of the foot. Beginning at the little toe, move your finger along the edge of the foot until you feel a depression. Press this point with the tip of your finger for one minute.

Diet: Sweet basil, peppermint, spearmint, rosemary, green onion, radishes, watermelons, bananas, and spinach are recommended to help ease headaches. It is also important to drink an adequate amount of water every day.

Naturopathy

Diet: Eat whole foods that are low in refined sugars and food additives, which can contribute to headaches. Headaches can also be linked to constipation, so eat foods that are high in fiber, such as fresh vegetables and fruits, beans, and whole grains, and drink 8–10 glasses of water a day as a preventive measure. Consuming calcium and magnesium can also prevent against headaches. Good sources are green leafy vegetables, beans, almonds, walnuts, and wheat germ. Salmon and mackerel are high in omega-3 fatty acids, which may also help in preventing headaches. Be mindful of foods that trigger headaches and eliminate them from your diet. The most common food allergens are wheat, dairy, eggs, corn, citrus fruits, soy products, chocolate, alcohol, pork, and yeast. Additives such as monosodium glutamate (MSG) can trigger headaches as well as artificial flavoring and nitrates, which can be found in cold cuts and hot dogs. Avoid sugary foods and junk food at all costs.

Supplements: Take 250 mg of magnesium three times a day as it has been shown to alleviate headaches and prevent them. Take 50 mg of vitamin B6 a day. It is partially involved in the synthesis of serotonin, a neurotransmitter found to be deficient in those that suffer from migraines. Take 400 mg of riboflavin (vitamin B2) a day and 100 mg of 5-hytroxytrptophan (5-HTP) three times a day, both of which have been shown to be effective in preventing migraines. Take 5 g of fish oils daily for their anti-inflammatory effect, and 1,000 mg of calcium a day for its ability to relax the nervous system and muscles.

Herbs: Feverfew has been shown to reduce the duration and frequency of headaches. Take 250–500 mcg daily of a product standardized to contain parthenolides. You can also try applying peppermint and menthol cream to the temple area to relieve tension headaches. Take 60–120 mg of white willow bark a day as it is an effective pain reliever. Ginger has anti-inflammatory benefits and relieves pain. Take 1–2 g or 1–2 ml of a tincture three times a day.

Tip: PEPPERMINT OR LAVENDER OIL COMPRESS

Peppermint or lavender oil can help relieve pain in some patients. Add 2 drops of peppermint or lavender oil to 1 cup of water. Soak a cloth in the solution and apply it as a compress to the head.

Homeopathy

The following remedies can help a recent, mild to moderate headache that has set in as a response to an obvious trigger. To treat recurrent, severe conditions, consult a professional homeopath.

Nux vomica: If a headache has symptoms of a hangover, whether too much alcohol has been consumed or not, try Nux vomica. Classic symptoms include pain that may lodge at the back of the head and neck, or radiate over one eye, queasiness and nausea, and a general sense of feeling "toxic." Pain and discomfort is more intense and distressing when getting up and moving around, while some relief is gained from resting in a quiet room, or holding the head still.

Bryonia: Consider using this remedy if headaches have been set off by low-grade dehydration, which is often accompanied by constipation. Pain tends to lodge at the front of the head, often setting in above the right eye and radiating to the back of the neck. Discomfort is made worse by the slightest movement, and bending forward. Pain feels eased by cool air and cool compresses, by applying firm pressure, and when resting in one position.

Pulsatilla: Cluster (several simultaneous) headaches may respond well to this remedy, especially if they are associated with hormonal changes that occur premenstrually. Symptoms, which include dizziness and nausea, are worse when in stuffy, overheated surroundings, while taking gentle exercise in fresh air helps.

Tip: RELAX

If stress and tension levels are high, try to keep your face and jaw muscles relaxed. Loosen your neck and shoulders to avoid tight back muscles. If trying to consciously let go and relax these areas isn't enough, try taking up yoga, T'ai chi, or Pilates.

Herbalism

Pain-relieving tea or tincture: Sitting for hours at a desk, daily stress, poor diet, and lack of exercise and sleep all result in inflammation and spasm in the muscles of the back, shoulders, neck, and scalp, which can lead to a headache. A combination of several herbs in tea or tincture form can relax the muscles and provide anti-inflammatory relief. Valerian is an effective anti-inflammatory, antispasmodic, and analgesic which helps to relieve pain and tension associated with headaches. It is also a sedative herb, which can help to relieve any associated insomnia. Willow bark contains mildly anti-inflammatory salicylates, which are similar to those found in aspirin. Willow bark is used to relieve pain related to muscle and joint inflammation. Other herbs with pain-relieving properties include meadowsweet and turmeric. A blend of all of these herbs might be recommended by your herbal expert, as an infusion or a tincture.

To treat headaches due to insomnia: If stress and insomnia are the causes of the headache, create a soothing blend of herbs to stop the mind chatter and allow you to let go of the day's events. Chamomile can be used to treat nervous irritability and mental restlessness. Lavender relieves muscle spasms, which result in headaches, and calms nervous exhaustion. Skullcap is a bitter, cooling plant from the mint family used to relieve fear, anxiety, and restless sleep. Again, a blend in the form of an infusion or tincture might be recommended by your herbal expert. Lavender aromatherapy is also effective for tension and insomnia.

Migraine

Diagnosis

A migraine is a headache that is so severe that it prevents you from continuing with your normal everyday activities. Migraines are believed to be caused by the release of the chemical serotonin into the bloodstream, resulting in changes in the neurotransmitters and blood vessels in the brain. Exactly what causes this to happen is still uncertain; however, various factors have been identified that may trigger attacks in susceptible people, including stress, poor diet, environmental issues, fatigue, and hormones such as estrogen. For most people it is not just one trigger, but a combination of several aggravating factors that cause an attack.

Symptoms

- Intense throbbing pain on one side of the head
- Visual disturbances such as distorted vision and flashing lights
- Nausea, vomiting, and/or diarrhea
- Increased sensitivity to light, smells, and sounds
- Stiff neck
- Lack of concentration

Treatment Goal

To reduce the severity of attacks. Treatment aims to relieve symptoms and identify triggers to prevent future episodes.

Conventional Medicine

The goal of conventional treatment is to prevent headaches from occurring or to reduce the frequency of attacks. A severe migraine that does not respond to treatment should be evaluated by a doctor.

Medication: Once a migraine has occurred, it is treated by acetaminophen or non-steroidal anti-inflammatory drugs (NSAIDs). Trials show that these medications are more effective than a placebo, but they are not specific for migraine headaches. A more appropriate first-line migraine treatment is a class of drugs called triptans. Sumatriptan and naratriptan are in this category. Ergotamines can also be used to treat severe headaches, unless the patient has a history of coronary artery disease. Sometimes anti-emetic drugs are added to treat the nausea and vomiting that can accompany a migraine. Prophylactic treatment, which protects those prone to migraines, includes beta blockers, tricyclic antidepressants, gabapentin, and verapamil.

Prevention: Eliminate foods that trigger migraines (these may include caffeine, alcohol, nitrites, coffee, and cheeses) and reduce your stress levels as much as possible. Magnesium aspartate and B vitamins, especially riboflavin, along with the herbs butterbur and feverfew, have been shown to be effective in treating migraines. Acupuncture and chiropractic treatment may also be worthwhile.

Traditional Chinese Medicine

Herbs: For each formula, make a decoction. Mix the herbs in a ceramic pot and add 3 cups of water. Bring to a boil and simmer for 30 minutes. Strain and drink 1 cup twice a day.
• **Formula one:** Mix 12 g of Tian Ma (gastrodia rhizome), 12 g of Guo Teng (stem and thorns of gambir vine), 10 g of Du Zhong (eucommia bark), 10 g of Zhi Zi (cape jasmine fruit), 15 g of Niu Xi (achyranthes root), 8 g of Chai Hu (hare's ear root), 12 g of Bai Shao (white peony root), 10 g of Dan Pi (cortex of tree peony root), and 10 g of Chuan Xiong (Szechuan lovage root).
• **Formula two:** Mix 10 g of Huang Qi (milk-vetch root), 10 g of ginseng, 12 g of Bai Zhu (white atractylodes rhizome), 12 g of Chuan Xiong (Szechuan lovage root), 6 g of Sheng Ma (bugbane rhizome), and 12 g of Bai Shao (white peony root).

Acupressure: The Shuai Gu point is located on the head directly above the top of the ear, 1½ inches past the hairline. Use your thumb to apply pressure to this point for one minute and then repeat. The Tai Yang point is situated at the temple, in the depression between the lateral end of the eyebrow and eyelid. Apply medium pressure to this point with the tip of your finger. The Yang Bai point can be found on the forehead, 1 inch above the eyebrow and in line with the pupil. Press this point for one to two minutes with the tip of your finger.

Diet: Sweet basil, radish, watermelon, banana, spinach, orange squash, green onion, and spearmint are recommended foods.

Naturopathy

Diet: Be mindful of foods that can trigger migraines and eliminate them from your diet. The most common culprits are wheat, dairy, eggs, corn, citrus fruits, soy products, chocolate, wine, alcohol, pork, tea, and yeast. Additives such as monosodium glutamate (MSG) can trigger headaches, as can artificial flavorings and nitrates, which can be found in cold cuts and hot dogs. Avoid sugary foods and junk food at all cost, and cut out cold foods and drinks since they may trigger headaches. Instead, eat whole foods that are minimally processed and low in refined sugars. Constipation is linked to migraines, so guard against this by eating foods that are high in fiber, such as fresh vegetables and fruits, beans, and whole grains, and by drinking 8–10 glasses of water every day. Consuming good sources of calcium and magnesium, such as green leafy vegetables, beans, almonds, walnuts, and wheat germ, and foods high in omega-3 fatty acids, such as salmon, can also prevent migraines.

Supplements: Take 250 mg of magnesium three times a day as it has been shown to alleviate and prevent headaches. Take 50 g of vitamin B6 a day. It is partially involved in the synthesis of serotonin, a neurotransmitter that is deficient in those that suffer from migraines. Take 400 mg of riboflavin (vitamin B2) a day, and 100 mg of 5-hytroxytrptophan (5-HTP) three times a day; both have been shown to be effective in preventing migraines. Also take 5 g of fish oil a day for its anti-inflammatory effect and 1,000 mg of calcium a day to relax the nervous system and muscles.

Herbs: Feverfew has been shown to reduce the duration and frequency of migraines. Take 250–500 mg daily of a product standardized to contain parthenolides. White willow bark is an effective pain reliever and can be taken at 60–120 mg a day. Also take 1–2 g of ginger, or 1–2 ml of a tincture, three times a day for its anti-inflammatory benefits and ability to relieve pain. Do not take more than 1 g of ginger a day if you are pregnant.

Tip: TRY TO REDUCE STRESS

Massage the upper neck and back for a few minutes for instant relief, and take deep breaths to make sure your body is getting an appropriate amount of oxygen.

Homeopathy

Any of the remedies listed below may help to ease the acute symptoms of a migraine and promote recovery. Recurrent, severe migraines will benefit most from treatment by a practitioner.

Nux vomica: If migraine has developed in response to stress, too little sleep, too much alcohol, or too much junk food, try Nux vomica. It can also be helpful to treat migraines triggered by an overreliance on painkillers or sleeping tablets. As well as feeling sick and hungover after waking, sufferers are likely to be hypersensitive to noise. Additional, symptoms include constipation and queasiness.

Lachesis: Consider this remedy when a migraine is felt on the left side of the head, or moves from above the left eye to the right. It is also appropriate for women who suffer from migraines mid-cycle to the onset of a period. Symptoms include feeling aggravated when waking up, and bursting or constricting pains. There may be disorientation that is more intense when the eyes are closed. An episode may be a response to overexposure to sunshine, or becoming overheated.

Sulphur: This remedy is helpful for a migraine that has been triggered by low blood-sugar levels. Symptoms include a throbbing sensation in the crown of the head, where the brain feels constricted, and dizziness that is made worse by bending forward. Eating a small snack at frequent intervals eases symptoms.

Tip: REGULATE YOUR SLEEP PATTERNS

It is often easy to overlook the importance of regular, refreshing sleep, especially when life is demanding. Burning the candle at both ends can lead to stress-related migraines. To prevent this from occurring, avoid engaging in demanding mental work just before going to bed, and using caffeine and alcohol to stay awake. Instead adopt a regular sleep routine.

Herbalism

Migraines can be very debilitating and, at times, difficult to treat. Symptoms associated with migraines include nausea, vomiting, dizziness, and tinnitus. In addition to adding herbs to your migraine repertoire, also consider identifying and avoiding potential food intolerances and environmental allergies, and take supplements of particular minerals (e.g., magnesium) and vitamins (e.g., B2 and B6) that are often found to be deficient in migraine sufferers.

Feverfew: Although very useful to treat and prevent migraines, other traditional uses of feverfew are for healing colds, coughs, fever, and dyspepsia. The active constituents found in feverfew are sesquiterpene lactones such as parthenolide, which are thought to contribute to its anti-inflammatory action; flavonoids, which are antioxidant and heal and stabilize vascular tissue; essential oils; and small amounts of melatonin, which promotes the release of growth hormone, the body's natural rejuvenator. Clinical studies have shown feverfew to effectively treat and reduce the frequency of migraines when 100 mg of the dried herb, standardized to contain at least 0.6 mg of parthenolide, is taken twice daily. Side effects are rare, but include mouth ulcers (from fresh leaves), indigestion, and diarrhea. Traditionally, fresh leaves are used and seen as more effective in treating migraines. Due to the side effect of fresh leaves causing mouth ulcers, it is often recommended to roll 2–3 leaves in a little bread before taking, to reduce contact with the mucous membranes of the mouth.

Skullcap: This herb helps to relieve migraines due to its anti-inflammatory and antispasmodic properties. It is also a nervine herb that aids relaxation and relieves nervous tension; which is particularly beneficial for stress-triggered migraines. Skullcap tincture may be taken 2–4 ml three times daily. An infusion may also be made by infusing 2–3 g in a cup of boiling water for 10 minutes. Drink three times daily.

Neuralgia

Diagnosis

Neuralgia is a type of nerve pain that is often described as a burning or shooting sensation. The most common forms are trigeminal neuralgia and post-herpetic neuralgia.

Trigeminal neuralgia affects the face. Symptoms include severe face pain, which can be triggered by a simple action such as swallowing or brushing the teeth. The frequency of attacks is variable, but pain can sometimes strike several times a day. Once the condition has been diagnosed, individual triggers must be identified and avoided.

Post-herpetic neuralgia is associated with the virus that causes chickenpox and shingles. After the scabs have resolved, the area where the rash was becomes painful. The condition can last from a few weeks to several months.

Symptoms

- Stabbing, burning, or lancing pains
- Pains may last from a few seconds to over a minute
- Pains are brought on by touching a trigger point, or activities such as chewing or brushing the teeth

Treatment Goal

It is necessary to identify and avoid triggers as much as possible. Treatment also aims to develop ways of managing the pain when an attack occurs.

Conventional Medicine

Neuralgia can have many causes and ultimately treatment depends on identifying the source of the pain. This may involve an in-depth assessment from a neurologist or general practitioner. Some conditions that may cause neuralgia are metabolic disease such as diabetes or vitamin deficiency, inflammatory disease such as swelling around the nerves, infections, tumors, a reaction to medication, and toxins such as pesticides.

Medication: There are numerous medications used to treat this condition. A category of drugs called tricyclic antidepressants can be used. Paxil, a newer antidepressant, is also used to treat neuralgia. A class of drugs called anti-eleptics, which includes carbamazepine (Tegretol®), gabapentin (Neurontin®), topiramate (Topamax®), and lamotrigine (Lamictal®) are often prescribed. Analgesic pain-relieving drugs may be used as well. Tramadol, morphine, and oxycodone are sometimes needed to treat the serious pain of neuralgia. Topical anesthetics such as a lidocaine patch can also ease symptoms.

Other types of therapy: Patients may need to begin counseling, since psychological issues can make neuralgia worse. Also, physical therapy may be helpful, as well as stress-reduction techniques.

Traditional Chinese Medicine

Herbs: According to traditional Chinese medicine theory, the numbness, tingling, and pain of neuralgia are caused by poor circulation. To treat this mix 12 g of Huang Qi (milk-vetch root), 12 g of Fang Fen (ledebouriella root), 12 g of Qiang Huo (notopterygium root), 12 g of Chi Shao (red peony root), 10 g of Chen Xiang (aloeswood), 12 g of Dang Gui (Chinese angelica), 8 g of fresh ginger, and five pieces of Da Zhao (Chinese jujube). Place these herbs in a ceramic or glass pot and add 3 cups of water. Bring to a boil and simmer for 30 minutes. Strain and drink 1 cup twice a day.

Acupressure: Gently massage the area that is numb and aching. Press the Xue Hai, Yin Ling Quan, and Jie Xi points to treat the upper extremities, and the Qu Chi and Wai Guan points to treat the lower extremities. The Xue Hai point is on the inside of the leg, in the depression just above the knee. The Yin Ling Quan point is in the depression on the inside of the lower leg, about 3 inches below the kneecap. The Jie Xi point is found on the crease between the foot and the leg, in the depression between the tendon of the big toe and the smaller toes. With the elbow flexed, you will find the Qu Chi point on the outside of the elbow at the lateral end of the crease. The Wai Guan point is on the top side of the lower arm, about 1 inch above the center of the wrist. Apply pressure to these points for one to two minutes at a time.

Diet: Eat foods that help circulation, such as spinach, bamboo shoots, ginger, and green onions.

Naturopathy

Diet: Eat foods that are high in B vitamins, which are healing to the nervous system. These include wheatgerm, brewer's yeast, eggs, and whole grains. Brightly colored fruits and vegetables such as squash, carrots, berries, and oranges have high amounts of bioflavonoids and vitamins C and A, which will help resolve inflammation and blisters of the skin, and increase the efficiency of the body's immune system. A freshly pressed green vegetable juice a day will give you essential nutrients to alkalinize the body and boost immunity. Avoid meat, fried foods, sugar, chocolate, and sodas, which suppress the immune system and interfere with the healing process.

Supplements: Take 1,200 IU of natural vitamin E (mixed tocopherols and tocotrienols) a day to help treat neuralgia, and 400 IU a day to help prevent it. Vitamin C helps to support the immune system and reduces stress damage to nerves. Take 1,000 mg four times a day. Also take 30 mg of zinc a day to help support the immune system. Take 200 mg of selenium a day to help with viral infections, and 500 mg of L-lysine twice a day to help with healing. B vitamins are essential for nerve health.

Take 100 mg three times a day. Vitamin B12 injections, administered by a qualified practitioner, are also essential to help the body recover more quickly and reduce pain associated with neuralgia. Proteolytic enzymes are thought to benefit cases of neuralgia caused by the herpes zoster virus by decreasing the body's inflammatory response and regulating immune response to the virus. Take 2–3 capsules on an empty stomach twice a day.

Tip: DO NOT SCRATCH

Keep blistered areas clean using soap and water. This will help prevent any bacterial infections from developing. Although it may be difficult, do not scratch. Scratching increases the risk that the blisters will become infected from dirt under the fingernails.

Herbs: Take 500 mg of olive leaf extract four times a day for its potent anti-viral benefits. Lomatium root, which can be taken at 500 mg four times a day, is used for immune support and anti-viral effects. St. John's wort also has anti-viral properties. Take 300 mg or 4 ml of tincture three times a day. Capsaicin cream is available in two strengths: 0.025 and 0.075%. Both preparations are indicated for use in neuralgia and should be applied sparingly to the affected area three to four times daily. Treatment should continue for several weeks as the benefit may be delayed. Capsaicin creams are approved over-the-counter drugs and should be used as directed. You may feel a burning or stinging sensation when this cream is first applied, but the pain will subside.

Homeopathy

Any of the following remedies can help ease a recent, mild to moderate episode of neuralgia. More severe symptoms are best treated by a homeopathic practitioner, possibly in combination with conventional treatment.

Aconite: Consider this remedy if symptoms of facial nerve pain have been triggered by exposure to cold, biting winds. Symptoms include a feeling of being pierced with hot wires, or a sensation that icy water is traveling along the pathway of the affected nerves. There may also be a feeling of crawling on the surface of the skin of the face.

Arsenicum album: This remedy can help ease symptoms of neuralgia associated with high anxiety levels, which are likely to be the most severe at night and in the early hours of the morning. Pains lodge in the area around the right side of the face. There may also be a sensitive, sore scalp, and discomfort is aggravated by exposure to cold, and temporarily eased by warmth.

Lachesis: This remedy can also be useful to treat pains that have been triggered by exposure to cold winds, especially if the pains are more intense on the left side, and worse on waking from sleep. Pains are most likely to be at the back of the head, and soreness is intensified from the pressure of the pillow when lying down.

Colocynthis: If neuralgic pains come in waves and affect one side of the face in the area of the jaw or around the eye socket, use Colocynthis. Pain is eased by applying pressure and heat. Resting is more uncomfortable than moving.

Mag phos: This remedy is helpful when symptoms are similar to those described for Arsenicum album. However, pains are not burning in nature, and symptoms may come on after extreme mental effort, resulting in poor concentration and exhaustion.

Herbalism

St. John's wort: Nerve irritation and pain may respond to a few drops of St. John's wort, either blended with ½ tsp of olive oil and directly applied to the affected area on the face, or in a warm compress applied to the area. Some practitioners find St. John's wort more successful if the symptoms are described as stinging, burning, or shooting. This wonderful nerve tonic can be helpful whenever there is nerve injury or irritation, especially when this pain leads to nervous exhaustion, inability to sleep, and a depressed mood. For internal use, a tincture or a standardized extract might be recommended. This herb may cause photosensitivity with long-term use, and may react with medications, so consult a doctor or herbal practitioner before taking St. John's wort orally if you are taking pharmaceutical medications.

Chili pepper: This can be applied topically to provide pain relief. Capsicum, found in chili pepper, is available in health food stores in cream or ointment formulation. Most preparations contain 0.025–0.075% capsaicin and can be applied to the affected area three to four times daily. Capsicum causes very few side effects, the most prevalent being a slight burning and itching of the application area. This treatment may make symptoms worse for one to three days until improvement occurs. If your neuralgia still is not better after a week of therapy, discontinue use and consult your herbal expert.

Wintergreen oil: This can be used topically by diluting in a base oil, or cream base. It is typically applied three times daily to ease pain from neuralgia, painful joints, or muscle inflammation, and acts as a counter-irritant. Those with salicylate hypersensitivity should avoid wintergreen.

Repetitive Strain Injury

Diagnosis

Repetitive strain injury (RSI) is mainly caused by work that involves performing small repetitive tasks and movements. It affects the musculoskeletal system, particularly the neck, shoulders, arms, and hands. Tenosynovitis (inflammation of the tendon sheath) of the wrist associated with typing is the most common repetitive strain injury. RSI can be painful, and may eventually result in the loss of function in a limb. A variety of movement is important: While you are working, flex your fingers, stretch your arms, and do exaggerated backward shoulder rolls. Take regular breaks to stretch, walk around, and shake tension out of your arms. Stretch your fingers and press your palms together. Early detection and treatment is essential, as chronic RSI is often irreversible.

Symptoms

- Pains in the neck, shoulders, arms, and hands
- Localized tenderness in the affected area
- Tingling sensation like pins and needles
- Aching
- Stiffness
- Muscle spasms
- At the outset, symptoms may only be experienced toward the end of the day
- Eventually they may progress, and affect the sufferer all day

Treatment Goal

Prevention through correct exercises and using the right equipment at work is essential to RSI treatment. Treatment aims to relieve any discomfort and discourage RSI from developing into a chronic condition.

Conventional Medicine

Rest: Rest Initial treatment is to immobilize the affected area and rest it from the trigger activity. However, a shoulder should not be immobilized as it may become "frozen." Applying ice to the affected site for 15–20 minutes is often helpful.

Exercise: Exercise or physical therapy may serve to strengthen the surrounding tendons and prevent recurrence of RSI. Ergonomic training should be carried out to learn different postures to avoid further strain. Hydrotherapy may also be a particularly effective form of physical therapy.

Vitamin D3: Ask your health care provider to check your vitamin D3 level. If it is low, repletion through the use of vitamin D3 supplementation can improve pain.

Medication: Non-steroidal anti-inflammatory drugs (NSAIDs) such as Motrin® are commonly used for pain relief. Steroid injections into the area of the injured tendon in combination with lidocaine can also cause notable pain relief.

Supplements: Fish oil can be used in amounts of about 4 g a day to reduce inflammation, as can ginger root in the amount of 1 g a day. Curcumin and boswellia also reduce inflammation.

Surgery: Surgical procedures may be helpful for chronic pain, but it is not appropriate for all cases of RSI. The benefits depend on the individual injury and the area of the body that is affected. Splints and assistive devices and supports may be necessary, and therapeutic ultrasound may be helpful for healing if chronic pain is present.

Traditional Chinese Medicine

Herbs: Take Du Huo Ji Shen Wan pills to strengthen the soft tissue and prevent recurring injury. To treat existing pain, try taking Yuan Hu Suo Zhi Tong Pian or Shan Qi Shen Pian pills for relief. All of these patent Chinese herbal pills are available from Chinese pharmacies or Chinese medicine clinics.

Acupressure: Press the acupressure points around the injured area. Usually you can press each point for one to two minutes twice a day.

Diet: Eat a balanced diet that includes fresh vegetables and fruits such as cranberries, blueberries, pears, and bananas. Mung beans, red beans, bamboo shoots, and purslane are also recommended.

Naturopathy

Diet: An anti-inflammatory diet is essential in helping an RSI to heal. Eat anti-inflammatory foods such as deep-water fish, which are a rich source of the polyunsaturated fats called omega-3 fatty acids. Originally praised for their heart-healthy actions, the omega-3s have also been shown to fight inflammation. All fish contain omega-3s, but the cold-water varieties—such as salmon, sea bass, tuna, trout, and mackerel—contain especially high amounts of these beneficial fats. Pineapple contains bromelain, a powerful enzyme that has been shown to have an anti-inflammatory effect on muscle and tissue. Bromelain breaks down fibrin, a blood-clotting protein that can impede circulation and prevent tissues from draining properly. It also blocks the production of certain compounds that cause swelling and pain. Apples and onions are high in quercetin. With its proven anti-inflammatory properties, quercetin can help reduce inflammation in the joints and muscles. Include anti-inflammatory spices such as turmeric and ginger in your meals and drink eight glasses of water a day to flush clean your system of waste material and metabolites that increase inflammation and inhibit the healing process. Whole grains, fresh fruit, and vegetables should be a staple for providing the muscles with all the nourishment they need to assist in the healing process.

Supplements: Proteolytic enzymes destroy free radicals, which inhibit healing, and proteins involved in the inflammatory process. Take three tablets or capsules between meals. Vitamin C is required for the formation of connective tissue and to combat free radicals. Essential fatty acids such as flaxseed and fish oil reduce inflammation and promote tissue healing. Take 5 g of fish oils a day or 1–2 tbsp of flaxseed oil. Take 1,500 mg of glucosamine sulfate a day to provide the raw material for the body to manufacture ligaments and tendons.

Herbs: Ginger has anti-inflammatory properties that help with pain. Try taking 100–200 mg of the standardized extract in pill form three times a day. You can also take ½–¾ tsp of fresh powdered ginger every four hours or up to three times a day. Try drinking several cups of ginger tea a day. It is available in prepackaged bags or can be prepared by

Tip: IMPROVE YOUR POSTURE

Good body positioning is essential in preventing RSI. Nature did not intend the body to sit for long periods, and sitting over a keyboard tends to force the head down and weaken the neck muscles. The best position for typing is with your feet flat on the floor, your ribs centered over the pelvis, and your head balanced on top of your spine, so that your ears, shoulders, and hips are in alignment. Also remember to take regular breaks. Sitting combines awkward positioning and poor posture with static loading (holding still while tightening muscles) and is unnatural to the body. Mix sit-down work with rest and stretching for the best results.

steeping ½ tsp of grated ginger root in 8 oz of very hot water for 5–10 minutes. A cup of tea, when steeped for this amount of time, can contain about 250 mg of ginger. Alternatively an 8 oz glass of ginger ale, which can be drunk several times a day, contains approximately 1 g of ginger. However, be sure to select products that are made with real ginger. Ginger is also available in crystallized form; eat two 1-inch-square, ¼-inch-thick pieces a day to obtain about 500 mg of ginger. Do not take more than 250 mg of ginger four times a day during pregnancy without consulting your obstetrician. Bromelain also has natural anti-inflammatory effects; take 500 mg three times a day between meals. Also take 1,500 mg of boswelia three times a day for its strong anti-inflammatory properties. Make sure this product contains 60–65% boswellic acids. Arnica oil reduces swelling and pain and can be applied to the injured area twice a day. White willow bark is a natural pain reliever without the side effects of over-the-counter aspirin. Take 30–60 mg a day of an extract standardized to salicin.

Homeopathy

Established and severe symptoms associated with this condition are best treated by an experienced practitioner. The following practical suggestions may also be helpful in easing the condition.

Yoga: There is some evidence to suggest that practicing yoga regularly may be helpful in relieving some of the symptoms of RSI. In addition, yoga is a very helpful therapy for stress relief. Since high levels of stress and tension may aggravate symptoms of RSI, regular yoga may bring benefits on both physical and psychological levels.

Evaluate your work station: Postural issues may also have an effect on RSI, and it is worth considering how healthy your workstation is, especially if you work for extended periods of time at a computer. Issues to consider include the height of your chair versus your desk, whether you need to use a foot and/or hand rest, and the maximum amount of time you can safely spend engaged in one activity at a time.

Herbalism

Arnica: The topical use of arnica flowers calms the swollen and inflamed tissue associated with RSI. After icing the site for three to five minutes, you might be advised to place a poultice or oil of arnica on the affected area, and repeat this several times daily. Place gauze or bandages in the infused oil and wrap the injured area. Arnica should not be placed over open wounds or taken internally.

Valerian: This root is used as an anti-inflammatory, mild pain reliever, and antispasmodic in cases of RSI. An added benefit is that it is a nervine, anxiolytic herb, which may help to alleviate the added stress and tension caused by the pain. A tincture can be taken as 1–3 ml three times daily, but may cause sedation. The root is also used as a cold infusion or decoction. Valerian doesn't work well for everyone, in terms of its sedative properties, and instead can leave some feeling more restless.

Castor oil: This oil can be massaged into the affected area, or applied to a washcloth that is then wrapped around the injury. The washcloth should be wrapped with a thin plastic wrap to contain the oil and covered with a hot towel for 20–30 minutes. The castor oil pack can also be placed on the site before going to bed and, once well covered, left on all night to decrease inflammation.

Anti-inflammatory oils: There are several essential oils that can be diluted in base oil or cream and rubbed either singly or in combination over the site of an RSI. These oils soak into the tissue and relieve inflammation. For example, peppermint essential oil contains menthol, which desensitizes nerves that conduct pain messages to the brain, leading to a decrease in pain. Camphor yields a cooling oil that acts locally as a counter-irritant and numbs sensation, thereby relieving pain. Camphor is safe when used in the short term in lotions or ointments of low concentrations (0.1–11%) on intact skin. Wintergreen and arnica oils are other topical treatments that can be massaged onto the area of an RSI.

Carpal Tunnel Syndrome

Diagnosis

Carpal tunnel syndrome (CTS) is triggered when pressure is applied to the median nerve located in the wrist, causing tingling, burning, and aching in the fingers. Passing through a narrow channel called the carpal tunnel, this nerve transmits impulses that allow feeling in the fingers. Compression of the median nerve can also occur in the forearm just below the elbow. This is known as pronator teres syndrome and has symptoms similar but not identical to CTS. CTS can develop as a response to a repetitive manual activity or it can accompany conditions such as rheumatoid arthritis. Hypothyroidism and diabetes can also predispose patients to symptoms. The cessation of the trigger activity usually results in the rapid resolution of symptoms.

Symptoms

- Deep, dull throbbing pain, localized in the wrist and hand
- Occasionally, the pain radiates up along the arm and even to the shoulder
- Numbness and tingling
- Sensory symptoms often develop at night, causing loss of sleep
- Inability to "pinch grip"
- Difficulty manipulating or maneuvering objects

Treatment Goal

To eliminate the physical cause of the condition and to prevent any further deterioration. If a medical cause is suspected, appropriate screening tests are carried out.

Conventional Medicine

Rest: Try to minimize any factors that contribute to the condition, such as repetitive motion. This may require a temporary rest. A wrist splint can also be used to inhibit movement that aggravates the condition. It is also helpful to examine how a trigger activity is carried out, and to try using a different angle of wrist flexion and extension as a preventive measure.

Diet and supplements: An anti-inflammatory diet that excludes dairy and gluten may be helpful. Also try to include a high-dose fish oil, ginger, curcumin, and turmeric in your diet. Decreased vitamin B6 levels have been associated with CTS, and vitamin B6 and B12 supplements are recommended.

Medication: Non-steroidal anti-inflammatory drugs (NSAIDs) such as ibuprofen, diclofenac, or naproxen can be used to relieve pressure and pain. A local injection of steroids is another therapy that often has successful results.

Surgery: Surgical therapy includes decompressing the inflamed nerve by sectioning the flexor tendon. The flexor tendon is separated from the nerve tunnel to make more room and thereby relieve pressure in the area. This is now frequently done by endoscope, which is a less invasive procedure.

Traditional Chinese Medicine

Herbs: In general, herbs are not taken internally for this condition, but you can try applying some Chinese medicinal ointments topically to the affected area. For example, Wan Hua oil, available from Chinese pharmacies or online, can be applied to the wrist two to three times a day. It helps relieve pain and may reduce inflammation.

Acupressure: Press and knead the Yang Chi and Yang Xi points with the thumb. The Yang Chi point is on the back of the hand at the crease of the wrist in the depression on the ulna (the bone of the outer forearm) side of the tendon. Press and knead in the direction of the ulna. The Yang Xi point is on the edge of the wrist below the thumb. When the thumb is tilted upward, it is in the depression between the tendons.

Diet: Green onion, purslane, taro, honey, lychee, spearmint, squash, and bitter gourd can help to manage the pain. A healthy diet of fresh fruits, vegetables, and grains is also recommended.

Naturopathy

Diet: To combat fluid retention, drink 1 glass of water every couple of hours. Eat foods that are high in vitamin B6, including beans, brewer's yeast, green leafy vegetables, and wheat germ. Eliminate sources of sodium, which contribute to fluid retention and aggravate symptoms.

Supplements: A high-quality multivitamin will provide the proper nourishment to encourage tissue healing. Follow the instructions on the pack. Vitamin B6 has been shown in studies to reduce nerve inflammation. Take 100 mg three times a day. A calcium and magnesium combination reduces nerve irritation and muscle tightness. Take 500 mg of calcium and 250 mg of magnesium.

Herbs: Take 500 mg of bromelain three times a day for its natural anti-inflammatory effect. Take a white willow product that is standardized to include 240 mg of salicin, or take 5 ml of a tincture, three times a day to relieve pain. Also take 1–2 g of ginger, or 1–2 ml of tincture, three times a day for its anti-inflammatory benefits and ability to relieve pain. Ginkgo biloba, taken at 120 mg twice a day, can help improve circulation. Make sure the product is 24% flavone glycosides.

Hydrotherapy: Hot and cold water can be used to improve blood flow and provide pain relief. Submerge the affected hand and wrist in hot water for 3 minutes then in cold for 30 seconds. Repeat this sequence three times.

Tip: REGULAR BREAKS

When working on a computer, take breaks every 30–60 minutes. Also use a wrist rest when typing.

Homeopathy

The following remedies can be very effective in treating mild or intermittent symptoms of carpal tunnel syndrome. However, if symptoms begin recurring, or become permanent, consult an experienced homeopathic practitioner for advice and treatment.

Aconite: Use this remedy to relieve pain, discomfort, and tingling sensations that are especially noticeable at night. Symptoms may be severe enough to wake the sufferer, and trigger distress, restlessness, and anxiety.

Arnica: If there is a sense of bruising and pain, as well as localized soreness or cramping, consider using Arnica. This remedy is especially helpful for easing recent flare-ups of pain and tenderness that have been triggered by overuse, injury, or trauma.

Ruta: If Arnica is initially helpful in easing the symptoms described above, but the benefits are not sustained, use Ruta. Symptoms include a sensation of lameness, stiffness, and pain that is troublesome even when resting the affected area.

Rhus tox: If stiffness and pain is aggravated by initial movement, but eased by moderate exercise, try Rhus tox. Symptoms become more intense following contact with damp and cold, and overexertion. There is also likely to be a strong sensation of weakness in the arms and wrists, and discomfort causes restlessness when trying to sleep at night.

Herbalism

Carpal tunnel syndrome is traditionally treated by splinting the wrist, stretching the hands and wrists, manipulating the carpal bones in the hand, or surgery. Herbal medicines can be used to alleviate swelling and pain.

Hot and cold compresses: Hot water promotes circulation, which brings needed healing nutrients to the affected area. Cold water flushes out excess fluid and toxic metabolites created by inflammation. Apply a hot compress to the area for three minutes, followed by a cold compress for 30–45 seconds.

St. John's wort: Although this herb is most well known for being of use in depression, St. John's wort is also an effective nerve anti-inflammatory. This herb is commonly used by herbalists for nerve pain, and may be taken in tincture, capsule, or infusion form or used topically as an infused/macerated oil. It is best to apply topically three times daily, or more if required. When using St. John's wort, consult a practitioner if any medication is being taken. Photosensitivity may also occur with sun exposure while taking St. John's wort.

Capsicum oil: Capsicum acts locally as a counter-irritant and numbs sensation, thereby relieving pain. It is safe when used dilute in the short term in low concentrations of 2–5% on unbroken skin.

Castor oil: Place 5–10 ml of castor oil onto a washcloth and wrap this around the wrist. Cover the cloth with thin plastic wrap and place a heated towel over the area for 20–30 minutes. This can help to relieve the pain.

Back Pain

Diagnosis

Back pain or stiffness can be caused by damage to the muscles or nerves. Most back pain is caused by strains or a minor injury. The pain may start a day or two after an injury occurs, or it may build up gradually over many years. Some of the more common causes of stress and strain on the spine are: poor posture; lifting items incorrectly; sleeping on a mattress that doesn't give the correct support; being unfit; and generally overdoing it. Pain generally lasts just a few days or a week. Back pain lasting longer than four weeks can be an indicator of something more major, so you should see a doctor.

Symptoms

- Pain and stiffness on waking up
- Pain and stiffness at the end of the day
- Pain and stiffness after sitting
- Pain in the buttocks and legs
- Weakness and fatigue

Treatment Goal

To establish the cause of the back pain and take remedial action. Often the best way to reduce stress and strain on your back is to stay in good physical condition. Exercise can also play a role in treating back pain.

Conventional Medicine

Treating back pain involves first diagnosing the cause of the pain. For example, back pain caused by a pulled muscle is treated differently to that caused by a herniated vertebral disc. The goal of treatment is to make sure a serious problem is not present, and to relieve symptoms.

To treat back pain caused by muscle strain:
This is the most common type of back pain. Treatment may involve ergo-dynamic education (learning how to lift correctly), exercises to strengthen abdominal muscles, and weight loss to decrease strain on back muscles. Massage therapy, heat therapy, and chiropractic adjustments may also be helpful. Muscle relaxation with magnesium aspartate

as a nutritional supplement usually helps to relieve muscle spasms, as does valerian root. Medication usually consists of non-steroidal anti-inflammatory drugs (NSAIDs) to help back pain and decrease swelling. Narcotic analgesics can be used in appropriate individuals for 48 hours prior to using NSAIDs. Skeletal muscle relaxants such as cyclobenzaprine (Flexeril®) may be helpful for severe spasm. Local and epidural injections sometimes alleviate chronic back pain.

Vitamin D3: Ask your health care provider to check your vitamin D3 level. If your level is low, repletion through the use of vitamin D3 supplementation can improve pain.

Traditional Chinese Medicine

Herbs: In general, you do not have to take herbal medicine for a backache. However, if you have persistent backache and you also experience weakness in your back, along with fatigue, try the following formula: Mix 12 g of Sang Ji Sheng (mulberry mistletoe stem), 12 g of Shu Di Huang (cooked Chinese foxglove), 15 g of Niu Xi (achyranthes root), 12 g of Tu Si Zi (Chinese dodder seed), 12 g of Sang Shen Zi (mulberry fruit-spike), 10 g of Shan Zhu Yu (Asiatic cornelian cherry), 12 g of Chuan Xiong (Szechuan lovage root), 12 g of Xu Duan (Japanese teasel root), and 10 g of Du Zhong (eucommia bark). Place the herbs in a ceramic pot, add 3 cups of water, and bring to a boil.

Tip: USE TUI NA

Tui Na is a Chinese medicine therapy similar to deep-tissue massage and/or chiropractic treatment. It is one of the most effective therapies for back pain. Consult with a well-trained practitioner regarding Tui Na treatment.

Simmer for 30 minutes, then strain the liquid into a container. Drink 1 cup twice a day.

Acupressure: Use the base of the palm to press on the back muscles with gentle to medium pressure five times, following the muscle line straight up and down. Also press and massage the Shen Shu, Shang Jiao Shu, and Da Chang Shu points. The Shen Shu points are ½ inch to either side of the back, below the second lumbar vertebra (just below the top of the hipbone). The Shang Jiao Shu and Da

Chang Shu points are at the same location, just below the first and fourth lumbar vertebrae.

Diet: Try boiling 20 g of cinnamon stick with 30 g of fresh ginger in 2 cups of water. Boil until only half the liquid is left. Drink 1 cup three times a day. You can also take 30–60 g of hawthorn fruit wine at bedtime for pain management.

Naturopathy

Diet: Eat small light meals throughout the day. This will help you keep at a sensible weight and avoid toxic build-up that can aggravate back pain. Eat plenty of fiber to avoid constipation, which may aggravate back pain. Drink at least eight glasses of water a day to keep your body hydrated. This will also help move your bowels more efficiently. Eat plenty of foods high in essential fatty acids for their anti-inflammatory effects. These include walnuts, salmon, mackerel, and ground flaxseeds. Avoid caffeine, alcohol, and refined sugars. They promote inflammation and interfere with weight loss. Green tea or green tea extract though, may help with weight loss.

Supplements: A high-quality multivitamin will provide the proper nourishment to prevent joint destruction. Follow the instructions on the container. Take 4,000–8,000 mg of methylsulfonylmethane (MSM) a day for its natural anti-inflammatory properties and ability

to reduce pain. Fish oil also reduces inflammation and provides joint lubrication; take 4–6 g a day, but allow two to three months for significant effects to emerge. Take 500 mg of calcium and 250 mg of magnesium a day to alleviate muscle spasm. Also take 1–3 g of vitamin C to strengthen connective tissue, and 1–2 capsules of protease enzyme on an empty stomach to reduce inflammation.

Herbs: Take 500 mg of bromelain three times a day for its natural anti-inflammatory effects. Apply cayenne cream to the affected area two to four times a day as it depletes the nerves of a neurotransmitter that transmits pain messages to the brain. Take 1,500–2,500 mg of devil's claw three times a day to help with pain in the joints, but do not take it if you have a history of gallstones, heartburn, or ulcers. Take a white willow product standardized to contain 240 mg of salicin or 5 ml three times a day to relieve pain. Ginger has anti-inflammatory benefits and also relieves pain. Take 1–2 g or 1–2 ml of tincture three times a day.

Massage: Find a reputable therapist in your area for a therapeutic massage to help alleviate pain. Try an essential oil mixture that contains arnica oil.

Hydrotherapy: Hot water treatments can alleviate pain. Let the hot water hit you in the affected area for 20 minutes. You can also try using a hot water bottle for the same purpose.

Homeopathy

The following homeopathic remedies may be helpful in easing mild to moderate symptoms of back pain that have developed recently and that are not due to an underlying mechanical cause. The latter type of condition is best treated by other forms of therapy, such as osteopathy, chiropractic therapy, physiotherapy, or surgery, depending on the nature and severity of the problem.

Tip: ALEXANDER TECHNIQUE

If muscle tension and poor postural habits are aggravating or setting off problems with back pain, it may be helpful to have a regular neck, shoulder, and back massage and to consider learning the Alexander Technique. The latter can be an extremely effective way of teaching you good posture and encouraging better postural alignment.

Gelsemium: If backache is combined with a heavy, weak sensation in the legs and feelings of unsteadiness, try Gelsemium. Discomfort tends to be most distressing at night and moving around after lying still feels uncomfortable. Damp, cold weather aggravates problems, while gentle, continuous movement may relieve the pain.

Hypericum: This remedy is appropriate for back pain that is more intense when sitting, when pains feel sharp, shooting, and burning. Numbness may follow, and the left side may be more affected than the right. Pain may have set in following a fall that has jarred the coccyx at the base of the spine, or at the site of an epidural injection.

Rhus tox: If back pain is muscular and pain and stiffness are most intense when resting, use Rhus tox. Pain may be eased by moderate movement, provided it is not overdone. A warm bath or shower also provides temporary relief, while cold, damp conditions aggravate.

Herbalism

Chronic back pain should be evaluated by a doctor to rule out any underlying serious structural abnormalities.

Arnica: Begin treatment by applying topical arnica to the affected area in gel or lotion form. Arnica is specific for trauma or injury to skin, muscles, tendons, and ligaments, and acts as an anti-inflammatory and circulatory stimulant with mild analgesic properties. Arnica is safe when used topically; however, using it internally or on an open wound is potentially toxic and must be supervised by a qualified practitioner.

Essential oils: These oils are a wonderful way to alleviate muscle spasms and strain, while soothing the senses and relieving pain. Wintergreen and peppermint contain volatile oils that act as analgesics and counter-irritants when placed on the skin. Add 5 drops of each to a ½ tsp of olive or massage oil and apply it to the affected area. Combine these oils with alternating hot and cold towels. Ginger, black pepper, rosemary, and frankincense essential oils may also be beneficial.

Tip: CREATE A PAIN-RELIEVING TINCTURE

Combine herbs that sedate and soothe with herbs that relieve muscle spasms and improve circulation to the area. When the muscles in the back are injured, they tend to swell and begin "guarding" against any further movement, leading to pain and stiffness. Both valerian and passionflower are wonderful examples of herbs that relieve the anxiety and muscle spasm that can accompany back pain. These can be puchased as tinctures (either alcohol or glycerin-based) and combined in equal parts. Take a dropperful of the combination twice or three times daily while the back pain is acute and severe. The passionflower slightly tempers valerian's strong taste. Consult a medical herbalist for other treatment ideas; for example, some people use kava kava to treat cases of back pain, but this should only be taken under strict medical supervision.

Sciatica

Diagnosis

Sciatica is a common condition in which pain radiates along the sciatic nerve, located in the lower spine. The pain may be continuous or only be felt when in certain positions; typically, symptoms are only felt on one side of the body. Sciatica is generally caused by the compression of a nerve root in the lumbar spine, which can be triggered by a herniated disk, spinal stenosis, infection, or a fracture. Risk factors include a sedentary lifestyle, gardening, sports (particularly if not played regularly), being overweight, and wearing high heels.

Usually the pain goes away without treatment, but this will depend upon the severity of the condition. Rest in bed for up to 48 hours, then get up and move about as soon possible.

Symptoms

- Numbness down one side of the body
- Tingling
- Pain in the lower back, buttocks, and legs
- Throbbing pains
- Sharp, shooting pains
- Weak legs
- Occasionally, problems with bladder or bowel function

Treatment Goal

To ease pain and restore mobility to the affected area. Symptoms of sciatica usually begin to feel better within one week of the initial injury.

Conventional Medicine

Conservative treatment should be attempted first, as 95% of patients improve without resorting to more complicated treatment. Rest for 48 hours. Serious possible causes, such as cancer, infection, or severe trauma, should also be excluded.

Medication: Use non-steroidal anti-inflammatory drugs (NSAIDs) for pain relief and to reduce inflammation. Corticosteroids, including prednisone, may be helpful for short-term use, and muscle relaxants such as cyclobenzaprine (Flexeril®) and carisoprodol (Soma®) may also be helpful in managing pain. However, caution should be exercised, as these drugs are sedating and may be addictive.

Steroid injections: Epidural steroid injections may give good short-term relief, and repeated injections into the epidural space around the spinal cord may be necessary.

Surgery: Surgical intervention is sometimes needed in people who have severe symptoms that do not respond to the above treatments.

Lifestyle modifications: If you are overweight and suffer from sciatica, begin a weight-loss program to help ease symptoms. Nutrition should be based on a high-protein diet, with plenty of whole grains, fruits, and vegetables. Cut out processed foods and sugar, and drink plenty of water. Exercise is important, but heavy lifting, twisting, bending, and exposure to vibrations should be limited.

Traditional Chinese Medicine

Herbs: The following decoction can be taken to relieve pain and keep the condition from worsening. Combine 12 g of Ji Shen (jilin root), 15 g of Niu Xi (achyranthes root), 12 g of Du Huo (pubescent angelica root), 12 g of Ru Xiang (frankincense), 8 g of Hong Hua (safflower flower), 15 g of Bai Shao (white peony root), 12 g of Yan Hu Suo (corydalis rhizome), 5 g of Gan Cao (licorice root), and 10 g of Huang Bai (phellodendron) in a ceramic pot. Add 3 cups of water, bring to a boil, and simmer for 30 minutes. Strain the liquid and drink 1 cup twice a day. You may take this formula for five to seven days.

Acupressure: While lying down so that the painful side is facing up, have someone press the Huan Tiao and Yang Ling Quan points with deep and strong pressure for one to three minutes, once or twice a day. The Yang Ling Quan point is on the outside of the lower leg, parallel to the knee, in the depression on the head of the fibula. The Huan Tiao point is on the outside of the thigh, in a depression just behind the top of the femur.

Diet: Foods that are cooling, such as spinach, lettuce, apples, barley, tofu, loquat, mandarin oranges, mangoes, and peppermint are recommended.

Naturopathy

Diet: Extra weight and constipation can aggravate sciatica. Sciatica sufferers should eat a diet that will enable them to lose weight if necessary and have regular bowel movements. Eat light, frequent meals throughout the day. Big, heavy meals slow digestion and decrease overall gastric function within time. Apples, fresh vegetables, and whole grains have high fiber levels. Eat several portions a day to relieve constipation. Stay hydrated by drinking eight glasses of water a day, as dehydration aggravates sciatic pain. Eat foods that are high in essential fatty acids, such as walnuts, salmon, and flaxseeds to help relieve constipation and reduce inflammation.

Supplements: Vitamin C helps with inflammation and strengthens connective tissue in your lower back. Take 1,000 mg three times a day. Take 2 protease enzymes on an empty stomach between meals twice a day to reduce inflammation and help with pain. Take

Tip: TRY VERTEBRAL AXIAL DECOMPRESSION (VAX-D)

VAX-D may reduce pain and improve function in patients with chronic lower back pain and sciatic pain. The procedure is thought to alleviate pain and enhance healing by relieving pressure within the discs, and promoting the in-flow of oxygen, fluids, and nutrients to the spinal column. Some chiropractors, naturopathic doctors, or osteopaths may have this type or equipment.

2,000 mg of methylsulfonylmethane (MSM), a natural anti-inflammatory that also alleviates pain, three times a day. Take 250 mg of magnesium twice a day as it also alleviates muscle spasm. Glucosamine sulfate is helpful for sciatica caused by a herniated disc. Take 1,500 mg a day.

Herbs: Take 500 mg of bromelain three times a day for its anti-inflammatory effects. White willow relieves pain in the lower back and throughout the body. Products should be standardized to contain 240 mg of salicin or take 5 ml of a tincture three times a day. Ginger has anti-inflammatory benefits and relieves pain. Take 1–2 g or 1–2 ml of a tincture

three times a day. Dimethyl sulfoxide (DMSO) is a sulfur-containing substance derived from wood pulp. It may relieve pain, stiffness, and inflammation in the lower back. Talk to your doctor about whether this is appropriate and about dosage options. Curcumin, the yellow pigment of turmeric, has a significant anti-inflammatory action. Curcumin has been shown to be as effective as cortisone or phenylbutazone in certain models of inflammation. Curcumin also exhibits many beneficial effects on liver functions. The typical dosage of curcumin is 400–600 mg three times a day.

Homeopathy

The following remedies can provide complementary pain relief for a mild, recent attack of sciatica. Any mechanical problem that has caused the sciatica will also need to be dealt with by the appropriate therapist, whether a doctor, chiropractor, or osteopath. Chronic conditions should be referred to a homeopathic practitioner.

Hypericum: This remedy can ease shooting pains that can develop into burning, tingling sensations that radiate into the affected leg. Pains may be restricted to the left side, and can be set off by a fall that has jarred the base of the spine. Discomfort may be aggravated by damp, cold conditions and jarring movements, while massage or lying on the belly may give relief.

Kali carb: When this remedy is indicated there may be a general sense of weakness in the affected leg, with tearing pains radiating from the hip to the knee. Throbbing pains are made more intense when lying on the affected side.

Colocynthis: Try this remedy when shooting pains extend from the top of the leg to the foot on the affected side. Symptoms include sharp pains that are followed by a numb sensation. The latter can be temporarily eased by applying pressure to the affected area.

Tip: USE ARNICA OR HYPERICUM CREAM

Applying arnica cream to the affected area may soothe aching pains, while hypericum cream or oil may help ease shooting pains. For maximum effect, apply when the skin is warm either after a bath or shower. The muscles will be relaxed by the heat and the warm skin will absorb creams or oils more readily.

Herbalism

Inflammation of the sciatic nerve, or sciatica, can occur anywhere along the length of the nerve and causes a variety of symptoms. The underlying cause needs to be addressed, following recommendations from your doctor. Herbs can be used to calm the pain and inflammation, providing relief until the situation resolves. See Back Pain (p. 366) for other herbal treatments relevant to sciatica.

Anti-inflammatory herbs: See Arthritis (p. 310) for details about anti-inflammatory herbs such as turmeric and Indian frankincense. These herbs act on some of the same physiological systems as pharmaceutical medications, although they may not act as quickly.

St. John's wort: Although this herb is most well known for being of use in depression, St. John's wort is also an effective nerve anti-inflammatory. This herb is commonly used by herbalists for sciatica for this reason, and may be taken in tincture, capsule, or infusion form,

or used topically as an infused/macerated oil. It is best to apply topically three times daily, or more if required. When using St. John's wort, consult a practitioner if any medication is being taken. Photosensitivity may also occur with sun exposure while taking St. John's wort.

Willow: This plant contains mildly anti-inflammatory salicylate compounds. Many species of willow have medicinal effects, with specific varieties and concentrations of the active medicinal compounds. Willow bark is used to relieve pain related to muscle and joint inflammation, and can help with the symptoms of sciatica. A tea can be made from high-quality willow bark (it should contain at least 7% total salicin compounds), as advised by your herbal medicine practitioner. Several cups of this tea can be ingested daily. The more finely ground the bark, the better the extraction of the active compounds. As with aspirin itself, there is the possibility of stomach upset with repeated use of willow bark.

Hernia

Diagnosis

A hernia is formed when the intestine pushes against a weak spot in the abdominal wall and slips through it to form a lump. It can be caused by being overweight or pregnant, lifting heavy items, coughing, and straining when constipated.

The most common hernias are those found in the groin. Occasionally baby boys can be born with an indirect inguinal hernia. Although surgery can be performed immediately after birth to repair the hernia, some surgeons prefer to wait until the child is older. Femoral hernias occur near the groin and affect mostly middle-aged and overweight women. Incisional hernias develop in the abdomen, particularly around the navel. The treatment, again, is surgery.

DANGER: A hernia can be dangerous if it becomes trapped in the weak spot in the abdominal wall. This is known as a strangulated hernia. Gangrene and peritonitis, which can be life-threatening, may occur as a result. This is an emergency requiring urgent surgery.

Symptoms

- A bulge in the abdomen
- Vomiting and nausea (if the hernia becomes strangulated)

Treatment Goal

A hernia in itself is harmless. Treatment aims to correct the hernia where possible and prevent complications from occurring.

Conventional Medicine

Conventional medicine focuses on reducing the hernia to prevent strangulation, which arises when the hernia cannot be pushed back through the defect in the abdominal wall. It also aims to immediately repair the defect if strangulation has already occurred.

Truss or hernia belt: These devices can be used to hold the reduced hernia in place. They can help to improve discomfort and are generally used while the patient is waiting for an operation, or is unfit for surgery. A truss, however, is not a cure. It is a temporary measure and does not replace the need for surgical evaluation.

Surgery: The only definitive cure of a hernia is surgical repair through a herniorrhaphy.

Immediate surgical repair is needed if the hernia cannot be reduced. Surgical techniques include open repair and laparoscopic repair. Sometimes mesh gauze is used during the operation to reinforce the abdominal wall. An antibiotic such as cefoxitin can be prescribed if infection is suspected.

Modify your lifestyle: Several lifestyle changes can prevent hernias from occurring and recurring. These primarily include weight loss and exercise to increase abdominal muscles. Consult a doctor before beginning an exercise regime if a hernia is present.

Traditional Chinese Medicine

Herbs: To treat a hernia, Chinese herbal medicine is usually accompanied by acupuncture. Consult a doctor of traditional Chinese medicine for a Chinese herbal medicine treatment that is appropriate for your condition.

Acupuncture: Consult an experienced practitioner to see if acupuncture is suitable to treat your type of condition. It is usual to have treatment for a few months or longer, beginning with one full course of 12 treatment sessions. Treatment may be needed once or twice a week.

Acupressure: Use the tip of your finger to press the Bai Hui point for about one minute, and repeat. The Bai Hui point is found on the top of the head, at the midpoint along the line running up and over the head from ear to ear.

Diet: To ease the pain of a hernia, crush 60 g of lychee seeds and 15 g of caraway seeds, boil them in water, and drink the liquid once a day. You can also boil 30 g of dried peaches and mango in water. Eat these twice a day to help relieve pain.

Naturopathy

Diet: Inflammation is one of the main causes of the pain and discomfort of hernias. There are some foods that contribute to inflammation more than others, such as gluten, dairy, and corn. Eliminate these from your diet for three weeks and then reintroduce them one food at a time for one week. Take note of how you feel on a daily basis to identify any triggers. Eat spices such as ginger, tumeric, and garlic. These have anti-inflammatory effects and help strengthen the immune system. Salmon, mackerel, and walnuts have high levels of essential fatty acids, which also have anti-inflammatory properties. Eat these foods two to three times a week. Eat vegetables and fruits that are high in vitamin C and bioflavonoids, including berries, citrus fruits, green leafy vegetables, and carrots, as they strengthen the ligaments and tendons. Also drink 8–10 glasses of water a day and 1–2 freshly squeezed vegetable juices a day to stay hydrated and provide nutrients to nourish the surrounding tissues.

Supplements: A high-quality multivitamin will provide the proper nourishment to prevent further deterioration and strengthen surrounding ligaments. Follow the instructions on the container. Take 4,000–8,000 mg of methylsulfonylmethane (MSM) a day for its natural anti-inflammatory benefits. Taking 4–6 g of fish oil a day also reduces inflammation, but allow two to three months to see significant effects. Protease enzymes also reduce inflammation. Take one to two capsules on an empty stomach.

Herbs: Take 500 mg of bromelain three times a day for its natural anti-inflammatory effects. Cayenne cream can deplete the nerves of a neurotransmitter that transmits pain messages to the brain. Try applying the cream to the affected area two to four times a day. Take a white willow product standardized to contain 240 mg of salicin to relieve pain, or take 5 ml of a tincture three times a day. Ginger, taken at 2–4 g or 1–2 ml of tincture three times a day, has anti-inflammatory benefits and relieves pain. Do not take more than 1 g of ginger a day if you are pregnant. Dimethyl sulfoxide (DMSO) is a sulfur-containing substance derived from wood pulp. It may relieve pain, stiffness, and inflammation. Talk to your physician about this option.

Homeopathy

Although surgical intervention is the most common treatment for a hernia, homeopathy can still have a useful role. Homeopathic remedies can help prevent the problem from recurring, and can provide pre- and postoperative support. The advice here is given with the latter in mind.

Arnica: This remedy can encourage the body to heal efficiently, and help with the psychological trauma and shock of surgery. It is especially valuable in promoting the reabsorption of blood, healing bruising, tenderness, and swelling around the site of surgery.

Staphysagria: Consider this remedy to treat pain and sensitivity that remains around the site of the wound once superficial healing has taken place. When it is appropriate, there will be an excruciating sensitivity to touch or pressure, and some relief is gained by contact with warmth.

Nux vomica: This remedy can be used in the short term to relieve some of the discomfort of a hernia while waiting for surgery. Symptoms include spasmodic, shooting pains and a sensation of heaviness that triggers irritability. Following surgery, Nux vomica can be a helpful remedy in easing nausea, retching, or stubborn constipation.

Herbalism

Be advised to avoid any activity that will increase pressure in the intra-abdominal cavity, such as heavy lifting or straining while having a bowel movement. After surgical repair, prevention of additional ruptures includes reducing risk factors such as losing weight, treating constipation, and strengthening connective tissue by taking the herbs below.

Gotu kola: The tissue that normally holds our abdominal contents in place is weakened after a hernia, therefore it is important to strengthen this tissue. Gotu kola, a spicy, cooling herb from the parsley family, is used to build and strengthen connective tissue. However, this is not its only medicinal ability. Gotu kola also calms the nervous system, supports adrenal fatigue from daily stress, and acts as a mild laxative. Whether used topically or internally, gotu kola hastens recovery periods and

reduces scar formation. Drink an infusion of 1 tbsp of the whole plant per cup of water, or take 2 ml of a 1:1 tincture or 60 mg in capsule form three times daily.

Horsetail: This is a slightly sweet, cooling, and astringent plant, closely related to ferns. The early spring stems are used to make medicine, as the mature plant contains higher levels of potentially irritating silica. Horsetail increases the tone and strength of connective tissue, while also acting as a mild diuretic. Infuse 1 tbsp per cup of fresh stems in cold water for 12 hours, or take 2 ml of a 1:1 tincture in water and drink throughout the day. Be aware that long-term use of horsetail will deplete vitamin B1 (thiamin) and potassium levels in the body due to the diuretic effect. Take 30 mg of vitamin B1 and 40 mg of potassium daily as a preventive measure.

Knee Pain

Diagnosis

Knee complaints are very common and arise from a variety of causes. Pain, swelling, bruising, or tenderness in or around the knee is usually an indication that you have injured it in some way. The knee joint often takes the full weight of the body, and is therefore vulnerable and susceptible to injury. Problems may occur in the knee bones, joint, or ligaments.

The causes of pain in the knee can be divided into several different categories. Pain can result from diseases such as arthritis and other bone problems; mechanical problems such as tendonitis and bursitis; and/or direct traumas such as sports injuries, accidents, or falls, which can lead to a fracture, dislocation, sprain, strain, or torn ligaments.

Symptoms

- Swelling
- Redness
- Tenderness
- Soreness
- Pain

Treatment Goal

To establish the cause of the pain in the knee and treat it accordingly. To relieve any pain and discomfort and restore full mobility.

Conventional Medicine

The cause of the knee pain must first be established to determine an appropriate treatment. Some sources of pain require surgical intervention, while others, such as knee fracture, dislocation, ligament tears, or infection, require immediate medical evaluation.

To treat patellofemoral joint pain: One of the most common causes of chronic and acute knee pain is patellofemoral joint pain. This occurs when the knee cap tracks improperly on the thigh bone during movement, leading to pain around the knee cap. This is generally treated with rest from strenuous activity, although weight-bearing, physical exercises to strengthen the muscles and ligaments around the knee are encouraged. Exercises focus on hamstring stretching and on strengthening the thigh muscles. Pain can also be relieved by taking non-steroidal anti-inflammatory drugs

(NSAIDs). Orthotics (supportive braces and splints) can also be helpful. After the knee has healed and the patient can resume physical activity, a patellar band (which can be purchased at drug stores) can be worn around the knee to prevent further injury.

To treat a meniscal injury: A meniscal injury involves the cartilage within the knee. To treat this type of injury, rest the knee and take NSAIDs to manage the pain. If there is no resolution, surgical intervention to repair the cartilage and to remove damaged cartilage may be needed.

To treat bursitis of the knee: This type of injury is usually treated with rest, NSAIDs, and cortisone injections, as well as applying ice packs.

Traditional Chinese Medicine

Herbs: Combine 12 g of Ji Shen (jilin root), 15 g of Niu Xi (achyranthes root), 12 g of Chi Shao (red peony root), 12 g of Yu Jin (turmeric tuber), 10 g of Yan Hu Suo (corydalis rhizome), 10 g of Ru Xiang (frankincense), 12 g of Du Zhong (eucommia bark), and 18 g of Ji Xue Teng (millettia root). To make a decoction, place the herbs in a ceramic pot and add 3 cups of water. Bring the liquid to a boil and simmer for 30 minutes. Strain the liquid and drink 1 cup twice a week.

Acupressure: The Du Bi point is located on the knee, in the depression just to the outside of the kneecap when the knee is flexed. Apply pressure to this point with the tip of your finger.

Diet: Take 30–60 g of hawthorn fruit wine before bed to manage the pain. Also add green onion, purslane, taro, honey, lychee, spearmint, squash, and bitter gourd to your diet to help relieve pain.

Naturopathy

Diet: Knee pain can be caused by several factors, but inflammation is generally involved. Eat an anti-inflammatory diet, avoiding refined sugars, hydrogenated oils, and glutens. Gluten is a protein found in some grains, especially wheat, that has been shown to be an allergen to some people, causing inflammation. Other common allergens include soy, dairy, egg, and corn. Foods that contain essential fatty acids, such as salmon, mackerel, and walnuts, also have anti-inflammatory properties. Eat vegetables and fruits high in vitamin C and bioflavonoids, such as berries, citrus fruits, green leafy vegetables, and carrots. These substances strengthen ligaments and tendons therefore, decreasing the occurrences of sprains.

Supplements: A high-quality multivitamin will provide the proper nourishment to prevent further deterioration and strengthen the ligaments. Follow the instructions on the container. Glucosamine sulfate, which is usually combined with chondroitin sulfate, reduces knee pain and rebuilds cartilage. Take 1,500 mg of glucosamine daily with 1,200 mg of chondroitin. Take 4,000–8,000 mg of methylsulfonylmethane (MSM) a day for its natural anti-inflammatory benefits. Niacinamide has been clinically reported to help arthritis, which can present as knee pain. Take 500 mg three times a day. Higher doses should be supervised by a doctor. Methionine is a sulfur-containing amino acid that is important for cartilage structure, and has also been shown to have benefits in arthritic patients. Take 250 mg four times a day.

Herbs: Cayenne cream can deplete the nerves of a neurotransmitter that transmits pain messages to the brain. Try applying the cream to the affected area two to four times a day. Devil's claw, taken at 1,500–2,500 mg three times a day, helps with pain in the knee joints. However, it should not be taken if you have a history of gallstones, heartburn, or ulcers. Ginger, taken at 2–4 g or 1–2 ml of tincture three times a day, has anti-inflammatory benefits and relieves pain. Do not take more than 1 g of ginger a day if you are pregnant. Dimethyl sulfoxide (DMSO) is a sulfur-containing substance derived from wood pulp. It may relieve pain, stiffness, and inflammation. Talk to your physician about this option.

Always Discuss Allergies and Medication
If you have existing allergies you must discuss these with your practitioner so that they may safely prescribe a treatment. If you have any medical conditions or are taking any type of medicine, it is imperative that you inform your practitioner, who will be able to advise you on safe use of complementary treatments.

Homeopathy

The following remedies may help with knee injuries that are caused by sprains or other minor injuries. Also see Arthritis (p. 309).

Arnica: When an injury has been sustained, this remedy can help the body deal with the systemic shock. It will also help to ease pain and encourage reabsorption of blood from engorged tissues.

Bryonia: If Arnica has been initially helpful in reducing pain and swelling, but does not improve the injury any further, try Bryonia. Pain may be aggravated by movement, and there is an obvious improvement when keeping the knee firmly supported and rested.

Rhus tox: If pain and stiffness is made much worse from resting, and obviously improves through gentle movement for a limited period of time, take Rhus tox. This remedy can follow Arnica if the latter has provided initial relief.

Herbalism

It is important to distinguish between acute injuries to the knee and pain due to chronic injuries, as they may be managed differently. Herbal medicines can be used to support the healing of knee tissue and improve circulation in an area that is normally known to have decreased blood flow. Herbs work best when combined with physical therapy and other nutritive support such as glucosamine sulfate.

Compresses: You can quickly relieve swelling and pain in acute injuries by applying ice to the knee over a thin cloth for three to five minutes, as often as can be tolerated, over the first 24–48 hours.

Anti-inflammatory tincture: A combination of anti-inflammatory herbs, such as licorice, willow bark, boswellia, ginger, and curcumin might be suggested by your herbal medicine practitioner, in a tincture. If it is expected that you will be using a tincture long term for pain, the licorice component may be left out, or its use monitored. Cramp bark may also help to relieve spasms. Topically, oils of rosemary, cayenne, frankincense, ginger, and wintergreen may offer relief. One, or a blend of a few of these oils, is often used diluted in base oil, or mixed into a cream base.

7

Personal Complaints

Premenstrual Syndrome

Diagnosis

Premenstrual syndrome (PMS) involves various physical or psychological changes in the body that precede a period. Common symptoms include mood swings, depression, cravings, cramping, and water retention. A small proportion of women experience severe symptoms. The cause of PMS is uncertain. Symptoms such as bloating, tender breasts, and headaches are thought to be linked to the fluctuating levels of female hormones that occur just before menstruation. Lower than normal levels of serotonin, a chemical in the brain, may explain some of the nonphysical symptoms such as irritability, depression, and mood swings. Symptoms tend to be worse in the week leading up to a period, and usually disappear as soon as a period starts.

Symptoms

- Fatigue
- Mood swings and/or irritability
- Loss of confidence and weepiness
- Poor memory and difficulty concentrating
- Cravings for sweet/salty foods
- Tender breasts
- Bloating
- Weight gain
- Headaches, sometimes severe

Treatment Goal

Treatment depends upon the nature of the symptoms. The focus is on relieving acute symptoms and developing long-term strategies for dealing with symptoms.

Conventional Medicine

The choice of therapy when treating PMS is largely determined through trial and error, beginning with the simple therapies and moving on if one fails. Most commonly, B vitamins, evening primrose oil, and oral contraceptives are used to suppress the menstrual cycle.

Lifestyle modifications: Losing weight and stopping smoking, when applicable, are primary lifestyle modifications that can alleviate PMS. Other strategies include daily exercise and limiting your caffeine and alcohol intake. Diets that are high in lignans (found in flaxseed and soy), fiber, and whole grains, low in fat, and free from processed foods and dairy products seem to alleviate symptoms.

Supplements: Supplements that have shown promise in helping PMS are magnesium aspartate dosed at 400 mg daily, calcium hydroxyapetite at 1,500 mg daily, and vitamin B6 at 50 mg daily. Chaste tree (which should not be used if you are trying to become pregnant), rhodolia root, licorice, ground flaxseed, and St. John's wort can also help to relieve symptoms.

Medication: Generally oral contraceptives and antidepressants (selective serotonin reuptake inhibitors, SSRIs) are prescribed. Progesterone and/or estrogen can also alleviate symptoms when administered transdermally (through the skin). Other medications, such as non-steroidal anti-inflammatory drugs for pain relief, bromocriptine for breast tenderness, and beta blockers and anxiolytics for anxiety, are used as needed for severe symptoms.

Traditional Chinese Medicine

Herbs: To prepare a formula, place the raw herbs in a ceramic pot and add 3 cups of water. Bring the mixture to a boil, simmer for 30 minutes, and strain. Drink 1 cup twice a day.
• **To treat Qi stagnation:** Symptoms include irritability, mood swings, and tender breasts. Mix 10 g of Chai Hu (hare's ear root), 15 g of Bai Shao (white peony root), 12 g of Dan Gui (Chinese angelica root), 12 g of Chuan Xiong (Szechuan lovage root), 15 g of Fuling (poria), 15 g of Bai Zhu (atractylodes rhizome), 6 g of Bo He (field mint), and 12 g of Xiang Ru (aromatic madder).
• **To treat Qi stagnation and spleen deficiency:** Symptoms include those above plus stomach bloating, diarrhea, and swelling. Add 5 g of Chen Pi (tangerine peel), 15 g of Shan Yao (Chinese yam), 25 g of Yi Yi Ren (seeds of Job's tears), and 10 g of Mu Xiang (costus root) to the ingredients above. Take this formula for one to

three months, and consult a TCM doctor if your condition does not improve.

• **To treat blood stagnation:** Symptoms include headaches, disturbed sleep, cramps, and dark bleeding. Combine 12 g of Chuan Xiong (Szechuan lovage root), 12 g of Chi Shao (red peony root), 15 g of Dan Gui (Chinese angelica root), 12 g of Yan Hu Suo (corydalis rhizome), 15 g of Niu Xi (achyranthes root), and 12 g of Dan Pi (cortex of tree peony root).

Acupressure: Pressing the Di Ji and San Yin Jiao acupressure points may help reduce some PMS symptoms. The San Yin Jiao point is on the inside of the leg, about 3 inches above the center of the anklebone. The Di Ji point is on the inside of the lower leg in the depression about 3 inches below the knee. Apply pressure to these points with the tip of the finger for one to two minutes, and repeat twice a day.

Diet: Eat foods that are light and neutral, including apricots, beef, beetroot, black sesame seeds, Chinese cabbage, castor beans, celery, duck, grapes, honey, beef, liver, oysters, pineapple, and soybeans.

Naturopathy

Diet: Reduce your intake of sugar, red meat, and salt. These foods cause hormones to fluctuate and will augment common PMS symptoms including bloating and swelling of the hands and feet, tender breasts, and dizziness. When you do eat red meat, make sure it is organic, grass-fed beef as this will not interfere with estrogen levels in the body. Keep insulin and blood sugar levels balanced by eating frequent small meals throughout the day. Imbalanced insulin levels aggravate PMS and promote mood swings and tension. Restrict or eliminate caffeine, which can aggravate anxiety, depression, and tender breasts. The most common sources of caffeine are coffee, chocolate, soft drinks, and some pain-relieving pills. Increase your intake of fruits, vegetables, beans, nuts, and seeds. They contain fiber and nutrients that may help balance blood sugar, regulate bowel movements, and provide nourishment. Avoid alcohol, especially during the first two weeks before your period. Its dehydrating effects worsen PMS symptoms and blood sugar levels.

Supplements: Take 50 mg of vitamin B6 a day to assists in the production of progesterone to counterbalance estrogen. Take 250 mg of magnesium twice a day; it benefits women with cramps, mood swings, depression, fatigue, breast tenderness, and water retention, and is involved in prostaglandin metabolism and vitamin B6 activity. Evening primrose oil contains gamma-linolenic acid (GLA), which is involved in the metabolism of hormone-like substances called prostaglandins that regulate pain and inflammation in the body. Take 2,000–3,000 mg of an oil that includes omega-3 fatty acids such as flax oil or fish oil. Calcium may be beneficial for women with premenstrual cramps and moodiness. Take 500 mg of calcium citrate, the most easily absorbed form of the supplement, twice a day. Also take 15 mg of zinc a day as part of a multivitamin, as it has been shown to be low in women with PMS. Take 400 IU of vitamin E mixed tocopherol, which may reduce breast tenderness and relieve PMS. D-glucarate assists in the metabolizing of estrogen and can be taken at 500 mg twice a day, while indole 3 carbinol helps in the breakdown of estrogen in the liver and can be taken at 300 mg a day.

Herbs: One of the main causes of PMS is estrogen dominance—which occurs when estrogen levels are too high. One way of treating PMS is to decrease estrogen levels by increasing progesterone. Licorice is believed to lower estrogen levels while simultaneously raising progesterone levels. Take 500–1,000 mg of the freeze dried form a day, or 1–2 tsp of a tincture a day. Chaste tree berries are highly regarded for all menstrual problems, especially those associated with premenstrual syndrome. Do not take it if you are on birth control medication, as it can potentially decrease the effects, otherwise take 240 mg of a capsule standardized to 0.6% aucubine, or 1 tsp twice a day of the tincture. Passionflower relaxes the nervous system and improves some PMS symptoms. Take 300 mg two to three times a day. Milk thistle improves liver function, important in the metabolism of hormones. Take 250 mg three times a day an 80–85% silymarin extract.

Homeopathy

Any of the following homeopathic remedies may be helpful in easing mild to moderate, infrequent symptoms of PMS. More established problems are best treated by a homeopathic practitioner.

Lycopodium: If PMS symptoms are associated with a craving for sweet foods and a bloated stomach, use Lycopodium. Leading up to a period there may be gastric disturbance that alternates between constipation and diarrhea. Sufferers also tend to experience mood swings and feelings of anxiety, irritability, and lack of confidence.

Lachesis: When PMS symptoms build in intensity from mid-cycle until the onset of the period, use Lachesis. Disturbed sleep, left-sided headaches, and mood swings all become most intense just before a period starts. Symptoms are relieved as soon as the period starts.

Sepia: If PMS has a negative effect on optimism, motivation, and energy, try Sepia. Mood changes can occur rapidly, from feeling irritable to complete indifference. Symptoms are relieved by brisk, aerobic exercise.

Pulsatilla: If sufferers feel weepy, and PMS symptoms are eased after a good cry, Pulsatilla is a strong choice. Physical symptoms include premenstrual headaches that feel worse in hot, stuffy conditions, irregular periods, persistent indigestion, a sensitivity to rich, fatty foods, tender, enlarged breasts, and premenstrual thrush. All symptoms may become more intense following pregnancy or approaching menopause.

Herbalism

An excess of estrogen is thought to contribute to the development of PMS symptoms. To rid the body of excess estrogen, herbal medicines are used to support the liver and digestion and to balance internal hormonal production. Herbal medicine treatment for hormone related ailments may be best used with practitioner guidance.

Liver support formula: The liver is one of the main organs that removes internally and externally derived hormones (such as those found in birth control pills). If you have a poor diet, poor digestion, and excess hormones, the liver becomes overwhelmed and cannot detoxify the body as well as it should. The following herbs regenerate and heal the liver, improve the flow of bile (needed to break down fats), and encourage bowel movements. This is important because excess estrogen that is broken down by the liver must be moved out of the intestines in a timely manner, or it will be re-absorbed. Combine equal parts of dried dandelion leaf and root, yellow dock root, nettle, artichoke, and milk thistle. Decoct 1 tbsp of the combined herbs per cup and drink, or take 2–3 ml of a combined tincture three times daily. This blend may be best used with practitioner supervision.

PMS prevention tonic: These following herbs support liver function, decrease uterine spasm, and stabilize emotions. Combine equal parts of the following dried herbs: chaste tree, Dong Quai, dandelion, and cramp bark. Drink an infusion made from 1 tsp per cup of water or take 2 ml of a combined tincture three times a day one week before menstruation begins as a preventive measure. To ease symptoms, drink an infusion made from 2 tsp per cup of water, or take 2–4 ml of a combined tincture three to four times a day. Skullcap may also be of use to relieve spasms and nervous tension.

Period Pains

Diagnosis

Many women experience uncomfortable cramping pains (known as dysmenorrhea) at the time of their period. It is a common problem and not generally a cause for concern. These pains are caused by contractions in the muscle of the uterus that result from the release of prostaglandins, which are hormones produced by the lining of the womb. For most women the pain is manageable. However, some women experience such severe pain that it affects their daily routine, or forces them to stay in bed for a couple of days. Lifestyle changes can help to improve symptoms. Try to eat a healthy, balanced diet, take daily exercise, get plenty of sleep, and avoid stressful situations. If period pains are more than an just inconvenience, it is wise to consult your doctor, who may wish to perform a pelvic examination to rule out any underlying conditions, such as pelvic inflammatory disease, endometriosis, or fibroids.

Symptoms

- Cramping sensations in the abdomen
- Pain in the lower back
- Dragging pains
- Heavier blood loss than usual
- Headaches
- Dizziness and fainting

Treatment Goal

To isolate the cause of the pain to rule out a serious underlying condition. Treatment involves relieving symptoms of pain and discomfort.

Conventional Medicine

A thorough medical history is taken and a physical examination performed to make sure there a serious disease is not causing the pain. An ultrasound is also usually carried out to check for fibroids or cysts. Once it has been established that there is not a serious problem, therapies can be initiated.

Compresses: Applying warm compresses to the abdomen can be helpful in relieving pain. Add castor oil to a warm washcloth and place it over the painful area.

Diet: A dairy-free diet has reportedly helped relieve menstrual cramping.

Medication: Taking non-steroidal anti-inflammatory drugs (NSAIDs) such as ibuprofen (Motrin®) or naproxyn (Naproxyn® and Alleve®) two days before a period begins until the second day of bleeding can help to ease pain. Taking oral contraceptive pills may also help.

TENS machine: Transcutaneous electrical nerve stimulation (TENS) has been shown to have some effect. A TENS machine gives out tiny pulses of electrical energy which prevent pain signals from reaching your brain.

Surgery: If all else fails, a procedure called laparoscopic presacral neurectomy, which involves interrupting nerve tissue that goes to and from the uterus, may be effective.

Traditional Chinese Medicine

Herbs: To prepare a formula, place the herbs in a ceramic pot with 3 cups of water. Bring the mixture to a boil, simmer for 30 minutes, and strain. Drink 1 cup twice a day.
• **To treat sharp pains in your lower abdomen and cold hands and feet:** Symptoms also include feeling chilly and looking pale. Mix 10 g of Wu Zhu Yu (evodia fruit), 12 g of Dang Gui (Chinese angelica), 12 g of Chuang Xiong (Szechuan lovage root), 10 g of ginseng, 10 g of Gui Zhi (cinnamon), 8 g of Xiao Hui Xiang (fennel fruit), 10 g of Ai Ye (moxa), and 3 g of Gan Cao (licorice root).

• **To treat period pains associated with strong mood swings:** Mix 12 g of Dang Gui (Chinese angelica), 12 g of Chuan Xiong (Szechuan lovage root), 12 g of Chi Shao (red peony root), 10 g of Zhi Ke (bitter orange), 12 g of Yan Hu Suo (corydalis rhizome), 12 g of Xiang Fu (nut grass rhizome), 12 g of Dan Pi (cortex of tree peony root), and 3 g of Gan Cao (licorice root).

Acupressure: Press the Xue Hai, Feng Shi, Susanli, and San Yin Jiao acupressure points. The Xue Hai point is on the inside of the leg in the depression just above the knee. Locate the

Feng Shi point along the outside of the leg at the end of the fingers when the arm is hanging straight down at the side. The Susanli point is found on the lower leg, about 1 inch to the outside of and 3 inches below the kneecap. The San Yin Jiao point is located in the center of the inside of the leg, about 3 inches above the anklebone.

Diet: Drink plenty of water. Eat fresh fruits and vegetables, and food that promotes blood circulation, such as black soybeans, brown sugar, chestnuts, peaches, and sweet basil. Eat less fatty and greasy food since they create stagnation that will worsen the pain.

Naturopathy

Diet: Constipation is often linked to menstrual pain. Eat a high-fiber diet to guard against this. Vegetables, fruits, whole grains, nuts, seeds, and beans all contain high levels of fiber. Ground flaxseeds, also high in fiber, can be sprinkled on salads and cereals. If you eat meat, stick to organic, hormone-free beef and chicken to avoid hormonal imbalances in your body. Diets low in inflammatory foods are essential for the relief of pain with periods. These foods include hydrogenated fats, sugar, processed carbohydrates, wheat, and dairy products. Also eat oily fish such as salmon, sardines, and mackerel, and flaxseed to obtain omega-3 fatty acids, which can help reduce inflammation. Drink at least eight glasses of water a day, and cut down on the amount of alcohol and caffeine you consume to protect against dehydration, which contributes to period pain.

Supplements: Take 50 mg of vitamin B6 a day, as it has been shown to help with painful periods and premenstrual syndrome (PMS). Magnesium is required for the metabolism of estrogen, and also works synergistically with vitamin B6 to reduce pain; take 250 mg a day. Muscles that are calcium-deficient tend to be hyperactive and therefore might be more likely to cramp, so take 1,000 mg of the citrate form of calcium a day. Niacin has been shown to be helpful in treating menstrual cramps as it dilates the blood vessels to improve blood flow to the contracting uterus. Take 100 mg every three hours during episodes of menstrual cramping, and 100 mg a day for prevention, but make sure you use the non-flushing type of niacin. Vitamin C appears to work synergistically with niacin in people suffering from painful periods. Take 3,000 mg a day with 1,500 mg of bioflavonoids, which help the body to absorb vitamin C and also have other general health benefits. Take 400 IU a day of a natural vitamin E with a blend of mixed tocopherols to relieve menstrual pain and breast tenderness. Evening primrose can counter the inflammatory hormones causing pain. Take 2,000–3,000 mg of evening primrose oil with 200–300 mg of gamma-linolenic acid (GLA) a day.

Herbs: Black cohosh has a history as a folk medicine for relieving menstrual cramps. Take 250 mg three times a day of a dry powdered extract. Tinctures can also be taken at 2–4 ml three times per day. Blue cohosh has also been used traditionally for easing painful menstrual periods. Blue cohosh, which is generally taken as a tincture, should be limited to no more than 1–2 ml taken three times per day. False unicorn was used in the Native American tradition for a large number of women's health conditions, including painful menstruation. Generally, false unicorn root is taken as a tincture at 2–5 ml three times per day. It is typically taken in combination with other herbs that support the female reproductive organs.

Homeopathy

If you experience severe period pains, consult a homeopathic practitioner. The acute homeopathic remedies listed below can help as a stop-gap measure and as complementary support in providing pain relief.

Belladonna: If violent, abrupt pain is accompanied by a bright red flow and some clotting, use Belladonna. Sufferers also tend to be irritable and short-tempered.

Arsenicum album: Use this remedy if exhausting period pains are associated with a sense of chilliness, restlessness, nausea, diarrhea, and possibly vomiting. There may also be severe anxiety and a fear of feeling ill. Applying a hot water bottle to the abdomen feels soothing.

Lachesis: To ease period pains that are most severe immediately preceding the onset of a period, use Lachesis. The flow tends to be dark in color, and large clots are usually present. Cramping pains build in intensity from around mid-cycle until the onset of a steady flow. Other symptoms include premenstrual left-sided headaches, migraines, disturbed sleep, night sweats, hot flashes, palpitations, and anxiety.

Colocynthis: If waves of cramps come on and then subside rapidly, consider using Colocynthis. The pain may leave you feeling weak and cause you to instinctively double over. Firm pressure provides some relief, but it is usually difficult to find a comfortable position.

Cimicifuga: When this remedy is helpful, period pains become proportionally more severe as the flow increases. Symptoms include flitting, shocklike pains that often radiate from the belly down to the thighs. Walking around, moving your bowels, and warmth provide some temporary relief.

Herbalism

Painful menstruation is typically caused by excessive uterine tone and spasm. Elevated pro-inflammatory chemicals (prostaglandins and leukotrienes) are commonly found in uterine tissue of women with this condition. Many herbal medicines can reduce uterine tone and spasm quite effectively.

Motherwort: This herb relieves painful uterine cramping, as well as heart palpitations and high blood pressure brought on by stress. Take 1 tbsp of the above-ground parts as an infusion, or 2 ml of a tincture three times daily. The best results are seen when this herb is taken in the long term.

Cramp bark: This is a wonderful uterine and intestinal antispasmodic. Clinical studies have shown that two active constituents, scopoletin and viopudial, have a strong antispasmodic effect on uterine tissue. Cramp bark also has anti-inflammatory properties, can calm the nerves, and may help to lower blood pressure. For many, 5 ml of tincture in a little water three times daily is sufficient, but depends on the severity of cramping.

Lady's mantle: This herb is high in tannins, which account for its astringent effect on the uterus, and is ideal for treating heavy menstrual bleeding. Flavonoids within this herb also provide anti-inflammatory and nutritive properties to the uterus. Drink an infusion made from 2 tsp of dried herb in 1 cup of water, or take 30 drops of tincture, three times daily.

Seek Professional Advice
The information in this book is a not a substitute for professional medical advice or health care. Consult a qualified health professional when there is any question regarding the presence or treatment of any health condition.

Yeast Infection

Diagnosis

A vaginal yeast infection is caused by the yeast fungus, Candida albicans. Infection is caused by a reduction in the acidity of the vagina, which allows too much yeast (tiny organisms that live on the skin and inside the vagina) to grow. The acidic balance can be changed by menstruation, pregnancy, diabetes, some antibiotics, oral contraceptives, and steroids. Clothing that is too tight or made of synthetic materials that trap heat and moisture can also lead to infections, as yeast thrives in this type of environment.

Yeast infections are extremely common and will affect three out of four women at some point in their lives. Many women will also suffer from repeated infections, which become more common after menopause. Although they are particularly uncomfortable, they are not usually serious and are easy to treat. However, it is important to consult a doctor to get an accurate diagnosis since other infections, such as some sexually transmitted diseases, can cause similar symptoms but require different treatments.

Symptoms

- Itchiness and burning in the vagina and around the vulva
- A white vaginal discharge
- Pain during sexual intercourse
- Swelling of the vulva
- Burning sensation when urinating

Treatment Goal

To relieve symptoms and restore the balance of bacteria in the vagina. It is important to identify the cause of the yeast infection to avoid recurrence, and to rule out diabetes as raised glucose levels can trigger candida overgrowth.

Conventional Medicine

Conventional treatment of a vaginal fungal infection involves a proper diagnosis and pharmacological therapy. A diagnosis is usually made after a pelvic exam and swab. A yeast infection has a discharge that gives a typical pattern, and is easily identified under a microscope.

Suppositories and creams: Women familiar with the symptoms of a yeast infection and may opt to use an over-the-counter product such as miconazole (Monistat®) suppositories, which are taken for three to seven days. Alternative treatments include boric acid suppositories or tea tree oil suppositories, which are both made by a compounding pharmacist. Nystatin cream and suppositories can also be used. These have a cure rate of about 80% and cause few side effects. Clotrimazole, taken in the form of a 200 mg vaginal tablet, can be used for three to seven days as prescribed. Butoconazole, another cream, is usually used for three days and also has a good cure rate.

Fluconazole: Other pharmacologic therapy includes fluconazole, which is a pill that is taken in one dose. This can be associated with nausea, headaches, and stomach pain. Fluconazole (Diflucan®) can be used orally once a month for prevention.

Oral probiotics: The oral probiotics bifidus, acidophilus, and S. boullardii species are recommended to help prevent recurrence of a yeast infection, as is a diet that is low in processed food and sugar.

Traditional Chinese Medicine

Herbs: To make a decoction, combine the herbs in a glass or ceramic pot and add 3 cups of water. Bring to a boil, simmer for 30 minutes, and strain. Drink 1 cup twice a day.
• For symptoms of fatigue, poor appetite, a bloated stomach, loose stools, and a clear vaginal discharge: These symptoms are considered to be related to spleen deficiency. Mix 12 g of Huang Qin (baical skullcap root), 12 g of Tai Zi Shen (pseudostellaria), 15 g of Bai Zhu (white atractylodes rhizome), 15 g of Fuling (poria), 5 g of Chen Pi (tangerine peel), and 12 g of Fa Ban Xia (pinellia rhizome).
• For symptoms of a bloated abdomen, yellow or thick vaginal discharge, itchiness, and thirst: Mix 12 g of Huang Qin (baical skullcap root), 15 g of Bai Zhu (white atractylodes rhizome), 15 g of Fuling (poria), 10 g of Zhi Zi (cape jasmine fruit), 10 g of Huo Xiang (agastache), and 10 g of Huang Bai (phellodendron).

Acupressure: Press the Nei Guan and San Yin Jiao acupressure points for two to three minutes, once a day. The Nei Guan point is located in the center of the wrist on the palm side, about 2 inches below the crease. The San Yin Jiao point is in the center of the inside of the leg, about 3 inches above the anklebone.

Diet: Eat rice instead of wheat. Also include food in your diet that helps eliminate dampness, such as daikon radishes, eggplant, celery, and. Avoid sweets and fatty, greasy food.

Naturopathy

Diet: The following measures are part of a standard diet to control candida, which causes yeast infections. Eat chicken, eggs, fish, yogurt, vegetables, seeds, oils, and lots of raw garlic (it has antifungal properties). Eliminate refined and simple sugars from your diet, and avoid added sugar of any kind, including white or brown sugar, raw sugar, honey, molasses, or grain sweeteners. Stevia is an allowed sugar substitute. Also avoid milk, alcohol, fruit or dried fruit, and mushrooms, which encourage fungal micro-organisms to grow. Avoid foods that contain yeast or mold, including all breads, muffins, cakes, baked goods, cheeses, dried fruits, melons, and peanuts. Take 1 tsp–1 tbsp of soluble fiber a day. Guar gum, flaxseeds, psyllium husks, or pectin can be mixed in an 8 oz glass of water and drunk twice a day on an empty stomach. Fiber helps to normalize bowel movements to expel fungal micro-organisms from the body, thereby preventing infections from developing.

Supplements: Take 1,000 mg of caprylic acid, a fatty acid that has been shown to have antifungal properties. Vitamin C, taken at 1,000 mg twice a day, helps to enhance immune functions. Also take a high-potency multivitamin to obtain many nutrients that will support immune function. Take a probiotic product that contains about four billion micro-organisms twice a day 30 minutes before each meal. These micro-organisms provide acidophilus and bifidus, which are friendly bacteria that prevent yeast overgrowth and fight candida. Also take 200 mg of grapefruit seed extract two to three times a day for its anti-candida properties.

Tip: APPROPRIATE CLOTHING

Wear cotton underwear and loose clothes. This will help to keep the area dry and reduce irritation.

Herbs: Oregano oil is known for its strong antifungal properties. Take 5 drops of oil under the tongue, or mixed with a glass of water if you find the undiluted drops to be too strong. You can also take oregano in capsule form at 500 mg a day. Take 500 mg of garlic to fight fungus and boost the immune system. Undecylenic acid, a derivative from castor bean oil, has been shown to have strong antifungal activity. Take 200 mg three times a day. Drink 2 cups of Pau d'Arco tea a day for its strong antifungal properties. Barberry also contains antifungal and antimicrobial properties. Take 250–500 mg three times a day.

Homeopathy

The remedies listed below can help to ease the severity and shorten the duration of a recent, mild to moderate vaginal yeast infection. A recurrent, severe, or established yeast infection should be treated by an experienced homeopathic practitioner.

Borax: To treat acute yeast infection symptoms that occur when ovulating (mid-cycle), take Borax. Symptoms include irritation and a swollen sensation in the vagina, with a thin discharge that may be bland or irritating.

Kreosotum: If symptoms include a smarting, burning sensation that travels deep into the vagina, Kreosotum may be appropriate. There may be a yellow discharge that eases symptoms, while sexual intercourse or being overheated is aggravating. Contact with cool air feels temporarily soothing, and eases irritation and burning.

Natrum mur: If symptoms of a yeast infection arise along with vaginal dryness, try this remedy. Persistent dryness and discomfort can alternate with the production of a thin, watery discharge. Symptoms tend to be more intense during or just after a period.

Tip: AVOID LOCAL ANESTHETICS

Creams that act as a local anesthetic do not support the body in dealing with a yeast infection. They also potentially mask an infection that may not be due to yeast. It is also possible to develop a sensitivity to the cream, which can further aggravate symptoms.

Tip: AVOID SCENTED BATH PRODUCTS

At the first sign of vaginal irritation, sensitivity, or itchiness, avoid using any bath products that are highly scented and/or contain harsh chemical detergents. Instead add a handful of sea salt, or a weak infusion of chamomile, to your bath.

Herbalism

Antifungal suppository: To treat vaginal yeast infections, create an anti-fungal suppository. Add 5 drops each of garlic oil, chamomile oil, and tea tree oil to a base of cocoa butter and vitamin A, which can then be put into vaginal suppository molds. Insert one suppository into the vagina at night for seven days. Calendula oil and goldenseal may also be added.

Douche: Make a vaginal douche by combining 2 tsp each of dried, chopped goldenseal root, calendula flowers, and garlic in 2 cups of hot water, and add 10 ml of vinegar. Let the mixture cool, and then douche with 1 cup of solution in the morning and 1 cup before bedtime. This treatment can be combined with vaginal antifungal suppositories.

Fibroids

Diagnosis

Fibroids are noncancerous growths of tissue that develop in the muscular wall of the uterus. There are four different types of fibroid. Submucosal fibroids grow on the inside of the womb; intramural fibroids grow within the uterine wall; subserosal fibroids grow on the outside of the womb on the lining between the uterus and the pelvic cavity; and pedunculated fibroids are stalklike growths that are attached to either the inside or outside wall of the womb. Many women with fibroids have no symptoms, while others experience heavy bleeding, pain, or incontinence. If fibroids become too large they can put pressure on other organs such as the bladder and the bowel, a condition known as compression syndrome. This can lead to backache, hip pain, and constipation.

Symptoms

- Often, no symptoms are present
- Painful periods
- Heavy periods
- Irregular periods
- Bowel or bladder discomfort
- Frequent urination/constipation
- Hip and back pain
- Infertility, if the fibroid is blocking the fallopian tube
- Miscarriage, if the fibroid is pressing on the cervix

Treatment Goal

Most fibroids do not require treatment. If the fibroids are causing complications, they may need to be removed. Treatment focuses on relieving the discomfort of symptoms.

Conventional Medicine

Conventional medical treatment involves reducing heavy bleeding, and relieving pain and pelvic discomfort. If a woman is approaching menopause, watching and waiting may be the extent of the treatment, as fibroids tend to shrink after this time due to reduced estrogen. If the fibroids are small and not causing significant symptoms such as anemia and pain, it is best to wait until they shrink on their own.

Medication: Non-steroidal anti-inflammatory drugs (NSAIDs) such as ibuprofen and mefenamic acid can help ease pain and, to an extent, the amount of heavy bleeding. Aminocaproic acid treatment, given either intravenously or orally, reduces heavy bleeding by affecting clotting. However, it should be used with caution in people with a history of thrombosis. Progesterone, when taken for 21 days of a woman's menstrual cycle, can also have an effect on bleeding; synthetic medroxyprogesterone or natural progesterone can be used. Oral doses should be used with caution in patients with a history of depression, and those with a history of progesterone receptor positive breast cancer should not take progesterone. Oral contraceptive agents may be used to reduce fibroid size, but in some women, they actually increase fibroid size as they increase synthetic estrogen in the body. However, they do reduce menstrual loss and regulate the timing of periods. Anti-gonadotropin agents, such as danazol, can be used to abolish ovulation, thus suppressing menstruation.

Surgery: Surgical procedures include a hysterectomy, where the uterus is removed, an endometrial ablation, which destroys the layer of cells that lines the uterus, a myomectomy to remove fibroids, and a laparoscopic myomectomy, which is key hole surgery to remove fibroids. Uterine artery embolization is a new non-surgical procedure that is rapid and has a good success rate.

Lifestyle modification: Many women who have fibroids have an excess of estrogen present in the body. Fat cells make more estrogen, so lifestyle changes that promote weight loss can help to decrease the chance of fibroids developing.

Tip: PROGESTERONE CREAMS

Under the supervision of a doctor, apply progesterone creams to the abdomen, thighs, neck, and arms to balance estrogen, regulate the menstrual flow, and relieve pain. An appropriate dose is ½ tsp applied twice a day, but do not apply the cream during the week of your menstrual flow.

Traditional Chinese Medicine

Herbs: Use herbs that are proven to remove blood stagnation and dispel phlegm, which are associated with fibroids according to traditional Chinese medicine. Combine 15 g of Xuan Shen (ningpo figwort root), 12 g of Chi Xiao Dou (adzuki bean), 15 g of Niu Xi (achyranthes root), 15 g of Dan Shen (salvia root), 12 g of Bai Jie Zi (white mustard seed), 12 g of Dang Gui (Chinese angelica), 12 g of Xiang Fu (nut grass rhizome), and 3 g of Gan Cao (licorice root). Place the raw herbs in a ceramic or glass pot and add 3½ cups of water. Bring to a boil and simmer for 30 minutes. Strain the liquid and drink 1 cup twice a day.

Acupressure: Press the Xue Hai, Feng Shi, Susanli, and San Yin Jiao acupressure points. The Xue Hai point is on the inside of the leg, at the depression just above the knee. Locate the Feng Shi point along the outside of the leg, at the tip of the fingers when the arm is hanging straight down at the side of the body. The Susanli point is found on the lower leg, about 1 inch to the outside of and 3 inches below the kneecap. The San Yin Jiao point is located on the inside of the leg, about 3 inches above the anklebone.

Diet: Eat food that is helpful for blood circulation like black soybeans, brown sugar, chestnuts, peaches, and sweet basil.

 # Naturopathy

Diet: Fibroids are affected by hormones, which are in turn affected by diet. Base your diet around whole grains, fruit, vegetables, fish, beans, and fermented soy products. It is important to eat organic products as much as possible because some of the chemicals used to fumigate foods mimic estrogen activity. If you have heavy periods, eat foods that have high amounts of iron such as blackstrap molasses, liver, and organic, grass-fed beef. Drink eight glasses of water a day to help flush out impurities. Soy products and flaxseeds are good sources of phytoestrogens, which are thought to help prevent fibroids. Avoid sugar, alcohol, caffeine, and foods that contain hydrogenated fats to avoid inflammation. These foods also depress your immune system.

Supplements: A high-potency multivitamin supplement supplies nutrients important in estrogen metabolism. Take them as directed on the label. B-complex vitamins are also necessary for estrogen metabolism. Take 100 mg twice a day. Take 400 IU of vitamin E to helps with inflammation. Essential fatty acids (EFAs) also help decrease inflammation and are nourishing to the female reproductive system. Take a daily combination of 2 tbsp of flaxseed oil a day, 500 mg of fish oils, and 300 mg of borage oil, all good sources of EFAs.

Herbs: Chasteberry balances estrogen/progesterone levels. Take 240 mg of a standardized extract that contains 0.6% aucubin. Do not use this herb if currently taking a contraceptive pill. Take 300 mg of indole-3-carbinol a day, a substance found in cruciferous vegetables such as broccoli that helps estrogen metabolism. D-glucarate is a plant chemical that assists the liver in estrogen breakdown. Take 500 mg a day. Drink 3 cups of red raspberry tea a day to help with uterine inflammation and pain.

Hydrotherapy: Regular sitz baths, where only the hips and buttocks are soaked in water or saline solution, will improve circulation to the pelvic region and help ease pain. You can add 10 drops of warming oils, such as rosemary or marjoram essential oils, to the bath to increase blood flow and relieve pain.

 # Homeopathy

Any of the following can be helpful short-term remedies to ease moderately heavy bleeding and pain that occur on an occasional basis as a result of fibroids. Severe or recurrent problems should be treated by a homeopathic practitioner.

Lachesis: If menstrual pain is accompanied by a clotted flow that is dark in color, try Lachesis. Cramping pains are relieved as soon as menstrual bleeding begins. Sufferers also experience mood swings and disturbed sleep from mid-cycle until the beginning of a period.

Phosphorus: To treat menstrual bleeding that is not heavy, but continues for an extended period and is bright red in color, use Phosphorus. Those who respond well to this remedy are anxious and fearful, but are calmed by reassurance and attention.

Silica: If heavy periods are combined with waves of icy coldness that travel through the body, use Silica. Menstrual cramps and pains are sharp and cutting in nature, and are aggravated when passing water. Classic symptoms include a profound sense of weakness and feeling stressed, nervous, and strung out when unwell.

Herbalism

There are many herbs traditionally used to help with one of the main symptoms of fibroids, uterine bleeding. These herbs have a variety of effects to control abnormal blood flow.

Lady's mantle: This herb is traditionally used in treating women with fibroids who experience heavy periods. It is rich in tannin content, and the herb is used as a styptic and to reduce menstrual flow. This herb may be taken as an infusion by steeping 2 tsp in freshly boiled water for 10 minutes. Drink 2–3 cups daily.

Dong Quai: The root of Dong Quai may help to normalize female hormones that contribute to the abnormal bleeding associated with uterine fibroids. The form and dose used is best assessed by a medical herbalist. Paeony may also be used in a variety of female hormone related issues to help balance the hormones.

Thuja and greater celandine: These herbs work effectively in combination in cases of fibroids, due to anti-mitotic properties and liver clearance actions. It is advised to consult a medical herbalist on how best to use these herbs, and on the dose to be taken.

Beth root: Beth root is rich in tannins and steroidal saponins. It can be effective in stopping uterine bleeding and has a hormone regulating effect. Make a tea of beth root from 2–4 g of the herb and drink daily; you can also take 60 drops of tincture three times a day to control excessive uterine bleeding. This herb should not be used if you have heart problems, or are pregnant or lactating. Sometimes beth root can cause stomach upset, nausea, and vomiting. Beth root is sometimes combined with other herbs for this condition.

Menopause

Diagnosis

Menopause marks the end of menstruation and a woman's reproductive years. On average this tends to happen around the age of 51, but there have been cases where periods have stopped in women in their 20s, while other women will continue to menstruate until their late 50s or early 60s. The perimenopause, the period leading up to menopause where periods start to become irregular, generally starts when a woman is in her 40s. Menopause can go on for many years, but once a woman has not had a period for one year she is considered to be postmenopausal.

Menopause is triggered when the ovaries no longer respond to the controlling hormones released by the pituitary gland. As a result, the ovaries stop releasing an egg each month and no longer produce the female sex hormones estrogen and progesterone. It is this decline of function in the ovaries and fall in hormone levels that give rise to the symptoms of menopause. Symptoms vary from woman to woman. Many only notice that their periods become irregular. Others, however, suffer from heavy bleeding, hot flashes, disturbed sleep, and emotional instability.

Symptoms

- Irregular periods
- Hot flashes
- Disturbed sleep, often with night sweats
- Emotional distress
- Vaginal dryness
- Dry skin
- Weight gain
- Low libido

Treatment Goal

To alleviate the symptoms of the menopause by adjusting hormone levels and introducing lifestyle changes. This should help to limit the physical and emotional impact that menopause can have on many women's lives.

Conventional Medicine

Menopause is a normal life transition, so there is no necessary medical treatment. It is possible, however, to ease symptoms through lifestyle modification and hormone replacement. For treatment of hot flashes, see p. 408.

Lifestyle modifications: A high-fiber, low-fat diet and reducing your intake of dairy and processed foods is recommended. Perform an aerobic exercise for 20 minutes every day to help with the weight gain that tends to occur with menopause. Stress-reduction techniques are also recommended.

Hormone replacement: Balancing the hormones can help the emotional challenges associated with menopause, as well as other troubling symptoms such as vaginal dryness, skin dryness, and low libido. Synthetic hormones have been shown to be detrimental to a woman's overall health, and they are now rarely recommended by doctors. Many doctors instead advocate the use of natural estradiol and estriol as well as progesterone and/or testosterone and DHEA, a steroid hormone. Blood levels can be taken to determine the amount of hormone needed and a pharmacist can make up an exact prescription. These hormones have not been studied to the same extent as synthetic hormones. They are thought to be safer due to their bio-identical compounding (they match the natural hormones of the body) and low dosage. Frequently, selective serotonin reuptake inhibitors (SSRIs) drugs such as Prozac® and Lexapro® are also prescribed to treat emotional difficulties, and may also alleviate hot flashes.

Traditional Chinese Medicine

Herbs: To prepare a formula, place the herbs in a ceramic pot and add 3 cups of water. Bring to a boil, simmer for 30 minutes, and strain the liquid. Drink 1 cup twice a day.
• **To treat perimenopause:** Mix 15 g of Sheng Di Huang (Chinese foxglove root), 10 g of Shan Zhu Yu (Asiatic cornelian cherry), 15 g of Shan Yao (Chinese yam), 15 g of Fuling (poria), 12 g of Ze Xie (water plantain rhizome), 12 g of Dan Pi (cortex of peony root), 12 g of Niu Zhen Zi (privet fruit), and 12 g of Wu Wei Zi (schisandra fruit).

• **To treat kidney Yang deficiency:** Symptoms may include chills, dizziness, cold hands and feet, and loose stools. Combine 15 g of Shu Di Huang (cooked Chinese foxglove), 12 g of Shan Zhu Yu (Asiatic cornelian cherry), 15 g of Shan Yao (Chinese yam), 12 g of Tu Si Zi (Chinese dodder seed), 12 g of Du Zhong (eucommia bark), 8 g of Rui Gui Zhi (inner bark of Saigon cinnamon), and 12 g of Dang Gui (Chinese angelica).
• **To treat Qi stagnation:** Symptoms include depression, loss of interest in life, and stress.

Mix 12 g of Chai Hu (hare's ear root), 15 g of Bai Shao (white peony root), 15 g of Bai Zhu (white atractylodes rhizome), 15 g of Fuling (poria), 5 g of Bo He (field mint), 6 g of Gan Cao (licorice root), 12 g of Xiang Fu (nut grass rhizome), and 12 g of Gou Ji Zi (wolfberry).

Acupressure: The Hegu and Fu Liu acupressure points may help to reduce hot flashes and perspiration. The Hegu points are located on the back of the hands in the depression between the thumb and the first finger. The Fu Liu point is on the inside of the leg, beside the ankle, in the depression 1 inch directly above the Achilles tendon. Use the tip of your fingers to press these points with moderate pressure for one to two minutes.

Diet: Eat a nutritious diet of fresh fruits and vegetables and grains to maintain good health. It is also important to drink plenty of water every day.

Naturopathy

Menopausal symptoms are related to falling levels of estrogen and progesterone, and the recommendations below may help to boost the levels of these hormones in the body.

Diet: Eat two to three servings of foods that contain phytosterols, which have hormone-balancing effects. These include whole grains, legumes, and fresh vegetables and fruits. Phytoestrogens, estrogen-like compounds that also have hormone-balancing effects, should be consumed as often as possible. Have one or two servings a day of miso, flaxseeds, or tofu, unless you are allergic to soy products. You can sprinkle 1–2 tbsp of ground flaxseeds, which also lower cholesterol, over cereal or salad, or add it to a smoothie. If eating meat, choose the organic, hormone-free kind to avoid hormonal imbalances.

Supplements: A high-quality multivitamin can nourish your body to keep hormones balanced. Follow the directions on the label. Take 1,000 mg of calcium and 500 mg of magnesium, both of which are essential for bone health. B-complex vitamins and vitamin C may all help to relieve hot flashes. Take 100 mg and 1,000 mg respectively three times a day. Take 1 tbsp of evening primrose oil three times a day. It can also help to relieve hot flashes and is excellent for the production of estrogen. Pregnenolone, which is involved in making estrogen and progesterone, can help with hormone imbalances. Take 30 mg twice a day.

Herbs: Take 80 mg of black cohosh twice a day; studies show that it alleviates hot flushes. Chaste berry has historically been used to prevent of hot flashes. Take 160–240 mg of an 0.6 % aucubin extract daily. Take 40 mg of red clover twice a day, as it has been shown to reduce some of the symptoms of menopause. Hops, taken at 250 mg three times a day, can help to reduce anxiety and tension, which are common menopausal symptoms, and has hormone-balancing effects. Soy protein powder has been shown in some studies to reduce hot flashes. Take 60 g a day mixed into a smoothie. Also take 4–6 g of sage a day to help control night sweats associated with hot flashes.

 # Homeopathy

Homeopathy can help ease symptoms, and may be helpful in treating the emotional distress that a difficult menopause can involve. Remedies can be used on their own, or alongside conventional treatment. The remedies below provide an overview of some of the strategies that practitioners will utilize when treating symptoms.

Calc carb: If symptoms include the feeling that the whole body system has slowed down, take Calc carb. Weight gain may be noticeable, coupled with low energy levels. Hot flashes come on with little physical effort, followed by a cold, clammy sensation.

Natrum mur: Symptoms that call for this remedy include dry mucous membranes, particularly of the vagina. The skin is also likely to show signs of dryness and sensitivity. Emotionally, sufferers tend to bottle up their feelings, resulting in low moods and depression.

Sepia: If menopause brings on exhaustion associated with feeling drained, take Sepia. The libido is very low and patients tend to feel irritable and emotionally flat. Flashes, which are likely to be a major symptom, sweep upward from the torso to the head, leading to profuse sweating that feels draining.

Pulsatilla: If changeableness is the key symptom of menopause, use Pulastilla. Moods are especially affected, and there is a tendency to be uncharacteristically emotional. Although sufferers feel chilly, sweats break out on the face due to waves of heat that are aggravated by being in stuffy surroundings, and when trying to sleep.

Tip: NIGHTWEAR CHOICE

If night sweats are a major issue, avoid wearing nightwear that is made from synthetic materials as it tends to hold in heat. Opt instead for natural fibers that allow air to circulate and the skin to sweat freely when the body needs to cool down.

Herbalism

Black cohosh: This herb is recognized for its ability to reduce or eliminate menopausal symptoms such as hot flashes, insomnia, fatigue, depression, irritability, and mood swings. Black cohosh also acts as an anti-spasmodic, anti-inflammatory, digestive stimulant, mild sedative, and blood pressure lowering agent by relaxing blood vessels in the extremities. Clinical studies show that black cohosh reduces symptoms of menopause in a similar manner to low-doses of estrogen replacement. Most importantly, these effects occur without increasing the lining of the uterus or estrogen levels in the body. The recommended dose is 40 mg per day of a standardized extract or 2 ml of tincture taken twp to three times daily

Sage: Used to reduce excess sweating, this herb is often employed for use in those experiencing night sweats and hot flashes due to the menopause. Sage is often also useful for those needing help with cognitive function during the menopause. An infusion is most often the recommendation. Steep 1-2 tsp, covered, in freshly boiled water, for 10 minutes. Strain and allow the infusion to cool. Drink three times daily.

Motherwort: Palpitations can be a symptom for many during the menopausal stage. Motherwort helps to relieve palpitations, and is also a calming anxiolytic herb. An infusion may be taken as 1 cup three times daily, by steeping 2 tsp of the dried herb in a cup of boiled water for 10 minutes. Tinctures are also available.

Liver and adrenal tonic: Because adrenal and liver stress exacerbates the symptoms of menopause, combine equal parts of the following herbs to support adrenal function and repair and detoxify the liver: licorice, wild yam, Dong Quai, black cohosh, milk thistle, burdock, and sage. Add cinnamon and spearmint to taste. Boil 2 tsp of the herb blend per cup of water and drink three times daily.

Hot Flashes

Diagnosis

A hot flash is the sudden unpleasant sensation of burning heat spreading across the face, neck, and chest. It is a side effect of menopause that affects many women, some long before menopause actually begins (this period is known as the perimenopause). A hot flash is triggered by a lack of estrogen, which causes irregularities in the body's cooling system. This can result in extreme discomfort, and disturbed sleep, particularly if flashes are accompanied by drenching night-time sweats. There is great variation in both the degree and the persistence of symptoms between different women. Some have no symptoms whatsoever, whereas others have severe problems that make a huge impact on their lives and last for years. Generally, however, the number of hot flashes women experience will subside over time.

Symptoms

- Sudden changes in body temperature
- Redness and blushing in the face, neck, and chest
- Increased sweating, particularly at night in bed

Treatment Goal

To relieve the distress and discomfort of hot flashes, and develop techniques for coping with episodes. Hormone replacement therapy (HRT) is effective at relieving hot flashes following menopause; however, HRT is not recommended for use for longer than five years. Discuss this treatment option with your doctor.

Conventional Medicine

HRT: Treating hot flashes involves stabilizing hormones during the menopausal period. Hormone replacement therapy (HRT), which involves increasing the levels of female hormones in the body, is the most effective way of achieving this, but it is currently a controversial form of treatment. Recent trials have shown that the use of combined synthetic estrogen-progestin therapy in postmenopausal women increases the risk of cardiovascular disease, stroke, breast cancer, venous thromboembolism, and probable dementia in women aged 65 years of age or older. Newer bio-identical hormones, which are natural, do not seem to share the same risk as synthetic hormones, but extensive tests have not yet been done. The severity of the hot flashes and other menopausal symptoms should be weighed against the risks of hormone therapy. In any case, the lowest amount of the most bio-identical hormone should be used to treat hot flashes. Estrogen should be combined with progesterone, rather than used by itself.

Other medication: Anti-depressant drugs, the selective serotonin reuptake inhibitors (SSRIs) drugs in particular (including Prozac®, Zoloft®, and Lexapro®), can be helpful in reducing episodes of hot flashes. Natural treatments such as vitamin E, taken at a dose of 400–800 IU daily, and black cohosh extract standardized to 5% triterpene glycosides, taken at 40 drops daily, are also recommended. Soy phytoestrogens as well as the phytoestrogens found in celery, parsley, whole grains (flax in particular), and alfalfa are weak estrogens that may be helpful. Plant medicine that contains estrogens includes Dong Quai, licorice root, chaste berries, and black cohosh.

Traditional Chinese Medicine

Herbs: Combine 15 g of Sheng Di Huang (Chinese foxglove root), 12 g of Shan Zhu Yu (Asiatic cornelian cherry), 15 g of Shan Yao (Chinese yam), 15 g of Fuling (poria), 12 g of Ze Xie (water plantain rhizome), 12 g of Dan Pi (cortex of tree peony root), 12 g of Di Gu Pi (cortex of wolfberry root), 12 g of Nan Sa Shen (glehnia root), and 5 g of Gan Cao (licorice root). If hot flashes are accompanied by heavy sweating, add 12 g of Fu Xiao Mai (wheat), and 15 g of Bai Shao (white peony root). Place the herbs in a glass or ceramic pot and add 3 cups of water. Bring the mixture to a boil and simmer for 30 minutes. Strain the liquid and drink 1 cup twice a day.

Acupressure: Press and release the Hegu point, located between your index finger and thumb, ten times on each hand and repeat. The Fu Liu point is on the inside of the leg, beside the ankle, in the depression 1 inch directly above the Achilles tendon. Place your index fingers on the depressions in each leg and apply gentle to moderate pressure, pressing and releasing ten times. Press these points once or twice a day to treat both acute and chronic conditions.

Diet: Add foods to your diet that tonify yin and clear out excessive heat, such as peppermint, mung beans, red beans, watermelon, string beans, black sesame seeds, and sword beans. Foods to be avoided are ginger, chilies, mustard greens, and mutton, because they are pungent, irritating, and increase heat in the body, which may make hot flashes worse.

Naturopathy

Diet: Eat two to three servings of foods that contain phytosterols, such as whole grains, legumes, fresh vegetables and fruits, since they have hormone-balancing effects. Phytoestrogens, estrogen-like compounds found in plant food, should be consumed as often as possible. Have one to two servings a day of miso, flaxseeds, or tofu. For example, 1–2 tbsp of ground flaxseeds can be sprinkled on cereal or salads, or added to smoothies. When eating meat, choose the organic, hormone-free variety to avoid hormone imbalances.

Supplements: A high-quality multivitamin can be helpful in nourishing your body to keep your hormones balanced. Follow the dosage directions on the label. Take 100 mg of B-complex vitamins three times a day, as they have been shown to relieve hot flashes. Vitamin C has also been shown to help relieve hot flashes and help women through menopause. Take 1,000 mg three times a day. Evening primrose oil is excellent for promoting the production of estrogen and alleviating hot flashes. Take 1 tbsp of the oil three times a day. Take 30 mg of pregnenolone, which is involved in making estrogen and progesterone, twice a day. Vitamin E complex may also help reduce hot flash symptoms. Take 400 IU a day.

Herbs: Take 80 mg of of black cohosh twice a day, which studies show alleviates hot flashes. Chaste berry has been used historically for prevention of hot flashes. Take 160–240 mg of a 0.6% aucubin extract daily. Hops can help reduce anxiety and tension, which are common menopausal symptoms, and have hormone-balancing effects. Take 250 mg three times a day. Soy protein powder has been shown in some studies to reduce hot flashes. Try mixing 60 g a day in a smoothie. Also take 4–6 g of sage a day, as it may help with controlling night sweats associated with hot flashes.

Tip: STOP SMOKING

Smoking can aggravate hot flashes and lead to premature menopause, so think about giving up if you smoke.

Homeopathy

Homeopathic remedies can be used on their own, or as complementary treatments to conventional support. The remedies listed below can provide short-term relief for mild to moderate, infrequent hot flashes. Consult an experienced homeopathic practitioner to treat severe, recurring episodes.

Belladonna: If hot flashes come on dramatically, triggering bright red, hot patches, consider using Belladonna. Skin remains dry, and sufferers feel irritable and cranky when feeling hot and bothered.

Sepia: If draining, exhausting, pulsating, sweaty flashes that sweep up the body are accompanied by feelings of anxiety, and preceded by a feeling of weakness, use Sepia.

Symptoms include low energy levels that improve after aerobic exercise, which stimulates the circulatory system.

Aconite: Also helpful for flashes that come on quickly, but those people helped by Aconite are more vulnerable to feelings of panic than irritability. Flashes emerge and fade quickly, but cause a great deal of emotional distress that manifests as trembling and palpitations.

Phosphorus: This remedy is helpful for burning hot flashes triggered by feeling anxious or excited, and eased by washing the face in cool water. Symptoms are most intense in the evening.

Herbalism

Black cohosh: The rhizome of black cohosh is well-known for treating menopausal and premenstrual symptoms. The most convincing studies have been on extracts standardized to the triterpene glycoside compounds, which are usually dosed at 40 mg twice daily. Most, but not all, of these clinical trials have shown a reduction in the frequency and severity of hot flashes. Black cohosh can also be taken as a decoction or tincture. To make a decoction, boil about 100 mg of the rhizome in 8 oz of water for 10 minutes, strain the herbs, and split the liquid into three amounts. Drink one of these

in the morning, one at noon, and one at night. Alternatively, you can take 2–3 ml of tincture twice a day.

Sage: Used to reduce excess sweating, this herb is often useful to those experiencing night sweats and hot flashes. An infusion is recommended. Make this by steeping 1–2 tsp in freshly boiled water for 10 minutes before straining. Allow the infusion to cool and drink three times daily.

Prostatitis

Diagnosis

Prostatitis is the inflammation of the prostate gland. It can occur as an acute or chronic condition. Acute prostatitis is commonly due to infection caused by bacteria that spreads from the urethra or bladder to the prostate. It is usually associated with lower urinary infection or with sexually transmitted diseases (STDs) such as gonorrhea or chlamydia. The main symptom is difficulty urinating, and the prostate can eventually become so swollen that it becomes impossible to pass urine. Contact a doctor immediately if this occurs.

Chronic prostatitis is rare and is usually associated with an infection elsewhere in the urinary tract. The main symptoms are genital or pelvic pain that comes and goes over a period of weeks or months, and intermittent urinary problems such as a sudden urge to urinate. The term chronic pelvic pain syndrome (CPPS) is now often used to describe this condition.

Symptoms

- Burning and discomfort when urinating
- Frequent urination
- Severe pain felt deep between the legs
- Fever
- Fatigue
- Pain in the lower back, scrotum, and rectum
- Discharge from the penis, if there is an STD present
- Problems with ejaculation

Treatment Goal

See a doctor to confirm that you have prostatitis. Treatment involves eliminating the bacteria that has caused the infection and relieving symptoms. Psychological therapy may also be needed to treat chronic conditions.

Conventional Medicine

Antibiotics: A broad spectrum of antibiotics such as Bactrim ® or ciprofloxacin is usually taken for four to six weeks to treat acute bacterial prostatitis. To treat chronic prostatitis, antibiotics are taken for an additional four to six weeks if a patient is asymptomatic, and for 12 weeks if he is symptomatic.

Other medication: If it is difficult to urinate, drugs such as doxazosin can be used to help improve urinary flow. Ibuprofen can also be taken to relieve pain and inflammation. Cernilton, which is a pollen extract, can help but may take several months to take effect.

Prostate massage: Chronic inflammation and swelling of the prostate can also occur with age. It is not caused by an infection, and repetitive prostate massage may help to relieve symptoms. Other lifestyle changes, such as cutting out caffeine and alcohol, may also help.

Traditional Chinese Medicine

Herbs: Mix 6 g of ginseng, 12 g of Mai Men Dong (ophiopogon tuber), and 6 g of Gan Cao (licorice root). Place the herbs in a ceramic pot, add 2 cups of water, bring to a boil, and simmer for 30 minutes. Strain and drink.

Acupressure: Press the Nei Guan point, found on the center of the wrist on the palm side, about 3 inches above the crease. The Susanli point is on the front of the lower leg in the depression about 3 inches below and to the left of the knee. Use the tip of a finger or thumb to press these points for one minute.

Diet: Drink plenty of water every day and eat fresh fruit and vegetables. Avoid hot chili peppers, beef, lamb, and deep-fried food since these create heat in the body.

Naturopathy

Diet: Eat whole, fresh, unrefined, and unprocessed foods. Include fruits, vegetables, whole grains, soy, beans, seeds, nuts, olive oil, and cold-water fish (salmon, sardines, halibut, and mackerel) in your diet. Eating organic food helps to reduce your exposure to pesticides, herbicides, and hormones. Avoid sugar, dairy products, refined foods, fried foods, junk foods, alcohol, and caffeine. These foods wreak havoc on hormones that affect the prostate and increase inflammation. Use an elimination diet to determine whether you have any food sensitivities. Cut out a common allergen, such as wheat, dairy, corn, oranges, and soy, for three weeks and then reintroduce it at the end of the third week to see if any changes occur. Flaxseeds contain phytonutrients that balance estrogen levels. Grind 2–4 tbsp and add them to your food daily. You can also take 1 tbsp of flaxseed oil a day, although it is not as beneficial.

Supplements: Take 400 mg of bromelain three times a day in between meals for its anti-inflammatory properties. Also take 500–1,000 mg of vitamin C three times a day to enhance immune function, inhibit the growth of E. coli, and make the urine more acidic. Probiotics such as acidophilus should be taken if you are on antibiotics as it can replenish the beneficial gut flora that antibiotics can kill. Take a product that has at least 4 billion organisms daily. Also take 500 mg of quercetin

twice a day for its anti-inflammatory properties. Selenium is an antioxidant, but may be more effective when taken with vitamin E. Take 200 mcg of selenium and 400 IU of vitamin E. Zinc is vital to the health of the prostate, which concentrates and secretes zinc, and also helps prevent infections. Take 100 mg daily along with 10 mg of copper for one month, then a preventive dose of 30 mg a day with 3 mg of copper.

Herbs: Bearberry acts as a diuretic and antiseptic for the urinary tract system. Take it standardized to arbutin at 250 mg of arbutin four times a day. Echinacea and goldenseal treat infections through their antiviral and antibacterial properties. Take 500 mg of the capsule or 4 ml of the tincture up to four times a day. Rye pollen extract has been used to improve symptoms of prostatitis, and can be taken as directed on the label.

Homeopathy

The following remedies can be used as a short-term, complementary measure to ease the pain and discomfort of a mild to moderate attack of prostatitis. However, severe or frequent attacks are best treated by a homeopathic practitioner.

Nux vomica: If symptoms have developed in response to "living in the fast lane" and escalating stress levels, use Nux vomica. Symptoms that are likely to respond to this remedy include spasmodic pains extending from the genitals to the thighs, with the right

side often more affected than the left. Pain and discomfort feels more intense when lying on the back, and slight incontinence may occur when sneezing or coughing.

Lycopodium: If the need to urinate becomes more frequent and urgent when traveling, try Lycopodium. Urine may leak or dribble from the penis when feeling stressed and anxious, and may have a dark-colored and murky appearance. Cool compresses may give temporary relief from pain and discomfort.

Herbalism

There are four types of prostatitis: acute and chronic bacterial prostatitis, nonbacterial prostatitis, and prostatodynia (a painful prostate without inflammation).

Prostate infection formula: The following formula treats infection in the prostate and urinary tract. The herbs included fight bacterial infection in the urinary tract, soothe and decrease inflammation, and support the immune system in assisting the elimination of bacteria. Combine saw palmetto, echinacea, buchu, goldenrod, uva ursi, and corn silk as dried herbs or tinctures. Saw palmetto, corn silk, and echinacea can make up the bulk of this formula, with lesser amounts of uva ursi, goldenrod, and buchu. Herbal combinations can also be put together by a herbalist, or at a local herbal store. Drink an infusion made from 1 tbsp of the dried herbs per cup of water, or take 2 ml of the combined tincture every three hours, even throughout the night, for up to three days. Then reduce the dose to three to four times per day for up to 10 days.

Inflamed prostate formula: When the prostate is inflamed but not infected, herbs that reduce inflammation and congestion around the prostate are indicated. Non-bacterial inflammation of the prostate is thought to be affected by increased levels of DHT (dihydrotestosterone), a potent form of testosterone that can stimulate growth of the prostate. Saw palmetto is a 5-alpha-reductase inhibitor, which prevent the conversion of testosterone to DHT. Stinging nettle root is anti-inflammatory, anti-histamine, and pain-relieving. Clinical studies show stinging nettles effectively relieve nonbacterial prostatitis. Cleavers is a gentle lymphatic herb moving congested lymph and swelling from the prostate; or calendula can be used as an alternative. Small flowered willow herb also has a long traditional use in treating those with benign prostate enlargement, and clinical studies have shown that it reduced PSA (prostate specific antigen) secretion levels, supporting its use in prostate diseases. Combine equal parts of the above as dried herbs or in tincture form. Drink an infusion made from 1 tbsp per cup of water, steeped for five minutes, or take 3 ml of the combined tincture, twice daily. You can also take 160 mg of saw palmetto twice daily.

Impotence

Diagnosis

Impotence (also known as erectile dysfunction) is the inability to get or keep an erection to allow for satisfactory intercourse. Men who suffer from erectile dysfunction are unable to get an erection at all, cannot get an erection that is firm enough for penetration, or cannot stay erect once penetration is achieved. It is generally due to a mixture of psychological and physical factors. In some cases, there is a problem with the blood vessels that carry blood into the penis. In younger males, the most common cause of impotence is anxiety about having sex, or drinking too much alcohol. Stress, tiredness, relationship issues, and emotional events, such as a death, are key triggers in middle age. Sometimes being overweight, unfit, and smoking can also lead to problems.

Symptoms

- Inability to attain an erection
- Inability to sustain an erection

Treatment Goal

Treatment involves first determining the cause of impotence, whether due to emotional or physical factors, or a combination of both. Treatment focuses on treating the cause, relieving psychological distress, and preventing further problems.

Conventional Medicine

The treatment of erectile dysfunction is dependent on a diagnosis of the cause. Possible treatment options are described below.

Medication: The most common drugs used are sildenafil (Viagra®), vardenafil (Levitra®), and tadalafil (Cialis®), all of which help sustain erection by increasing tissue levels of nitric oxide, a vasodilating chemical. These drugs should not be used by patients who are also taking nitrates to treat angina because of the potential for life-threatening low blood pressure. The lowest possible dose should be used first, as these drugs may have serious cardiac side effects in those who are already at risk. Intracavernosal alprostadil is a medication that is injected into the sides of the penis to treat impotence. This too has some potential cardiac effects and should not be used without a thorough evaluation.

Modify your lifestyle: Stop smoking, cut down on alcohol, exercise regularly, take adequate rest, and lower your stress levels. Exercises that may help improve erectile dysfunction include pelvic floor muscle exercises (also called Kegel exercises). These involve strengthening the same muscles one would use to stop the flow of urination. Exercises should be performed at least twice a day. Taking supplements of L-arginine, an amino acid that can increase blood vessel dilation, may also be helpful to treat cases of erectile dysfunction.

Mechanical instruments: A vacuum constriction device is a mechanical instrument that can be used to maintain an erection, which is relatively effective. If all of the above measures fail, surgery may be performed to insert a penile prosthesis, an artificial support for the penis.

Traditional Chinese Medicine

Herbs: According to traditional Chinese medicine, the common causes of impotence are kidney deficiency, spleen deficiency, and liver Qi stagnation. To prepare any of the formulas detailed below, place the raw herbs in a glass or ceramic pot and add 3½ cups of water. Bring to a boil and simmer for 30 minutes before straining. Drink 1 cup twice a day.
• **To treat kidney deficiency:** If kidney energy is low, you may have impotence accompanied by dizziness, tiredness, and lower back pain.

Mix 10 g of Rui Gui Zhi (inner bark of Saigon cinnamon), 15 g of Shu Di Huang (cooked Chinese foxglove), 12 g of Shan Zhu Yu (Asiatic cornelian cherry), 15 g of Shan Yao (Chinese yam), 15 g of Fuling (poria), 12 g of Ze Xie (water plantain rhizome), 12 g of Dan Pi (cortex of tree peony root), 12 g of Gou Ji Zi (wolfberry), 12 g of Du Zhong (eucommia bark), and 12 g of Ba Ji Tian (morinda root).
• **To treat spleen deficiency:** Symptoms include poor digestive function, loose stools, and fatigue. Combine 10 g of ginseng, 15 g of

Bai Zhu (atractylodes rhizome), 15 g of Fuling (poria), 15 g of Shan Yao (Chinese yam), 12 g of Yuan Zhi (Chinese senega root), 12 g of Wu Wei Zi (schisandra fruit), and 5 g of Gan Cao (licorice root).

• **To treat liver Qi stagnation:** Impotence is accompanied by depression, low motivation, loss of interest in life, and stress. Mix 12 g of Chai Hu (hare's ear root), 15 g of Bai Shao (white peony root), 15 g of Bai Zhu (atractylodes rhizome), 15 g of Fuling (poria), 5 g of Bo He (field mint), 6 g of Gan Cao (licorice root), 12 g of Xiang Fu (nut grass rhizome), and 12 g of Gou Ji Zi (wolfberry).

Acupressure: The Guan Yuan point is in the center of the abdomen, about 3 inches below the navel. The Tai Xi point is on the inside of the leg, in the depression between the Achilles tendon and the anklebone. Press these points for one to two minutes, release, and repeat. Repeat this two or three times a day.

Diet: To treat impotence, eat foods that strengthen kidney and yang energy, such as black sesame seeds, string beans, wheat, caraway seeds, chives, tangerines, walnuts, plums, chicken, egg yolk, shrimp, dates, lamb, and pork.

Naturopathy

Diet: Follow a diet high in vitamin E, which is essential for dilating blood vessels and improving circulation. Foods high in vitamin E include wheat germ, leafy green vegetables, almonds, avocado, and whole grains. Pumpkin seeds and sunflower seeds should be added to salads for their high zinc concentration, important for prostate health. Do not overeat before sexual intercourse, because this draws blood to your digestive tract, which may interfere with a healthy erection. Limit the amount of hydrogenated fats in your diet, found in margarine, baked foods, junk foods, and refined vegetable oils, as they can contribute to blocked arteries, which will impede with proper blood flow to the penis. Drink alcohol moderately, as over-consumption can lead to impotence.

Supplements: If tests show that your levels of DHEA, a steroid hormone, are low, take 50 mg daily under your doctor's supervision. Vitamin B3 or niacin is required to improve blood flow. Use the no-flush niacin found in most health food stores and take 250 mg three times a day. Zinc promotes health for the prostate and helps with testosterone synthesis. Take 30 mg twice a day, plus 3 mg of copper to avoid deficiency.

Tip: EXERCISE

Regular exercise is crucial for stimulating blood flow, reducing stress, and unclogging arteries, all of which increase sexual performance. Find an exercise that you enjoy and practice it four times a week.

Herbs: Panax ginseng improves energy, sexual function, and libido in men. Take 100 mg three times a day of a product standardized to 4–7% ginsenosides. Ginkgo biloba has been shown in some research to benefit sexual function and increase circulation. Take 120 mg twice a day of the standardized form of 24% flavone glycosides and 6% of the terpene lactones. Take 500 mg of potency wood, which has been historically used in South America to increase sexual vigor, three times a day. Also take 500 mg of puncture vine, which may increase testosterone levels and is a folk remedy for improving libido and erectile function, three times daily. Damiana, a traditional remedy for increasing libido and potency, can be taken at 400 mg three times a day, and yohimbe, which increases blood flow to the penis during an erection, can be taken at 10 mg three times a day under a doctor's supervision. This latter herb should be avoided if patients have high blood pressure, a heart condition, kidney disease, or psychological disorders.

> *Tip:* USE ESSENTIAL OILS
>
> Some essential oils relieve stress and at the same time stimulate sexual desire. Add 10 drops of ylang ylang, sandalwood, and/or jasmine oil to a bath or a massage oil mix.

Homeopathy

Men who are experiencing established problems with achieving and maintaining an erection are likely to be under a great deal of psychological pressure, which can itself contribute to further problems. Due to the complex nature of this condition, it is best treated by a homeopathic practitioner who will prescribe at a constitutional level. The following lifestyle recommendations can provide further support in improving the situation.

Relaxation techniques: Make it a priority to address high stress levels. Psychological tension and anxiety are known to contribute to a significant number of cases of erectile dysfunction where a physical cause has been ruled out. Consider taking up relaxation techniques, meditation, or yoga.

Avoid alcohol: If stress levels are high, it may be tempting to drink alcohol as a way of relaxing. However, bear in mind that this can have a negative effect on achieving an erection. Alcohol, as well as caffeine and some prescription drugs, may restrict efficient blood flow.

Counseling: If unresolved tensions exist within a relationship, counseling may help by allowing sensitive issues to be aired and discussed in a neutral environment.

Herbalism

As with many conditions, there are a variety of possibilities to take into consideration when deciding how to treat impotence and which herbs to use. It is important to consider any medication that could be in use, lifestyle, the potential for diabetes, or circulatory issues, and stress/emotional aspects. While some of these must be investigated, stress and emotional aspects are often not considered, but are of great importance. When using the herbs mentioned below, consider combining nervine, nourishing, and anxiolytic herbs (see Stress, p. 438).

Damiana: A herb known for its traditional use as an aphrodisiac, and for enhancing male sexual performance. This may be in part due to an alkaloid that acts in a similar way to testosterone. It may also be used for nervous exhaustion and anxiety, so may be beneficial from more than one aspect in impotence. One cup of damiana tea/infusion may be taken three times daily. Prepare by steeping 2 tsp of the leaf in a cup of freshly boiled water for 10 minutes. Alternatively, 2–3 ml of tincture could be taken three times daily.

Ginkgo: This herb is used for those with impotence when circulatory stimulation is required. This herb has vasodilatory and peripheral circulatory stimulant properties. Larger doses may be needed. Capsules of 80 mg (often standardized to 24% flavonglycosides) can be taken once daily. Strong herbal infusions may also be made of the dried leaves, or a tincture can be used.

Rectal Bleeding

Diagnosis

There are many conditions that can lead to rectal bleeding. Contact your doctor if you notice bright red blood coming from the anus or in the stools after a bowel movement. If the blood is accompanied by rectal pain and itchiness, you may have an anal fissure or hemorrhoids (see p. 234). If you have noticed a change in your bowel movements, for example if they have become infrequent, you may be constipated (see p. 210). Bleeding from the rectum can also be an indication of gastrointestinal disorders such as Crohn's disease and diverticulitis, particularly if accompanied by abdominal pain and mucus in the stools. Occasionally, rectal bleeding can also be a symptom of cancer of the colon. Contact your doctor if symptoms persist.

Symptoms

- Blood coming from the anus
- Blood mixed with stools
- Itchiness around the anus
- Rectal pain

Treatment Goal

Treatment involves establishing the underlying cause of the bleeding and treating it accordingly.

Conventional Medicine

Most episodes of rectal bleeding are not serious. If the blood is bright red, it usually comes from the anus or rectum; darker blood indicates a source of bleeding higher up in the intestines or stomach. If you experience repeated or severe episodes of rectal bleeding, you should be examined by a doctor. This usually involves an anoscopy, which allows a physician to view the anus, and sigmoidoscopy, an internal examination of the colon, to rule out malignant diseases. Treatment again depends on the diagnosis.

To treat a fissure: Bleeding that occurs with a bowel movement and that is accompanied by pain, is usually caused by a fissure, or crack, in the skin around the anus. This is treated by preventing constipation (see p. 211) so that stools are softer and easier to pass.

To treat hemorrhoids: A hemorrhoid can sometimes cause bleeding during a bowel movement. See p. 235 for advice on how to treat hemorrhoids.

To treat colitis: Bleeding that is accompanied by diarrhea may be caused by colitis. See Colitis (p. 221) for treatment options.

Traditional Chinese Medicine

Herbs:
• **To treat all kinds of rectal bleeding at all stages:** Mix 10 g of Bei Mao Gen (wooly grass rhizome) and 5 g of Jin Yin Hua (honeysuckle flower). To make a tea, put the herbs into a teapot, add boiling water, and let them steep for five minutes.
• **To treat chronic conditions:** Do not use this formula if you have loose bowel movements or diarrhea. Mix 12 g of Han Lian Cao (eclipta), 15 g of Xuan Shen (ningpo figwort root), 15 g of Zhi Mu (anemarrhena rhizome), 12 g of Di Gu Pi (cortex of wolfberry root), 12 g of Dan Pi (cortex of tree peony root), and 12 g of Mai Men Dong (ophiopogon tuber). To make a decoction, place the ingredients in a ceramic or glass pot and add 3 cups of water. Bring the mixture to a boil, simmer for 30 minutes, and strain the liquid. Drink 1 cup two to three times a day.

Diet: Include foods in your diet that are cooling such as purslane, mung beans, lotus, lettuce, mangoes, eggplant, spinach, pears, and cucumbers. Drink plenty of water every day and eat fresh fruits and vegetables. Avoid food that has warm properties, such as hot chili peppers, black pepper, beef, chicken, chives, spinach, cloves, ginger, red peppers, and lamb, as these will increase heat in the body. Also avoid deep-fried food, and eat less fatty and greasy food.

Naturopathy

Diet: One of the most common causes of rectal bleeding is an inadequate fiber intake. Base your diet on whole foods like fresh vegetables, fruits, whole grains, beans, nuts, and seeds. Sprinkle ground flaxseeds on your cereal, homemade shakes, or salads. Flaxseeds contain high quantities of fiber and essential oils that help with bowel movements. Eat five or six light meals throughout the day rather than two or three large meals. If you try to eat too much fiber at one time this may put excess pressure on your intestines. Drink plenty of water, 8–10 glasses throughout the day, so that stools can pass more easily. This will also protect against dehydration, which can worsen hemorrhoids and other causes of rectal bleeding. Avoid trans-fatty acids and hydrogenated oils. They slow down the digestive system and contribute to inflammation.

Supplements: Bioflavonoids are a type of plant compound that stabilizes and strengthens blood vessel walls and decreases inflammation of the rectum and the whole body. They have been found to reduce anal discomfort, pain, and discharge during an acute hemorrhoid attack. The major flavonoids found in citrus fruits, which include diosmin, herperidin, and oxerutins, appear to be beneficial. Take 1,000 mg of a bioflavonoid complex three times a day. Also take 500 mg of vitamin C three times a day to strengthen the rectal tissue. Probiotics contain friendly bacteria that help improve digestion and constipation. Take a product that contains at least four billion live organisms of lactobacillus and bifidobacterium.

Herbs: A witch hazel compresses, in the form of a cream, distilled liquid, or medicated pad, should be applied topically to the anal area. You can also add 1 oz to a sitz bath. Witch hazel decreases the bleeding of the rectum by acting as an astringent. It also relieves pain, itching, and swelling associated with hemorrhoids. Butcher's broom has a long history of use for rectal bleeding. Butcher's broom extract has anti-inflammatory and vein-constricting properties believed to improve the tone and integrity of veins and shrink swollen tissue. Take a standardized extract that provides 200–300 mg of ruscogenins daily. Horse chestnut is often recommended when there is poor circulation in the veins, or chronic venous insufficiency. It relieves symptoms such as swelling and inflammation, and also strengthens blood vessel walls. Take 100 mg of a standardized aescin daily. Bilberry improves circulation and strengthens capillary walls. Take a standardized extract containing 25% anthocyanosides at 160 mg twice a day. Stoneroot reduces hemorrhoid swelling and improves rectal bleeding. Take 500 mg three times a day.

Hydrotherapy: Take two or three sitz baths daily. Sit in a warm bath with your knees raised for 5–15 minutes. You can also alternate between hot and cold sitz baths to gain relief and improve circulation. Sit in warm water for one minute and in cold water for 30 seconds.

Homeopathy

The following advice is only appropriate for treating mild rectal bleeding that is bright in color and has been triggered by an obvious acute problem, such as hemorrhoids. If you have no previous history of rectal bleeding, the condition must be assessed by a doctor. This also applies if a change in bowel habit occurs that cannot be explained by an obvious cause, such as a major change in fiber or water intake, or an escalation of stress and anxiety levels.

Hamamelis: If hemorrhoids bleed very easily and quite profusely, try Hamamelis. Pain in the affected area is likely to feel stinging or prickling, and there also tends to be a general sensation of tension in the hemorrhoids. Moving about, making sudden jolting or jarring movements, and contact with cold air aggravates symptoms and increases pain and discomfort.

Nux vomica: If hemorrhoids that bleed easily have been triggered or aggravated by ineffectual straining when constipated, use Nux vomica. The affected area is likely to feel very sensitive to touch, and sharp pains radiate up the rectum.

Herbalism

Rectal bleeding may be due to hemorrhoids, but can be caused by a more serious medical condition, so an investigation is advised.

Hemorrhoid and venous support suppository or salve: Create a blend of astringent and tonifying herbs to support venous integrity. Witch hazel bark, which is astringent and cooling, is indicated for venous congestion that results in hemorrhoids. Butcher's broom strengthens and tonifies blood vessels, thereby reducing venous swelling and pain. St. John's wort is helpful for relieving nerve pain. Horse chestnut is anti-inflammatory, astringent, antispasmodic, and reduces swelling. Aescin, horse chestnut's main active constituent, reduces capillary permeability and improves venous tone, which results in smaller rectal veins. Calendula flowers speed the healing of connective tissue. Add 1–2 oz each of the powdered herbs to a base of 1 cup of olive oil or almond oil. Heat the herbs in a bowl over a pan of simmering water over low heat, stirring occasionally and being careful not to burn the mixture. Strain the herbs from the oil and add 1 oz of beeswax with added vitamin E and A over low heat. Pour the oil into small containers to use as a salve, or into suppository molds. Apply the salve topically or insert rectally once daily, usually in the evening.

Chlamydia

Diagnosis

Chlamydia is a sexually transmitted disease (STD) caused by the bacteria Chlamydia trachomatis. This infection can be contracted through unprotected oral, vaginal, or anal sexual contact with an infected partner. It is preventable and treatable. It often presents no symptoms, unless it leads to complications. In women, the infection can cause cystitis, urethritis, a change in vaginal discharge, or abdominal pain. More seriously, it can damage the fallopian tubes. In men, chlamydia can cause discharge from the urethra and mild irritation at the tip of the penis. More serious complications include inflammation of the testicles. Chlamydia can also lead to pelvic inflammatory disease (PID) in women if not treated.

Symptoms

IN WOMEN (sometimes)
- Cystitis
- A change in vaginal discharge
- Mild lower abdominal pain

IN MEN (sometimes)
- Urethral discharge from the penis
- Mild irritation of the penis, which often goes away

Treatment Goal

This condition is easily preventable by practicing safe sex. If the disease is contracted, the treatment aims to eliminate the bacteria and prevent further infection.

Conventional Medicine

Prevention: This is the best strategy for treating chlamydia. Always have protected sex by using condoms.

Antibiotics: If you do become infected, conventional medical treatment is to prescribe antibiotics. A first line of treatment is to take a one-time dose of 1 gm of azithromycin orally. This is usually given on site at the time of diagnosis. All sexual partners should also be treated to avoid reinfection. Alternately 500 mg of erythromycin can be taken four times daily for seven days. Those who are allergic to these medications, can take ofloxacin or levofloxacin as seven-day treatments. If infection occurs during pregnancy, ampicillin or erthromycin should be used. Ofloxacin and doxycycline cannot be used in pregnancy. Patients should be tested for the STD after treatment to make sure the infection is gone.

Traditional Chinese Medicine

Herbs: Consult a TCM practitioner for comprehensive herbal treatment for chlamydia.

Acupuncture: Consult with a doctor of Chinese medicine regarding acupuncture treatment for chlamydia. The doctor evaluating your condition can determine the number of treatments needed.

Diet: Eat a well-balanced diet that includes fresh food and make sure you drink plenty of water. Shrimp, beef, lamb, and chili pepper should be avoided as they may interfere with your herbal treatment and increase heat in your body.

Naturopathy

Seek the help of a holistic practitioner who can provide you with the proper treatment, whether drug based or complementary. Untreated chlamydia can cause long-term complications.

Diet: A diet that supports the immune system is appropriate. Include whole foods, fresh fruit and vegetables. Brightly colored foods and green leafy vegetables are helpful due to their high nutrient levels and bioflavonoids (plant chemicals with many health-supporting properties).

Supplements: Immune-supporting nutritional supplements are highly important in the treatment of chlamydia infection. Take a multivitamin/multimineral as directed on the container; 1,000 mg of vitamin C four times a day; 400 IU of vitamin E a day; 200,000 IU of beta carotenes a day; and 30 mg of zinc picolinate a day.

Herbs: Herbs that contain the natural antibiotic berberine are best suited to treat chlamydia, but should not be used if you are pregnant. Take 6–12 ml of a goldenseal tincture, or 250 mg in pills from a solid extract, three times a day. Take 250–500 mg of Oregon grape root extract three times per day, standardized to berberine or total alkaloid levels (approximately 5%). Continuous use should not exceed three weeks. Also take 2,000 mg of barberry in solid extract form three times a day.

Tip: MAKE A NATURAL DOUCHE

Add 3 drops each of lavender and tea tree essential oil—both have antimicrobial properties and lavender gives the douche a pleasant smell—to 3 cups of warm water and 2 tbsp of yogurt (packed with some healthy probiotics, which are important for the overall health of the vaginal area). Put the ingredients into a douche bag and slosh it around to mix them well. Use the douche once a day. If the problem does not clear up within five days, consult your doctor.

Homeopathy

This condition requires prompt conventional diagnosis and the relevant treatment, but homeopathy can provide complementary support once an initial conventional treatment has been given. In particular, the remedies listed below may be helpful if vaginal discharge is present. However, they are listed to give an idea of the range of potential remedies available to a practitioner, rather than to encourage self-prescribing.

Pulsatilla: If you feel emotional and weepy, Pulsatilla may be helpful. Localized symptoms include a cloudy discharge that is watery or thick and bland in texture. This triggers vaginal soreness that tends to be most troublesome when you are warm in bed, and premenstrually.

Sepia: This remedy is helpful if there is a general sense of feeling depressed, flat, and exhausted. Possible localized symptoms include bloating and distention of the belly. If a discharge is present, it is likely to smart and be yellow-tinged in appearance. There may also be an uncomfortable itchy sensation in the vulva.

Borax: If vaginal discharge resembles uncooked egg white and feels very irritating and possibly corrosive, Borax may help. The discharge may also irritate the top of the thighs. There may also be heat and inflammation in the vagina.

Herbalism

This is a serious infection with the potential to cause severe complications, especially in women. For that reason, it is extremely important to treat chlamydia infections with antibiotics as soon as possible; treatment should also be given to sexual partners. Herbs have a role only as adjunctive therapies, such as helping with urinary discomfort, until the antibiotics rid the body of infection. As well as the herbs listed below, see Urinary Tract Infection (p. 242) for other herbs that could be helpful for some of the symptoms associated with chlamydia.

Cleavers: The above-ground parts of cleavers have many helpful effects on the urinary system. It contains antioxidants, tannins, coumarins, and many other compounds that make it effective for kidney stone prevention, prostate problems, painful urination, and lingering symptoms from chlamydia infection. Purchase a tincture from a store that sells or makes herbal medicines, and take a ½ dropper (30 drops) twice a day until your symptoms have improved.

Marshmallow: This herb can soothe the urinary tract. To treat urinary symptoms of Chlamydia, use a tincture of marshmallow root, available from herbal medicines stores. The dose will depend on the severity of your symptoms, but an average dose is one dropper full (60 drops) three times daily.

Echinacea and goldenseal: These herbs may be taken to support the immune system, but not used instead of, or as an alternative to, antibiotics in the treatment of chlamydia. Care should be taken to ensure that any goldenseal used is from a sustainable source, as it is endangered due to overharvesting and poor growth away from its natural environment.

Herpes

Diagnosis

Genital herpes is an infection caused by the herpes simplex virus. It enters the body through a break in the skin and once you are infected it is possible for the virus to lie dormant in your system for months, and in some cases even years. During this time you will not have any symptoms. Stress can activate the virus, leading to an outbreak. After an initial phase of tenderness in the genital area, a rash of blisters appears. The blisters burst and turn into small ulcers, which crust over after two to three weeks. There are two types of herpes simplex virus. HSV-1 usually appears as cold sores on the mouth and lips, while HSV-2 affects the genitals. Some people experience just a few attacks of genital herpes or none at all, while others will have regular outbreaks.

Symptoms

- Prickling sensation in the genital area
- Redness and small watery blisters on the genitals
- Pain, itchiness, and burning
- Fever, aches and pains, and fatigue
- Discomfort during urination

Treatment Goal

Herpes is a preventable STD that can be avoided by practicing safe sex. Condoms reduce the risk of becoming infected or passing on the virus. If infection does occur, treatment involves resolving the infection and reducing the occurrence of further outbreaks.

Conventional Medicine

Medication: The first drug of choice to treat herpes is acyclovir, which is used for initial and recurrent episodes. The recommended dosage is five times a day for seven to 10 days to treat the first episode, and for five days to treat recurrent episodes. Usually a slow but steady improvement is seen. To treat viruses that are resistant to acyclovir, valcyclovir can be used. Famcyclovir is another option, and requires fewer daily doses. Some of these medications may also be used at lower doses to suppress the herpes virus and keep it in remission.

Local pain relief: Apply cool compresses of Burrow's solution four to six times a day to relieve local discomfort and promote healing. Additional measures include applying lidocaine gel, taking cool baths, and taking simple pain relievers.

Prevention: Avoid high-risk sexual behavior, fatigue, and stress to help keep herpes in remission. Some studies show that taking lysine supplements is also helpful.

Traditional Chinese Medicine

Herbs:
• To treat simplex Type 1 herpes or cold sores: Take Chuan Xin Lian Pian, a Chinese patent herbal pill. It contains the herbs Chuan Xin Lian and Bu Gong Yin, which have antiviral effects.
• To treat simplex Type 2 herpes or genital herpes, or herpes zoster or shingles: You can take the Chuan Xin Lian Pian herbal pill for this type of condition as well, or try washing the genital area with the following external formula. Mix 15 g of Ku Shen (sophora root), 15 g of She Chuang Zi (cnidium seed), 15 g of Huang Bai (phellodendron), 12 g of Xia Ku Cao (common self-heal fruit-spike), 15 g of Ma Zhi Xian (dried purslane), and 15 g of Ban Lan Gen (isatis root) in a ceramic pot. Add 3½ cups of water and bring to a boil. Simmer for 30 minutes and strain the liquid. Soak the area in the decoction for 15 minutes twice a day.

Diet: Eating foods that clean heat from the body may help this condition. Examples include mung beans, watermelon, purslane, towel gourd, crab, grapefruit, pears, red beans, cucumber, cabbage, watermelon, and tofu. Generally, light, fresh food is recommended such as celery, spinach, eggplant, and wax gourd. Avoid ginger, chilies, mustard greens, oranges, shrimp, baked potatoes, cheese, and mutton, because they are pungent, irritating, and increase heat in the body. Also avoid acidic, sweet, and greasy foods. .

Naturopathy

Diet: Consume foods that are high in the amino acid L-lysine, such as legumes, fish, turkey, chicken, and vegetables. Foods high in vitamin C and bioflavonoids such as peppers, broccoli, berries, and carrots help to heal the skin. Avoid foods high in the amino acid L-arginine such as almonds, peanuts, chocolate, and whole wheat, as they can stimulate herpes replication. Eliminate sugar and foods that contain sugars and hydrogenated fats; these suppress the immune system and interfere with the healing process. Acidic foods, such as tomatoes and citrus fruits, may aggravate symptoms during outbreaks and should be avoided.

Supplements: L-lysine, which has been shown to help with acute outbreaks of herpes, can be taken as a supplement at a dosage of 1,000 mg three times a day, or take 500 mg twice a day as a preventive measure. Take 1,000 mg of vitamin C with 500 mg of bioflavonoids three to four times a day to improve immune function and decrease the duration of the infection. Zinc reduces the severity of herpes and increases immune function. Take 30 mg daily with 3 mg of copper. Topical zinc sulfate can also be applied to the affected area two to three times a day. Taking 100 mg of B-complex vitamins twice a day can help to treat frequent herpes cold sore outbreaks. It is also

> **Tip:** MINIMIZE STRESS LEVELS
>
> Sufficient sleep is critical for maintaining an optimal resistance to herpes outbreaks and relieving stress. Keeping stress levels down minimizes the frequency and severity of episodes. Massage, exercise (particularly yoga), meditation, and breathing exercises can all help you to manage stress.

important to supply the gut with friendly bacteria to promote immune function. Take 4 billion active organisms 30 minutes after a meal.

Herbs: Lemon balm has been shown to help resolve the herpes virus and to heal cold sores. Apply a lemon balm cream, available from health food stores, to the affected area three times a day. Take 500 mg of lomatium root four times a day for its anti-viral and immune-enhancing properties. An anti-viral compound in St. John's Wort, called hypericin, helps kill herpes simplex and several other viruses to help heal sores. Brew a strong tea made from the herb, and, after it cools, dab it on the affected area. You can also take 300 mg three times a day of an extract standardized to contain 0.3% hypericin.

Homeopathy

The following remedies can be used as short-term, complementary therapies alongside conventional treatment to ease the discomfort and distress of an acute flare-up of herpes. For more extensive support, consult an experienced homeopathic practitioner, rather than trying to handle the situation through self-help measures alone.

Natrum mur: Consider using this remedy if the affected area feels dry and sore, leading to smarting, burning sensations. Symptoms tend to emerge when feeling emotionally stressed or physically run down, are sensitive to contact with heat, and soothed by contact with cool air and cool bathing.

Rhus tox: If the affected area feels sore and itchy, causing particular distress and restlessness at night, try Rhus tox. Cold and damp conditions can also trigger, or aggravate burning and itching sensations.

Petroleum: This can be a helpful remedy for herpetic eruptions that lead to violent itching, burning, and irritation. Sores may appear on the perineum, and between the scrotum and the thighs. Clothing and movement make the irritation more intense, while exposure to warm air may feel soothing.

> *Tip:* SOOTHING TINCTURE
>
> Applying a combination of diluted calendula and hypericum tincture can soothe sore, tender areas. One part of tincture should be diluted in ten parts of boiled, cooled water.

Herbalism

It is difficult to definitively treat a herpes infection, as it involves a virus that lives in a particular nerve, occasionally causing an "outbreak," or blister and pain in the skin served by that nerve. Herbs can, however, help with the skin symptoms, and facilitate the resolution of the pain and blisters. The immune system can also be supported by using a blend of immunomodulators, lymphatic herbs, and herbs with antiviral properties, such as echinacea, thyme, licorice, lemon balm, reishi, and St. John's Wort.

Aloe vera: To treat the blisters associated with a herpes outbreak, simply take the gel from a fresh cut leaf and apply it directly to the affected area. If fresh leaves are not available, there is a variety of gels and lotions containing aloe vera that can be purchased at your local health food store.

Licorice: Licorice root extracts, in creams, lotions, or ointments, can help provide pain relief and decrease healing time. Licorice, which has anti-viral properties, is a demulcent that coats and soothes the skin. Licorice, with research focused on one of its compounds, glycyrrhizin, works against the herpes virus.

St. John's wort: Topically, St. John's wort helps to relieve the pain and inflammation associated with herpes outbreaks. The oil can be applied topically, as required, or three to four times daily. Calendula oil may also be added, along with a few drops of garlic oil.

8

Mind
and
Spirit

Stress

Diagnosis

Stress generally describes feelings of frustration, anger, or anxiety. It tends to be an inevitable component of modern living, and affects everyone from time to time. Common triggers include work, study and exams, relationship problems, financial worries, and feeling unable to cope. When we find ourselves in a stressful situation, the nervous system goes on red alert. The brain sends signals to the adrenal glands to release more adrenaline into the system. This has multiple effects on the body, causing muscles to become tense, and the heartbeat and breathing rate to speed up. This rush of adrenaline also causes energy to flow away from the digestive system, which often leads to the nagging aches and upset stomach characteristic of stress. Stress is a normal part of everyday life, but learning how to control stress is important. Try to find ways of dealing with stress to neutralize the dangerous effects it can have on your health.

Symptoms

- Irritability
- No sense of humor and many negative thoughts
- Difficulty concentrating and memory loss
- Feeling defensive and constantly worrying
- Tightness in neck and shoulders
- Insomnia and sleep problems
- Sweating
- Breathlessness
- Loss of appetite and/or binge eating
- Stomach problems
- Constipation and/or diarrhea
- Headaches
- Cramps and spasms
- Loss of libido

Treatment Goal

Treatment involves examining your lifestyle and pinpointing any particularly stressful area. Treatment can help you to develop a strategy for dealing with stress to prevent long-term problems, such as depression.

Conventional Medicine

Treatment of stress involves learning techniques to modify your response to stressful situations and making lifestyle changes to reduce day-to-day stress. Stress affects the cardiac, immune, gastrointestinal, and hormonal systems greatly and, if any compromise in these areas exists, then evaluation by a health care professional is warranted.

Meditation: Formal stress reduction instruction has been initiated in several major hospitals. The most well known is Jon Kabat Zin's mindfulness based stress reduction program. This relaxation technique utilizes mindfulness meditation, which involves expanding one's consciousness to identify subtle emotions. Other forms of meditation are available, which help the mind to divert attention from problematic emotional responses and decrease mental chatter. Simple techniques such as relaxation breathing and repeating a focus word or mantra are forms of meditation that help to modify the stress response, not just while performing the meditation, but also during everyday activities. Meditation for 20 minutes a day is optimal.

Other therapies: Progressive muscle relaxation involves the systematic contraction and relaxation of major muscle groups, and can also be helpful for relaxation and stress reduction. Biofeedback involves the machine-based detection of tension responses, and can help a person learn to sense the physical signs of stress and modify them. Hypnosis uses verbal suggestions to relax the mind and body. A newer technique, known as Heart Math, uses heartbeat responses to emotions as a guide to reduce stress. Psychological counseling and behavior modification also have a role in the treatment of chronic stress.

Lifestyle modifications: Chronic stress depletes B-complex vitamins and magnesium in the body, so it is advised that you replace these through supplements during periods of stress. A practitioner who can measure adrenal hormones may also be helpful in evaluating the adrenal depletion that can occur with unremitting chronic stress. Adequate sleep and regular meals with little sugar or processed foods are mandatory during periods of stress to avoid physical side-effects. Regular exercise is one of the primary techniques to combat stress.

Traditional Chinese Medicine

Herbs: Mix 12 g of Chai Hu (hare's ear root), 15 g of Bai Shao (white peony root), 12 g of Yu Jin (turmeric tuber), 6 g of Bo He (field mint), 12 g of Gou Ji Zi (wolfberry), 15 g of Fuling (poria), 15 g of Bai Zhu (white atractylodes rhizome), and 5 g of Gan Cao (licorice root). Place the herbs in a ceramic pot and add 3 cups of water. Bring to a boil and simmer for 30 minutes. Strain the liquid and drink 1 cup twice a day.

Acupressure: To release stress, try pressing the Tai Yang points. With your eyes closed, put your thumbs on the depression at the temples. The Nei Guan point, located in the center of the wrist on the palm side, about 2 inches below the crease, can also be helpful. Each point can be pressed with moderate pressure for one to two minutes, released, and then pressed again. Repeat three to five times.

Diet: Eat foods that have a calming effect and help you to sleep, such as chamomile tea, peppermint, rice porridge, mandarin oranges, and pears. Eat plenty of fresh vegetables to keep bowel movements regular, and cut down on your caffeine intake. Fruits such as cranberries, blueberries, and bananas are recommended, along with mung beans, red beans, bamboo shoots, and purslane. Avoid food that is rich and fatty.

Naturopathy

Diet: Balance your blood sugar levels by eating small meals frequently throughout the day. Unbalanced blood levels can lead to a stressed stomach or aggravate an existing condition. Include whole grains such as oats, quinoa, or brown rice with every meal, which contain high levels of B vitamins and fiber, and increase your body's ability to make serotonin, which has a calming effect on the body and eases anxiety. B vitamins are also calming to the nervous system and the fiber keeps your bowels moving. Increase your B vitamin intake by consuming brewer's yeast, brown rice, and leafy green vegetables. Calcium and magnesium also have a calming effect on the body. Sea vegetables, green leafy vegetables, nuts, and yogurt can provide you with a good amount of these nutrients. Caffeine and refined sugars in alcohol can make symptoms worse, so avoid them. They will cause blood sugar imbalances and increase stressed stomach symptoms.

Supplements: 5-hydroxytryptophan (5-HTP) increases serotonin levels, to produce a calming effect in the body. Take 50–100 mg two to three times daily, but do not take 5-HTP if you are on antidepressant medications. Take 500 mg of calcium and 250 mg of magnesium a day to help calm the nervous system, and 200 mcg of chromium twice a day to help balance blood sugar. Digestive enzymes, such as lipases that digest fat, proteases that digest proteins, and amylases that digest starch, help you digest food more effectively to reduce irritation. Take two capsules or tablets of a full spectrum enzyme product with each meal. Betaine hydrochloride supports stomach acid levels and helps with digestion. Take one to two capsules with each meal. Probiotics also help digestion and prevent overgrowth of candida and other harmful microbes. Take a product containing four billion active organisms daily of Lactobacillus acidophilus and bifidus.

Homeopathy

The advice below is given with a view to helping ease mild stress-related symptoms that have developed recently. Severe, established problems should be treated by a homeopathic practitioner.

Arnica: If aching, tense muscles make it difficult to get to sleep, try Arnica. It can also be especially helpful for those who have decided to combat high stress levels by going to the gym and have overdone it, making every muscle achy and sore.

Arsenicum album: Perfectionists and high achievers can often benefit from this remedy. Symptoms include extreme restlessness at night and in the early hours of the morning, which interferes with sleep. When highly stressed, sufferers may become anxious about health issues, and show signs of becoming obsessive or compulsive. The digestive system is also affected by nausea at the thought or smell of food, and diarrhea may develop when feeling tense.

Nux vomica: This is a classic remedy for treating stress, especially in those who have relied on poor lifestyle choices to keep the pace. Symptoms include problems switching off mentally when trying to sleep, tension headaches, and feeling hungover on waking.

> *Tip:* USE AVENA SATIVA
>
> If a particularly stressful period at work and/or at home has left you feeling exhausted and strung out, take a diluted Avena sativa tincture to restore the nervous system. Consult a homeopath regarding the recommended dosage, which should be diluted in a small glass of water and taken daily for up to a month.

Herbalism

Herbs are best used in combination with lifestyle changes to address the fundamental causes of stress in your life. Herbal medicines can serve as sedatives and calmatives to ease the symptoms of stress, help to improve sleep, and decrease anxiety.

Herbal sedatives and calmatives: Chamomile is a gentle and safe herb that acts as a mild sedative. One of the active constituents in the flowers, apigenin, calms nerves and relieves anxiety. Drinking an infusion made from 1 tsp of flowers per cup of water several times a day can be very helpful. Allow the flowers to steep for 10 minutes while covered to prevent the loss of important volatile oils. Alternatively, take 2–5 ml of tincture two to three times daily for its calming effects.

Lemon balm and lavender: Lemon balm and lavender are two other mild sedatives. The entire herb and leaves of lemon balm can be infused with hot water. Use 2 tsp of plant material per cup of water and drink several times a day. Use an aromatherapy distiller to spread the calming scent of lavender essential oil throughout the air. With every breath, your tension will alleviate and stress levels will ease. Lavender lotions and oils can be purchased and massaged into the temples to achieve relaxation. Be careful not to get the oil or lotion in your eyes; if you do, flush with lots of water immediately.

Tonics: Herbal tonics, also called adaptogens, are often used to help strengthen the whole body and make it more resistant to the negative effects of stress. Common tonics are eleuthero (Siberian ginseng), rhodiola, and ashwaganda. See Post-Traumatic Stress Disorder for information on their use (p. 464).

Existing Conditions
If you have existing allergies you must discuss these with your practitioner so that they may safely prescribe a treatment. If you have any medical conditions or are taking any type of medicine, it is imperative that you inform your practitioner, who will be able to advise you on safe use of complementary treatments.

Insomnia

Diagnosis

Insomnia involves having problems falling asleep at night, waking up during the night, and erratic sleeping patterns. Transient or short-term insomnia lasts for a few days and can be triggered by a sudden change in your circumstances. You may find it difficult to sleep because it is too hot or too cold, too noisy, or too light in your bedroom. Sleep patterns can be affected by consuming too many stimulants, such as caffeine.

Learned insomnia is when people become apprehensive about going to bed because they fear they will not be able to get to sleep, setting off a vicious cycle. Other people are affected by "night terrors," which occur during deep sleep and may be caused by stress. Nightmares can also make people feel anxious about the thought of going to sleep.

Symptoms

- Difficulty falling asleep
- Waking up in the middle of the night and not being able to drift back to sleep
- Tiredness
- Feeling stressed and anxious about the thought of going to sleep

Treatment Goal

Try to determine the cause of the insomnia, and eliminate contributory factors. Treatment involves encouraging normal sleeping patterns and developing strategies to prevent insomnia from occurring.

Conventional Medicine

Sleep hygiene techniques: "Sleep hygiene" techniques involve looking at diet and medications, and identifying any factors that may be contributing to poor sleep, or an inability to sleep. It is also important to go to bed at a consistent time every night and avoid daytime naps.

Stimulant medications: Many stimulant medications, such as diet pills and drugs used to treat attention deficit hyperactivity disorder (ADHD), can cause insomnia. Children with ADHD are at particularly high risk of developing insomnia. Asthma medications, and all medications mixed with caffeine, can also cause insomnia. Some antidepressants, some blood pressure medications, and cold medicines can also lead to disturbed sleep.

Pharmaceutical sleeping aides: Medications can be used for a short period of time (a maximum of three weeks) to induce sleep.

These will generally make you sluggish in the morning, and all are potentially addictive. Temazepam (Restoril®), zolpidem (Ambien®), and zaleplon (Sonata®) are the most common sleeping aides prescribed.

Natural sleeping aides: These can be successful in treating insomnia. Natural sleeping aides include melatonin, at a dose of 3 mg, and 5-hydroxytryptophan, at a dose of 150 mg at bedtime. Plants such as valerian, kava, chamomile, and passionflower can also help you to sleep.

Traditional Chinese Medicine

Herbs: To prepare a formula, place the herbs in a glass or ceramic pot and add 3 cups of water. Bring the mixture to a boil and simmer for 30 minutes. Strain the liquid and drink 1 cup twice a day.
• **To treat insomnia associated with a deficient or weak constitution:** Mix 12 g of Yuan Zhi (Chinese senega root), 12 g of Suan Zhao Ren (sour Chinese jujube seed), 15 g of Fu Shen (poria spirit), 15 g of Bai Zhu (white atractylodes rhizome), 15 g of Ye Jiao Teng (fleece flower vine), and 6 g of Gan Cao (licorice root).
• **To treat insomnia associated with stress and anxiety:** Mix 10 g of Chai Hu (hare's ear root), 12 g of Bai Shao (white peony root), 12 g of Bai Zhu (white atractylodes rhizome), 15 g of Fuling (poria), 5 g of Bo He (field mint), 12 g of Dang Gui (Chinese angelica), 5 g of Gan Cao (licorice root), and 12 g of Zi Su Ye (perilla leaf).

Acupressure: The Nei Guan point is in the center of the wrist on the palm side, about 2 inches above the crease. The San Yin Jiao point is on the inside of the leg, about 3 inches above the center of the anklebone. Apply moderate pressure to these points with the tip of your finger.

Diet: Eat foods that have a calming effect and may help you to sleep, such as chamomile tea, peppermint, rice porridge, pears, and mandarin oranges. Foods that nourish the blood, such as black sesame seeds, red beans, black beans, spinach, fish, and carrots, are also good. In addition, food that is cooling, such as watermelon, green vegetables, tofu, and Chinese jujube dates, is recommended. Avoid hot, spicy food.

Naturopathy

Diet: Do not overeat at dinner and avoid having late meals. Also eliminate caffeine, including all caffeinated beverages such as colas and other carbonated drinks, as well as chocolate. If this is too difficult, limit your caffeinated beverages to the morning only. Helpful foods include turkey and tuna, which contain L-tryptophan to induce sleep.

Supplements: Take 1,200 mg of calcium at bedtime. Another supplement that can be helpful in promoting sleep is melatonin. Some researchers have found it to be as effective as tryptophan in promoting sleep, and it does not produce side effects. It is available in 2 mg capsules; take one a night for two weeks. Discontinue taking them if no results are produced.

Herbs: Try taking 2 capsules of valerian one hour before bedtime to help you sleep. You can also drink 1 cup of passionflower tea before bedtime.

Lifestyle modifications: Stop smoking, or at the very least do not smoke within a few hours of going to bed, as nicotine is a stimulant. It is important to avoid any form of stimulation before bedtime, including doing work, reading, or doing anything that is likely to cause anxiety. Do not take naps even if you are tired during the day. Instead develop regular sleep patterns by going to bed and getting up at virtually the same time every day. Get regular exercise, but avoid exercise in the evening close to bedtime. Finally, consult a doctor regarding any medications you may be taking, as some can cause insomnia.

Homeopathy

The remedies suggested below may be helpful in managing mild to moderate complaints of insomnia. If insomnia begins to disrupt your overall quality of life, consult a homeopathic practitioner.

Coffea: If a poor sleep pattern develops after drinking too many caffeinated drinks, try Coffea. Symptoms include feeling physically exhausted but mentally alert. Sleep, when achieved, is fitful and so light that you are woken up by the slightest sound.

Aconite: If sleep patterns have been affected by a recent traumatic incident, use Aconite. Symptoms include restlessness and frequently waking up feeling fearful, breathless, shaky, and panicky. Sleep is also likely to be disturbed by nightmares or very vivid dreams.

Lachesis: This remedy can help ease poor sleep patterns that are related to premenstrual syndrome. The difficulty of trying to sleep can produce a real aversion to going to bed, and sufferers tend to stay up late as a result. There is also an unpleasant jolting sensation just as you begin to lose consciousness.

Ignatia: If a previously healthy sleep pattern has been upset by bereavement, try Ignatia. Symptoms include repeated yawning, sighing, and muscle twitching.

Nux vomica: Try this remedy for easing sleep problems that set in as a result of living in the fast lane. Symptoms include tension in muscles that refuse to relax at night, an alert mind, and a tendency to fall into a sound sleep just before the alarm goes off. Additional triggers include relying on too much caffeine to keep going during the day, and alcohol to unwind at night.

Tip: AVOID ALCOHOL

Apart from the health risks associated with alcohol, it also has a negative effect on sleeping patterns. Alcohol tends to make you drift off into an artificially deep sleep, and then causes you to wake up shortly afterward feeling dehydrated and disoriented.

Tip: MAKE SURE YOUR BEDROOM IS CONDUCIVE TO SLEEP

Choose curtains or blinds that block out light adequately, ventilate the room so that it feels fresh but not too chilly or hot, and minimize noise as much as possible. Above all else, avoid the temptation to watch television when in bed.

Herbalism

Once any underlying medical conditions that may cause insomnia have been ruled out, a variety of herbal remedies can be used to improve sleep quality. Herbal medicines that are used to treat insomnia work by relaxing and calming the person so that he or she can reach a state that is conducive to sleep. Ideally, begin "preparing" for sleep 30–45 minutes before bed by taking calming herbs while sitting and reading, taking a bath, or doing deep breathing exercises.

Relaxing herbal formula: Lavender is a gentle sedative that is aromatic and cooling. Lavender flowers have antispasmodic, carminative, nervine, and anti-inflammatory properties. Oat seeds nourish and calm the body and spirit. They contain a variety of minerals that can improve the function of the nervous system, especially in times of exhaustion. Valerian will soothe and ground a person's energy with its sweet and earthy flavor, and is especially helpful if you are restless and irritated. Chamomile is excellent for individuals who are sensitive, restless, and irritable, making it a wonderful herb for fussy children. Chamomile's slightly sweet flowers will also soothe digestion and are mild sedatives. Catnip will also sedate and soothe. It is excellent for relieving restlessness and insomnia related to colds and flu, and is safe for use by children. Create a soothing tea or tincture by combining equal parts of each herb in dried or tincture form. Drink 2–3 cups of an infusion made from 1 tbsp of the combined herbs per cup of water before bed, or take 5–10 ml of a combined tincture 30 minutes before bedtime. Some people respond in an adverse way to valerian, and it can cause feelings of restlessness. In these cases, skullcap can be a useful alternative to add to the blend.

Tip: USE LAVENDER FLOWERS

Place ½ oz of lavender flowers in a packet and place it under your pillow. The scent will bring sleep more quickly and is thought to keep nightmares at bay.

Anxiety

Diagnosis

Anxiety is something that most people experience at one time or another. It usually results from anticipating and worrying about an upcoming event, such as an exam, a presentation, a sporting event, or a job interview. Lifestyle factors such as including too much caffeine and sugar in your diet, poor nutrition, recreational drug use, exhaustion, and stress, and the side effects of certain medications can also cause anxiety.

Becoming anxious under pressure can sometimes be a positive thing, as it can lead to increased performance levels. For most people, anxiety is a short-term problem and tends to disappear after the anticipated event has passed. If anxiety occurs on a regular basis and threatens to overwhelm you, however, it becomes a bigger problem. The psychological effects of anxiety include fear, tension, irritability, and an inability to relax or concentrate. You may have an overwhelming desire to seek the reassurance of others, making you clingy and dependent. You may start to have a pessimistic outlook on life, and always assume that the worst is going to happen.

Symptoms

- Rapid breathing and lightheadedness
- Feeling shaky
- Sweating profusely
- Dry mouth
- Heightened senses
- Feeling alert
- Increased muscular tension can cause discomfort and headaches
- Pounding heart
- Butterflies in the stomach
- Nausea and sickness
- Repeated urge to move your bowels and urinate

Treatment Goal

Treatment first involves eliminating any possible physical causes of the symptoms. It is then important to identify the cause of the anxiety, relieve acute symptoms, and introduce any necessary lifestyle changes to improve quality of life.

Conventional Medicine

Conventional treatment involves relieving the acute symptoms of anxiety to improve the quality of life and prevent harm from occurring to the self or others.

Diet and lifestyle modifications: Avoid caffeine, alcohol, nicotine, and taking cold remedies that contain ephedrine (which can cause rapid heartbeat and trembling). The amino acid phenylalanine seems to decrease anxiety and can be taken as a supplement. Taking 300 mg of magnesium aspartate daily divided into three doses can also be beneficial. Blackcurrant oil may provide fatty acids, which also improve anxiety levels. Environmental stressors should be identified and avoided to whatever extent possible. In some cases it is more effective to try to modify your response to stressors, as they cannot always be controlled. There are many meditation and relaxation techniques available to help you deal with stress, such as yoga or T'ai chi.

Benzodiazepines: Pharmacological treatment of anxiety depends on the severity of the symptoms. To treat cases of incapacitating anxiety, benzodiazepine drugs are used in low doses for as short a time as possible. These include alprazolam, which is short-acting and highly addictive. It should not be used for more than four to six weeks at a time. Clonazepam is a longer-acting and therefore generally less addictive drug that may also be effective. Diazepam, or valium, is one of the more well known benzodiazepines.

Other medication: SSRIs (selective serotonin reuptake inhibitors) can be used to treat anxiety, as can the antidepressant venlafaxine. Buspirone is an anti-anxiety drug that is as effective as the benzodiazepines, but takes longer to work. It is approved for use in case of generalized anxiety disorder. Beta blocker drugs can be used to resolve the physical effects of anxiety, such as shaky voice and racing heart.

Therapy: Therapy is advisable if any of the above drugs need to be used to treat an anxiety disorder. Cognitive therapy, psychotherapy, and support groups are useful tools that can help you deal with anxiety issues.

Traditional Chinese Medicine

Herbs: To make a decoction, combine the herbs of either formula in a ceramic pot and add 3 cups of water. Bring the mixture to a boil and simmer for 30 minutes. Strain and drink 1 cup twice a day.

• **Formula one:** Mix 10 g of Chai Hu (hare's ear root), 12 g of Bai Shao (white peony root), 12 g of Bai Zhu (white atractylodes rhizome), 15 g of Fuling (poria), 5 g of Bo He (field mint), 12 g of Dang Gui (Chinese angelica), 5 g of Gan Cao (licorice root), and 12 g of Zi Su Zi (perilla hips).

• **Formula two:** Mix 12 g of Tai Zi Shen (pseudostellaria), 15 g of Bai Zhu (white atractylodes rhizome), 15 g of Shan Yao (Chinese yam), 12 g of Yuan Zhi (Chinese senega root), 12 g of Suan Zhao Ren (sour Chinese jujube seed), 5 g of Chen Pi (tangerine peel), and five pieces of Da Zhao (Chinese jujube).

Acupressure: Press the Nei Guan point, which is located in the center of the wrist on the palm side, about 2 inches below the crease. The San Yin Jiao point is in the center of the inside of the leg, about 3 inches above the anklebone. Press these points for about one minute.

Diet: It is best to eat foods that are calming and nourishing, such as rice porridge, licorice (not the sweets since most do not have licorice in them), Chinese jujube, peppermint, chamomile, and chicken soup. Eat plenty of fresh vegetables and reduce your coffee intake. Avoid food that is rich and fatty.

Naturopathy

Relaxation movements: T'ai chi is a form of stress reduction and exercise that involves specific body movements and deep breathing. Yoga can also help with relaxation and stress reduction. It primarily involves deep breathing, stretches and meditation.

Biofeedback: This type of therapy operates on the notion that we have the innate ability and potential to influence the automatic functions of our bodies through the exertion of will and mind. Stress and anxiety affects your muscles by causing them to tense and tighten. This, in turn, can produce other aches and pains, such as headaches or backaches. By helping you to become more attuned to your internal body functions, biofeedback teaches you to control certain unhealthy conditions. Muscle biofeedback equipment, for example, can measure the tension of your muscles and relay this information to you. By focusing on this information, your mind becomes less preoccupied with the problems causing stress, which in turn causes fewer messages to be sent from your brain to your muscles telling them to stay tense. You can use the information from the biofeedback instrument to make connections between the information and the way you feel. This increases your awareness of your own muscle tension and helps you learn to recognize tension when it first begins. Biofeedback training also teaches you ways to control the tension before other symptoms have a chance to develop. In order to use biofeedback effectively, you need to be trained by a biofeedback professional.

Breathing exercises: Deep breathing relaxes the mind, calms the nervous system, and improves mental focus and energy. Deep breathing requires imitating the breathing patterns of a child—they breath from the belly not the chest. To deep breath properly, find a comfortable, quiet area. Stand with your knees slightly bent or sit straight with your buttocks touching the back of your seat. Breath in through your nose to a count of five, hold for two seconds, and exhale to a count of five. While breathing in, your stomach, rather than your chest, should expand outward. When breathing out, your stomach should flatten.

Aromatherapy: Plant essential oils can be added to baths, massage oil, or infusers to relieve symptoms of anxiety. A few drops of essential oils in a base oil can be massaged into the scalp and temples before bed. Essential oils that are used for anxiety and nervous tension are: bergamot, cypress, geranium, jasmine, lavender, melissa, neroli, rose, sandalwood, and ylang-ylang. Lavender is the most common and forms the base of many relaxing blends.

> *Tip:* EXERCISE
>
> Exercise is an effective method of managing anxiety. Cardiovascular exercise combined with calming exercise, such as walking several times per week, can be very beneficial.

Homeopathy

Any of the following remedies can help to relieve a single, mild to moderate episode of anxiety that has been triggered by an obvious cause. Severe and recurrent anxiety symptoms are best treated by an experienced homeopath.

Arsenicum album: This remedy can ease anticipatory anxiety that causes sufferers to become withdrawn and preoccupied. Symptoms develop slowly and insidiously, until they reach a point where the anxious state has become draining and exhausting. This leads to symptoms of profound weariness, indifference, and apathy, often coupled with painless diarrhea.

Lycopodium: If anticipatory anxiety particularly affects digestion, leading to tension in the stomach, try Lycopodium. The gut is also affected by bloating, noisy rumbling, and gurgling, and sufferers alternate between being constipated and having diarrhea. Patients tend to look deceptively calm and confident on the outside. Alternatively, sufferers may be sarcastic, critical, and domineering.

Nux vomica: When this remedy is helpful, anxiety is accompanied by addictive behavior, such as relying on stimulants to keep going, and depressants such as alcohol to unwind. As a result, sleep patterns suffer, aggravating feelings of irritability and impatience. Additional symptoms include muscle tension, tension headaches, and constipation.

Aconite: This is a fantastic remedy for treating anxious, panicky feelings that wash over you very quickly, making you feel terror-stricken. Symptoms are likely to be especially severe at night, waking you from sleep and making it very difficult to fall back asleep.

Herbalism

Skullcap: Historically, skullcap was used to cure people of hydrophobia, convulsions, mental agitation, and nervous system disorders including epilepsy. The sedative and antispasmodic properties of skullcap relieve restlessness leading to insomnia, nervous agitation, and fear, and have been shown to lower blood pressure related to anxiety. Skullcap's active constituents are antioxidant flavonoids, which are thought to induce brain-calming neurotransmitters; essential oils; lignans; and tannins, which give skullcap its astringent quality. Drink an infusion made from 1 tbsp of the aerial parts steeped 1 cup of water, take 3 ml of tincture, or take 1–2 g in capsule form up to three times daily. Large amounts of skullcap may cause drowsiness and should not be taken when driving or operating heavy machinery.

Passionflower: This herb relieves restlessness, insomnia, anxiety, and spasm within the muscles. Although not as potent as skullcap, clinical studies have shown passionflower to be effective at reducing symptoms of generalized anxiety disorder (GAD) and attention deficit hyperactivity disorder (ADHD). Recent studies have also shown some promising findings regarding passionflower's ability to relieve pain. The dried herb is used medicinally once the berries have matured. Drink an infusion made from 1–2 tsp of dried herb per cup of water or take 2–3 ml of a tincture three times daily.

Hops: As a tea or tincture, hops relieves anxiety, irritability, restlessness, and muscle tension. Drink an infusion made from 1 tbsp of dried strobiles (female parts) per cup of water or take 3 ml of a tincture three times daily. To treat insomnia, you may also place a packet of dried hops in your pillow to assist the onset of sleep. This herb is often avoided in cases of depression, so consult with a medical herbalist before use if this is something to be taken into consideration. 🌿

Depression

Diagnosis

It is normal to get a bout of the blues occasionally, but if these feelings start to interfere with your daily life and do not seem to subside, it could be a sign of clinical depression. Depression is a common problem. At least one in every six people will admit to feeling depressed at some point in their life, and one in 20 become clinically depressed. There is no one single cause of depression. In many cases, depression is first triggered by a traumatic event, such as the death of a loved one. It can also be caused by various health problems. Occasionally people become depressed in response to certain foods or poor nutrition, a lack of physical fitness, or an illness.

Symptoms

- Restlessness and agitation
- Sleeping problems, including waking up early and feeling tired
- Excessive smoking and drinking alcohol
- Poor appetite and weight loss
- Memory loss
- Feeling irritable or impatient, and getting no pleasure out of life
- Loss of libido
- Low self-esteem
- Preoccupation with negative thoughts, and feelings of emptiness and despair
- Cutting yourself off from others emotionally
- Thinking about suicide

Treatment Goal

To establish the cause and severity of the depression, and identify and avoid triggers to relieve symptoms. Depression is a serious condition that should be monitored by a health professional.

Conventional Medicine

Conventional treatment of depression involves protecting the patient from self-harm, relieving the symptoms, and preventing recurrence. A combination of therapy that includes psychotherapy, nutrition, and lifestyle changes, plus medication as needed, works best.

Diet and lifestyle modifications: Complete a 30-minute exercise routine daily and eat a diet that is high in protein and low in processed food. Supplements that have been shown to help relieve depression include omega-3 oils (eicosapentaenoic acid, EPA, and docosahexaenoic acid, DHA, in a 3:2 ratio) taken at a dose of 4 g daily of EPA and DHA combined, and B vitamins, particularly inositol, folate and B12. Take a B vitamin complex that provides about 1 mg of B12 and folate. SAM–e, a mood brightener, can be taken at 400 mg twice a day to increase the effects of the B vitamin. Taking the supplements 5-hydroxytriptophan (5-HTP) at 150 mg daily and St. John's wort at 300 mg three times a day can also be tried. St. John's wort interacts with several medications, so always consult a doctor before using it.

Medication: SSRIs (selective serotonin reuptake inhibitors), of which there are a wide variety, may be prescribed to treat depression. Common side effects affect the gastrointestinal system, the libido, and the nervous system. Venlafaxine (Effexor®), a combined SSRI and norepinephrine reuptake inhibitor, can lift the mood. Side effects include anxiety and insomnia, as well as the inability to achieve orgasm. Other drugs used to treat depression include duloxetine and bupropion. Several other categories of antidepressant drugs exist and these tend to have more severe side effects.

Other therapies: Psychotherapy, cognitive behavioral therapy, and support groups are helpful options. Electroconvulsive therapy, which involves passing an electrical current through the brain, is still used for severe depression that does not respond to medication.

Tip: EXERCISE

Exercise can be the most powerful antidepressant available. Its beneficial effects may be because exercise increases the levels of endorphins in the body, which are directly correlated with mood.

Traditional Chinese Medicine

Traditional Chinese medicine views depression as both a cause and a result of illness. Treatment for depression varies according to each individual patient's condition. Patients' physical conditions vary as well, and usually can be defined as excessive or deficient.

Herbs: To make a decoction, combine the herbs of either formula in a ceramic or glass pot and add 3 cups of water. Bring to a boil and simmer for 30 minutes. Strain the liquid and drink 1 cup twice a day.

• **To treat excessive depression:** Symptoms include feeling irritable and angry, a tightness in the chest, a bitter taste in the mouth, and sighing. Mix 12 g of Chai Hu (hare's ear root), 15 g of Bai Shao (white peony root), 10 g of Zhi Zi (cape jasmine fruit), 12 g of Dang Gui (Chinese angelica), 12 g of Xiang Fu (nut grass rhizome), 12 g of Fuling (poria), and 5 g of Gan Cao (licorice root).

• **To treat deficient depression:** Symptoms include fatigue, sleeplessness, decreased memory, and low motivation. Mix 12 g of Huang Qi (milk-vetch root), 10 g of ginseng, 12 g of Bai Zhu (white atractylodes rhizome), 12 g of Fu Shen (poria spirit), 12 g of Yuan Zhi (Chinese senega root), 12 g of Suan Zhao Ren (sour Chinese jujube seed), and five pieces of Da Zhao (Chinese jujube).

Acupressure: Press the Tai Yang and Nei Guan points. The Tai Yang point is situated at the temple, in the depression between the lateral end of the eyebrow and the eyelid. The Nei Guan point is in the center of the wrist on the palm side about 2 inches above the crease. Apply medium pressure to these points with the tip of your finger and repeat two to three times during the day.

Diet: Include foods in your diet that help you sleep and have calming effects, such as chamomile tea, peppermint, rice porridge, pears, and mandarin oranges.

Naturopathy

Diet: Nutrition is essential for proper brain chemistry. Eat a well-balanced diet consisting of whole grains, organic vegetables, and lean protein. Consume fish such as salmon and mackerel for their high content of essential fatty acids (EFAs), specifically omega-3 fatty acids, which have been shown to be helpful in treating depression. Flaxseeds are a good source of fiber and also contain EFAs. Sprinkle 1 tbsp of ground flaxseeds on salads, yogurt, or cereal. Cut out simple, processed carbohydrates, hydrogenated oils, and saturated fats, which increase fatigue and sluggishness, and contribute to depression. Also avoid alcohol, which is a known depressant.

Supplements: Take a good multivitamin/multimineral to obtain a base of nutrients for brain chemistry function. S-adenosylmethionine (SAM–e) seems to increase the concentration of neurotransmitters in the brain that are involved in regulating mood. Take 200 mg of an enteric-coated form twice a day on as empty stomach. Fish oils have been shown in some preliminary studies to be beneficial for depression. The eicosapentaenoic acid (EPA)

and docosahexaenoic acid (DHA) contained in fish oils, improve neurotransmitter function. Take 1,000 mg of of EPA/DHA a day. L-tyrosine is an amino acid that helps regulate brain function in depressed individuals. Take 500 mg a day, but do not take it in combination with other anti-depressive medications. Take 100 mg of 5-hydroxytryptophan (5-HTP), which is used by the brain to make serotonin, an important neurotransmitter in the regulation of mood, twice a day. Be sure to take it with 100 mg of a B-complex vitamin, as vitamin B6 is essential in the metabolism of serotonin, however, do not take it with pharmaceutical medications for depression.

Herbs: Ginkgo biloba improves blood flow to the brain. Take 60–120 mg twice a day. You can also take 1,000 mg of ashwagandha to improve stress hormone balance and relax the nervous system.

Tip: GET ASSESSED FOR HEAVY METAL TOXICITY

A naturopathic physician can determine the levels of heavy metals, such as mercury, in your system. These have a strong affinity with the nervous system and may contribute to depression.

Homeopathy

Feelings that will respond well to the remedies suggested below are more appropriately described as the blues. Clinical depression may be helped by an experienced practitioner. These remedies can be helpful as a first choice of treatment, or used alongside conventional treatment.

Ignatia: This remedy is helpful if depression follows a loss of any kind. Symptoms include rapid changes in mood, frequent sighing, and nausea, which is helped by eating a small amount.

Natrum mur: This remedy can help anyone who tries to keep a lid on their emotions and develops a depressed mood as a result. Symptoms include a strong dislike of crying in public, and an equal distaste of receiving sympathy and physical displays of affection. The blues may have developed in response to a long-term emotional strain or loss.

Sepia: If depressed feelings are related to major fluctuations in hormone levels, try Sepia. Symptoms include a feeling of being wiped out, and feeling aggressive one moment and indifferent the next. Although the idea of being in company is not appealing, being alone does not help either.

Lachesis: To treat premenstrual blues and mood swings that develop when ovulating and build in intensity until the onset of a period, use Lachesis. Symptoms include low, distressed, or anxious moods that are at their worst when you wake. As a result, a real dislike and fear of going to bed may develop.

Pulsatilla: This remedy can help to lift a mild bout of feeling blue that prompts you to feel much more emotional than normal. A good cry and being the object of attention helps to relieve symptoms.

Herbalism

Many herbal medicines can be used to elevate your mood and restore vitality. That said, depression is a serious condition that should be monitored by a health professional. Herbal medicines should be used in conjunction with treatments, such as counseling, that attempt to identify and treat any possible causes of the depression. Also be aware that many of these herbs should not be taken in high doses by those who are taking conventional medication for depression.

St. John's wort: Consider using this herb to treat depression associated with a sense of loss of connection with others, loss of self-worth, or depression due to chronic pain resulting in insomnia. Many clinical studies have demonstrated St. John's wort's effectiveness at relieving depression, while others have found it to be as effective as many of the pharmaceutical antidepressants, such as Prozac®, Zoloft®, and Paxil®. Its active constituents, hypericin and hyperforin, are thought to inhibit neurotransmitters in the brain, known as serotonin, dopamine, and norepinephrine. Small amounts of melatonin, the hormone responsible for sleep induction, have also been found within the herb. Take 300 mg three times daily, standardized to 0.3% hypericin content. St. John's wort is generally tolerated well; however, side effects include photosensitivity, photodermatitis, abdominal discomfort, and hypomania in those with bipolar disorder. Exercise caution if you are taking other medications as St. John's wort increases the liver's metabolism of many drugs. Do not take this herb with anti-coagulant medications. Due to the potential photosensitivity, avoid sun exposure while using St. John's wort.

Rhodiola: To treat mild depression, especially when combined with increased levels of daily stress and physical exhaustion, try rhodiola. Rhodiola is categorized as an adaptogen, recognized for its ability to improve physical performance, decrease fatigue and depression, and improve sleep. Rhodiola contains high amounts of antioxidant flavonoids, catechins proanthocyanidins, and rosavin, one of the main active constituents thought to impart rhodiola's adaptogenic ability. Rhodiola increases neurotransmitters in the brain (serotonin, dopamine, and norepinephrine) which are known to elevate moods. Take a 100 mg dose a day standardized to 2% rosavin, and increase to 300 mg daily if needed. Higher doses (above 200 mg) may cause irritability and insomnia.

A blend of calming, anxiolytic herbs taken alongside rhodiola and St. John's wort is often of use. These can include oat straw, lemon balm, lemon verbena, and lime flowers, among others. Also see herbs recommended for stress and anxiety on pp. 438 and 448.

Panic Attacks

Diagnosis

Panic attacks are feelings of intense fear and anxiety that come on without any warning, and often have no apparent trigger. They result from an exaggeration of the body's normal response to fear, stress, or excitement. Adrenaline floods the body, causing muscles to tense up, rapid breathing, the heart to pump harder, sweating, slow digestion, and a dry mouth. Panic attacks can be very frightening experiences.

In some people, attacks are linked to fear about an illness, a major life change, or being in a crowd or a confined space. In others, they are associated with extreme excitement. Attacks tend to come on suddenly and generally last between five and ten minutes.

Symptoms

- Feeling terrified, tense, and anxious
- Feeling detached, both from the body and surroundings
- Fear of dying or going mad
- Feeling out of control
- Feeling unable to breathe
- Rapid breathing
- Pounding heartbeat and pains in the chest
- Sweating
- Feeling faint, dizzy, or nauseous
- Tingling or numbness in the extremities
- Alternating sensations of being too hot or cold
- Weak bladder

Treatment Goal

Identifying triggers and confronting the emotional issues behind them. Coping strategies can be developed to prevent attacks from occurring, or to lessen their severity.

Conventional Medicine

The first step is to make sure that an underlying illness is not contributing to panic attacks. Specifically, hyperthyroidism can cause anxiety and panic. Drug abuse and heavy alcohol consumption can also lead to panic disorders, during active use or withdrawal. Some over-the-counter medications may also contribute to panic attacks. Consult a doctor to rule out these conditions.

Cognitive behavioral therapy: Most people benefit from cognitive behavioural therapy, which involves exposing the affected person to a feared situation, first in the imagination and then in reality, until he or she can tolerate the situation without symptoms. This should be conducted by a psychiatrist or counselor, and can be used in conjunction with medication. Psychodynamic psychotherapy is another treatment that can be offered by a psychiatrist or a counselor. It is based on the concept that mental processes outside of conscious awareness contribute to the panic attack and that dealing with these alleviates panic episodes.

Medication: Selective serotonin reuptake inhibitors (SSRIs) can be used to treat panic and depression. Escitalopram (Lexapro®) seems to be one of the best for helping with anxiety. Tricyclic antidepressants are also used, and benzodiazepines can be used as a secondary treatment. They are addictive but highly effective and sometimes necessary for treating severe panic.

Complications: Treatment programs should take into account co-existing diseases such as cardiac or respiratory illnesses. In these cases, a panic disorder may result in serious secondary damage during a full-blown attack. A strong therapeutic plan should be on hand to treat episodes of panic.

Traditional Chinese Medicine

Herbs: To prepare a formula, place the herbs in a ceramic or glass pot and add 3 cups of water. Bring to a boil and simmer for 30 minutes. Strain the liquid and drink 1 cup twice a day.
• **To treat Qi stagnation:** This formula can regulate energy flow to help patients who are unable to think clearly, and have stiff facial expressions. Mix 12 g of Fa Ban Xia (pinellia rhizome), 10 g of Hou Po (magnolia bark), 15 g of Fuling (poria), 12 g of Zi Su Gen (perilla), 6 g of fresh ginger, and six pieces of Da Zhao (Chinese jujube).

• To nourish and tonify the heart, spleen, and kidney: This formula can help those who suffer from panic attacks associated with fatigue, insomnia, excessive sleeping, diminished memory, or loss of appetite. Mix 10 g of ginseng, 15 g of Bai Zhu (white atractylodes rhizome), 15 g of Fuling (poria), 12 g of Yuan Zhi (Chinese senega root), 12 g of Dang Gui (Chinese angelica), 12 g of Long Yan Rou (longan), 15 g of Shu Di Huang (cooked Chinese foxglove), 12 g of Mai Men Dong (ophiopogon tuber), and 5 g of Gan Cao (licorice).

Acupressure: Press the Nei Guan and Tai Yang points while having a panic attack to help calm down the spirit, and reduce the sensation of panic. The Tai Yang point is situated at the temple in the depression between the lateral end of the eyebrow and the eyelid. The Nei Guan point is in the center of the wrist on the palm side, about 2 inches above the crease.

Diet: Eat food that is nourishing to the spleen, kidney, and blood, such as beef, polished rice, sweet potatoes, potatoes, string beans, wheat, red beans, black beans, spinach, fish, carrots, radishes, and black sesame seeds. Foods that have a calming effect such as chamomile tea, peppermint, rice porridge, mandarin oranges, and pears, are also recommended. Avoid hot, spicy food, such as chili peppers and garlic.

Naturopathy

Breathing exercises: Deep breathing relaxes the mind, calms the nervous system, and improves mental focus and energy. Deep breathing requires imitating the breathing patterns of a child—they breath from the belly not the chest. To deep breath properly, find a comfortable, quiet area. Stand with your knees slightly bent or sit straight with your buttocks touching the back of your seat. Breath in through your nose to a count of five, hold for two seconds, and exhale to a count of five. While breathing in, your stomach, rather than your chest, should expand outward. When breathing out, your stomach should flatten.

Bach flower remedies: The Bach flower remedies are a type of "vibrational, or energy medicine," developed in the 1920s by Edward Bach, an English doctor and homeopath. Because Bach flower remedies do not contain any of the original substance used, only its "vibrational pattern," they are considered to be different from homeopathic remedies (which contain minute amounts of the original substance). The most common types of remedies for panic attacks include cherry plum (to treat panic with loss of self-control), aspen (to treat vague, spooky fear that is not directed at anything specific), red chestnut (to treat fear for another's safety), star of Bethlehem (to ease fear related to a past trauma), and larch (to treat related issues such as lack of confidence).

Relaxation movements: T'ai chi is a form of stress reduction and exercise that involves specific body movements and deep breathing. Yoga can also help with relaxation and stress reduction. It primarily involves deep breathing, stretches, and meditation.

Tip: DRINK A HERBAL TEA

Mix ½ oz each of dried lavender, oats, linden flower, catnip, and lemon balm. Use 4 tsp of this mixture per quart of boiling water. Pour the water over the herbs and steep for about 10 minutes. Strain and drink while the tea is still warm. You can drink up to 6 cups of this drink per day after meals.

Homeopathy

The following remedies can help ease symptoms that develop in response to an obvious trigger. Severe and recurrent panic attacks are best treated by a practitioner. See also Post-Traumatic Stress Disorder (p. 463).

Phosphorus: If you experience "free-floating" panicky feelings that attach themselves to any focus of anxiety, use Phosphorus. Feeling tense can lead to exhaustion, but may be relieved by reassurance. Feelings of panic are especially noticeable in the early evening.

Argentum nit: If panic develops in connection with anticipatory anxiety, and is associated with mental and emotional restlessness that causes you to talk incessantly, use Argentum nit. Symptoms include palpitations and trembling, and a craving for sweet things. The stomach is also likely to be upset and be affected by diarrhea.

Gelsemium: This remedy is also a suitable choice to treat panic attacks associated with anticipatory nerves, especially if they cause you to become withdrawn and quiet. Symptoms build gradually, becoming more intense as the stressful event gets closer, making you feel exhausted, weak, and shaky.

Lycopodium: This is an appropriate remedy for those who can hide panicky feelings well. There tend to be strong feelings of anxiety in the stomach, causing acid to wash up into the throat when belching. Feelings of tension also lead to alternating bouts of diarrhea and constipation, as well bloating and loud rumbling sounds in the belly.

Herbalism

There are many herbs that can be useful for calming symptoms associated with panic attacks, including anxiety and an increased heart rate. In addition to the remedies below, any of the anti-anxiety, sedative, or relaxing herbs recommended in Anxiety (p. 448) and Insomnia (p. 443) may be useful.

Passionflower: This herb is used to calm many types of nervous hyperactivity, including panic attacks. It is available in capsule form, as a tincture, or as raw herbs that can be infused to make a tea. The recommended dose of passionflower varies, depending on the person and the severity of symptoms, and it may take several weeks before overall anxiety levels have improved and the frequency of panic attacks have lessened. Capsules are generally dosed at ½–1 g, tinctures at ½–2 ml, and a tea can be made from 1–2 g; all forms should be taken three times daily. Some people feel too sedated when taking passionflower, or any of the other herbs in this section. Be cautious if you are also taking psychoactive medications such as antidepressant medications, as these can increase the effect of passionflower.

Valerian: During a panic attack this herb is best taken as a tincture, for quick and easy use. It has anxiolytic properties, and works primarily on GABA receptors. This herb has a high volatile oil content, which can evaporate easily if the dried herb is boiled for too long. It is best to keep the mixture covered while simmering, or make a strong infusion. For a gentle, soothing touch, add some rose petal fluid extract.

Post-Traumatic Stress Disorder

Diagnosis

The term post-traumatic stress disorder (PTSD) is used to describe a range of psychological symptoms that may result from experiencing or witnessing a traumatic or life-threatening event. It can also occasionally follow a particularly difficult childbirth. Most survivors of trauma will go on to live normal lives once time has passed, but for others, just hearing news of shattering events can have a lasting impact. Indeed, people who have not been directly involved in a trauma may still experience high levels of distress. Sufferers may relive events through flashbacks or nightmares, and have difficulty sleeping as a result. Those with PTSD feel estranged or detached from those around them.

Symptoms

- Feeling numb
- Emotional and physical reactions
- Changes in behavior
- Nightmares
- Intense distress when reminded of the trauma
- Easily startled
- Disturbed sleep patterns
- Feeling irritable and aggressive
- Poor concentration
- Feeling guilty, as though responsible for the event
- Avoiding memories
- Feeling detached
- Feeling there is no point in planning for the future

Treatment Goal

It can be helpful for people to share their experiences with others who have been through similar problems. Treatment involves psychological therapy to come to terms with causes, and restore quality of life.

Conventional Medicine

Psychotherapy: The primary treatment for PTSD is psychotherapy. Specific techniques include anxiety and stress management with relaxation techniques, cognitive behavioral and exposure therapy (which involves exposing the affected person to a feared situation, first in the imagination and then in reality, until he or she can tolerate the situation without symptoms), group therapy, education, and play therapy for children.

EMDR: A technique known as eye movement desensitization and reprocessing (EMDR) is relatively new and promising. In this technique, a person focuses on the therapist's finger movement while visualizing the traumatic event. The goal is to maintain a deep state of relaxation while working through a traumatic event.

Lifestyle modifications: Avoid drugs and alcohol, as many people with PTSD have concomitant substance abuse disorder. A healthy diet and good nutrition also support other behavioral and medication therapies.

Medication: Selective serotonin reuptake inhibitors (SSRI), specifically Paxil® and Zoloft®, are used to treat this condition. Effexor®, another SSRI, has also been used for PTSD. Serotonin has a calming effect on the body and reduces feelings of aggression and anxiety. Anti-anxiety medication such as BuSpar® and benzodiazepines have also been used to treat PTSD.

Traditional Chinese Medicine

Herbs: The following formula can reduce the stress to your liver, which is the organ that is most sensitive to traumatic stress. Mix 12 g of Chai Hu (hare's ear root), 15 g of Bai Shao (white peony root), 12 g of Dang Gui (Chinese angelica), 8 g of Bo He (field mint), 15 g of Bai Zhu (white atractylodes rhizome), 12 g of Yu Jin (turmeric tuber), 12 g of Xiang Fu (nut grass rhizome), 12 g of Long Yan Rou (longan), and 8 g of Gan Cao (licorice root). To prepare the formula, place the herbs in a glass or ceramic pot and add 3 cups of water. Bring to a boil and simmer for 30 minutes. Strain and drink 1 cup twice a day.

Acupressure: Press the Shen Men, Hegu, Tai Yang, and Feng Chi points with moderate to heavy pressure for one minute and repeat. These points should be pressed when you feel an episode coming on. The Shen Men point is located on the inside of the wrist, just above the crease in the first depression at the base of the thumb. The Hegu point is located on the back of the hand in the depression between the thumb and first finger. The Tai Yang point is situated at the temple in the depression between the lateral end of the eyebrow and the eyelid. The Feng Chi point is at the back of the head at the base of the skull, about 2 inches from the center point.

Diet: Food that is calming and good for the liver, heart, and kidney is recommended, including chives, duck, plums, grapes, tangerines, egg yolk, celery, rice porridge, persimmon, adzuki beans, watermelon, black soybeans, lychees, and hawthorn fruit. Foods that nourish the blood will also help, as will cooling foods. Avoid hot and spicy foods.

Naturopathy

There are no natural cures for PTSD, but there are some natural recommendations that may help ease some of the symptoms of the condition, such as general restlessness, insomnia, aggressiveness, and depression.

Diet: Keep your blood sugar levels balanced by eating small, frequent meals throughout the day. Make sure to eat only when you are calm, however, as eating while depressed or angry may worsen symptoms. Include whole grains such as oats, quinoa, or brown rice with every meal. These foods contain high levels of B vitamins and fiber, and increase your body's ability to make serotonin (neurotransmitters have a calming effect on the body and ease aggression and anxiety). The B vitamins are calming to the nervous system and the fiber keeps your bowels movements regular. Calcium and magnesium also produce a calming effect. Sea vegetables, green leafy vegetables, nuts, and yogurt are good sources of these nutrients. Caffeine, refined sugars, and alcohol can make symptoms worse and should be avoided.

Supplements: 5-hydroxytryptophan (5-HTP) increases serotonin levels, which have a calming effect on the body. Take 50–100 mg two to three times daily, but do not take 5-HTP if you are on anti-depressant medications. Taking 500 mg of calcium and 250 mg of magnesium will also help calm the nervous system. Chromium can be taken at a dose of 200 mcg twice a day to help balance blood sugar. Those who suffer from PTSD often have symptoms that inhibit the production of digestive juices. Betaine hydrochloride supports stomach acid levels and helps with digestion. Take one to two capsules with each meal. Digestive enzymes also help your body to digest food more effectively, reducing irritation. The enzymes include lipases that digest fat, proteases that digest proteins, and amylases that digest starch. Take 2 capsules or tablets of a full spectrum enzyme product with each meal.

Herbs: Kava is an herb that is used widely in Europe to treat nervous anxiety, tension, agitation, and insomnia. Take 200–250 mg twice a day, but do not take pharmaceutical tranquilizers while taking kava. It is best to take this herb under the supervision of a doctor. Valerian is an herbal tranquilizer that is best known as a remedy for insomnia. It calms the nervous system, balances mood swings, and is not habit forming. Take 300 mg in capsule form or 0.5–1.0 ml of a tincture two to three times a day. People with serious health conditions, or who are taking prescription drugs for mood or neurological disorders, should consult a qualified professional before taking valerian. Passionflower relaxes the nerves and can be used during the day without causing drowsiness. Take 250 mg of a capsule or 0.5 ml of tincture three times a day. Lemon balm can be taken for its calming effect to help reduce anxiety levels. The standard oral dose is 1.5–4.5 g of dried herb daily. Extracts and tinctures should be taken according to instruction on the label.

Manage stress: Regular exercise, particularly cardiovascular activity combined with calming exercises, such as walking, can help you manage your stress levels. Massage therapy, shiatsu, and other forms of bodywork can also relax muscle tension, relieve stress, and improve sleep.

Homeopathy

Ideally, this condition requires a combination of professional homeopathic treatment and psychological support. However, the most appropriately selected of the following remedies can provide helpful temporary relief at an acute level while seeking medical help.

Aconite: This remedy can help to relieve feelings of terror or panic that are triggered by witnessing or being involved in a traumatic incident, or receiving very bad news. Symptoms such as trembling, breathlessness, and hyperventilation develop rapidly, with feelings of anxiety and fear that are so strong that sufferers are convinced they are about to die. Patients may also experience disturbed sleep.

Ignatia: To temporarily relieve a strong emotional reaction to an upsetting or traumatic event, try Ignatia. Symptoms include heightened emotions, and patients alternate between laughing and crying. Sighing and sobbing are also prevalent, and there is an associated irritability and a desire to be alone. This remedy is particularly suitable for providing emotional support for those who are grieving and coping with the early stages of loss.

Arnica: If you are in denial about an emotional or physical shock, try Arnica. Patients assert that everything is all right and reject help and support.

Herbalism

Herbs can help with some of the symptoms of this disorder while more definitive treatments, such as special psychotherapeutic therapies, are pursued. For example, any of the herbal hypnotics (see Insomnia, p. 443) would be effective to help people suffering from PTSD that affects sleep.

Tonics: Herbal tonics, also called adaptogens, are often used to help strengthen the whole body and make it more resistant to the anxiety and overall stress of this disorder. Common tonics are eleuthero (also called Siberian ginseng), ashwaganda, and rhodiola. Most herbal tonics have a variety of effects on several different body systems. For example, they may act as an anti-inflammatory and antioxidant, and affect hormones such as cortisol secreted by the hypothalamus, pituitary, and adrenal glands. A tincture of various herbal tonics is often dosed at 60–180 drops (1–3 droppers full) daily. Water-based infusions or decoctions of these tonics may be effective, though many of the important phytochemicals are not very soluble in water; standardized extracts and alcohol or glycerin tinctures are usually the most effective forms. Panax ginseng is often recommended, but is frequently found to be too stimulating when someone is depleted as a result of trauma or stress.

Seek Professional Advice
The information in this book is a not a substitute for professional medical advice or health care. Consult a qualified health professional when there is any question regarding the presence or treatment of any health condition.

Seasonal Affective Disorder

Diagnosis

Seasonal affective disorder (SAD) is a condition where sufferers experience seasonal changes of mood and behavior, such as depression. During the winter months, the change in the quality and quantity of light, specifically fewer daylight hours, has an effect on the outlook of some people. The exact causes of SAD are still unclear. Most research looks at the effect of light on the brain. When light hits the eye, particularly the retina, messages are passed to the hypothalamus gland, which releases serotonin and melatonin, which are neurotransmitters that control sleep patterns, appetite, libido, body temperature, mood, and energy levels. If we are not exposed to enough light, these functions slow down, leading to symptoms of fatigue, disturbed sleep, an inability to concentrate, and low libido. Around 20% of cases are fairly mild (known as the "winter blues," or sub-syndromal SAD), but 2–5% of cases are severe, and patients are unable to function without treatment.

Symptoms

- Lethargy or fatigue
- Sleep problems
- Depression and feeling sad and low
- Overeating, especially a craving for carbohydrates
- Irritability and tension
- Concentration problems
- Loss of libido
- Feeling under the weather
- Period problems

Treatment Goal

To develop strategies to compensate for lack of sunlight during winter months to relieve symptoms. Light therapy is the most effective treatment, and helps about 80% of patients.

Conventional Medicine

Light therapy: This type of treatment involves using a light box to expose patients to a full spectrum light at 2,500 lux (a measure of light intensity) or greater. Patients should receive treatment for two hours a day at 2,500 lux, or one hour a day at 10,000 lux. An alternative technique is known as dawn simulation, where a full spectrum lamp is used to create an artificial dawn for 60–90 minutes in the early morning.

Antidepressants: This type of medication is used in patients that are unresponsive to light therapy, or when light therapy is not acceptable to a patient. Selective serotonin reuptake inhibitors (SSRIs) are generally used. Serotonin has a calming effect on the body and reduces feelings of aggression and anxiety. No one SSRI seems to be more beneficial than another, but the atypical SSRI mirtazapine has the side effect of increasing appetite.

Lifestyle modifications: Eat a high-protein diet that excludes processed foods and is low sugar and caffeine. This can help to increase the effectiveness of other therapies. Winter holidays, or in extreme cases, relocation to a sunnier area may be advisable if possible. St. John's wort has been shown to be effective when taking 300 mg of a 30% hypericum extract; however, consult with a herbalist or doctor of integrative medicine before using this if you are taking other medication. Taking 2–4 g of fish oil a day also helps to combat depression. Stress management techniques, such as exercise or meditation, are also recommended as adjunct treatments.

Traditional Chinese Medicine

Herbs: To prepare a formula, place the herbs in a ceramic or glass pot and add 3 cups of water. Bring the ingredients to a boil and simmer for 30 minutes. Strain the liquid and drink 1 cup twice a day.
• To treat SAD associated with kidney deficiency: Mix 12 g of Ji Shen (jilin root), 15 g of Di Huang (Chinese foxglove), 15 g of Dan Shen (salvia root), and 12 g of Shan Zhu Yu (Asiatic cornelian cherry), 15 g of Shan Yao (Chinese yam), 15 g of Fuling (poria), 12 g of Sang Shen Zi (mulberry fruit-spike), and 12 g of Tu Si Zi (Chinese dodder seed).
• To treat SAD associated with fatigue and body weakness: Mix 10 g of ginseng, 12 g of Bai Zhu (white atractylodes rhizome), 15 g of Shan Yao (Chinese yam), 12 g of Huang Qi (milk-vetch root), 15 g of Fuling (poria), and 3 g of Gan Cao (licorice root).

Acupressure: Press the Hegu points with strong pressure and the Nei Guan point with moderate pressure for one to three minutes, and repeat. The Hegu point is located on the back of the hand between the thumb and first finger. The Nei Guan point is found in the center of the wrist on the palm side, about 2 inches above the crease.

Diet: Eat a well-balanced diet and foods that nourish the blood such as black sesame seeds, radishes, spinach, fish, and carrots. Also, choose food that is cooling, such as tofu, watermelon, green vegetables, and Chinese jujube dates. Avoid hot and spicy food.

Naturopathy

Naturopathic treatment involves normalizing serotonin and melatonin levels to regulate mood and sleeping patterns.

Supplements: The body creates vitamin D when it is exposed to the sun. Consequently, vitamin D levels in the body drop during the winter months. Taking 500–1,000 IU of vitamin D supplements daily may help to ease symptoms of SAD. Melatonin, a hormone produced in the pineal gland, plays a major role in regulating the daily biological clock, sleep patterns, and core body temperature at night. Taking low doses of melatonin (1–3 mg two to three hours before bedtime) has been shown to be effective in treating SAD. 5-hydroxytryptophan (5-HTP) is effective in increasing levels of serotonin in the body. Take 100–200 mg at night on an empty stomach or with a protein-free snack. Vitamin B6 is an important co-factor involved in the production of serotonin. Vitamin B6 deficiency should be considered when diagnosing SAD, particularly in the elderly, who may suffer from vitamin deficiencies. Take 250 mg daily early in the day. Do not take vitamin B6 within six hours of taking 5-HTP because it may interfere with the latter's conversion to serotonin. Eicosapentaenoic acid (EPA) and docosahexaenoic acid (DHA), which are omega-3 fatty acids, also play a role in the synthesis

Tip: CHANGE LIGHT BULBS

If you regularly suffer from seasonal affective disorder, consider placing full spectrum light bulbs all over your house, and, if possible, in your work area. Full spectrum light mimics sunlight and assists your body in the synthesis of serotonin.

> ***Tip:*** GO IN THE SUN EVERY DAY
>
> Get 15–30 minutes of natural light daily, especially in the morning so that your body stays in tune with its normal biological rhythms. Studies of patients with SAD indicate that bright light therapy in the morning has a greater therapeutic effect than evening light therapy.

on serotonin, and there is encouraging data about their use in depressive disorders. Take 700 mg and 500 mg a day respectively.

Herbs: St. John's wort has been shown to be effective in treating severe depression and the depressive symptoms of SAD. Take 300–900 mg daily on an empty stomach. St. John's wort can increase sensitivity to sunlight, so minimize your exposure to the sun when taking it to avoid getting a sunburn.

Essential oils: Various essential oils can be used to reduce stress and promote relaxation. Use 5 drops of all or some of the oils below in a steam inhalation, add them to your bath water, or incorporate them into a massage oil, using almond or apricot oil as a base. Petitgrain oil can be uplifting, balancing, calming, and refreshing. Bergamot oil has a fresh, sweet, fruity scent. It is often described as being like sunshine in a bottle, and has an uplifting, cheerful effect. Do not apply it directly to the skin. Neroli oil has a light, sweet floral fragrance. It has a balancing tonic effect on the nervous system and can be relaxing and uplifting. It is great for treating anxiety, nervous tension, and depression. Jasmine's heady aroma is considered emotionally warming and is useful for relieving sexual anxiety and fear.

Homeopathy

This problem appears to vary in its severity. Both severe and less severe conditions can benefit from homeopathic support. Since this is likely to be a recurring problem, it falls into a chronic category and is best treated by an experienced homeopathic practitioner. The remedies described below give an idea of some of the choices available, and are not intended to encourage self-prescribing.

> ***Tip:*** USE A LIGHT BOX
>
> If you cannot manage to take a vacation somewhere warm during the winter, invest in a portable full spectrum light box that can be used at home and at work.

Sepia: If symptoms of the blues are accompanied by mental, emotional, and physical exhaustion, nonexistent libido, and a general sense of indifference to things that would normally stimulate and excite, Sepia may be used. Patients may feel more positive after aerobic exercise.

Natrum mur: If you are feeling withdrawn and depressed, and also crave carbohydrates and salt, Natrum mur may be helpful. Patients may weep when alone, since crying in front of anyone else feels humiliating. Displays of affection and sympathy are not well received.

Tip: EXERCISE

Your body naturally produces feel-good chemicals called endorphins when engaged in aerobic exercise. Regular physical activity of this kind four times a week has been shown to lift low moods. Try cycling (use a stationary cycle if the weather is bad), running, or jogging.

Herbalism

See Depression (p. 454) for more details about St. John's wort and other herbs that may be helpful in treating SAD.

St. John's wort: St. John's wort can be useful for treating seasonal affective disorder. It seems to be most effective for mild-to-moderate depression rather than more severe cases. St. John's wort can be taken in many forms. It is possible to purchase tinctures, standardized extracts, tablets, or the dried herb (the above-ground parts) in order to make a tea. Many products will be standardized to one of the compounds, hypericin, that was originally thought to account for much of its antidepressant activity. Most clinical trials have used an extract standardized to 0.3% hypericin dosed at 300 mg three times daily. Herbal practitioners often use whole plant extracts, and not solely standardized extracts. For optimal effect in treating SAD, begin the daily use of St. John's wort two months before your symptoms usually start. This may be in late September or October, as the amount of daylight starts to wane. Be sure to avoid too much sun exposure when using this herb, due to potential photosensitivity.

9

First Aid

Insect Bites

Diagnosis

Insect bites are particularly common during the summer months. Insects that bite include mosquitoes, gnats, midges, horseflies, ants, spiders, fleas, and lice. The most obvious sign of a bite is a red bump on the skin, or several bumps that show up as a rash (fleas, for example, often bite several times). Bites tend to be itchy and are sometimes painful. The skin around a bite can also become red and swollen. Avoid scratching bites as much as possible as this can cause them to become infected. Bites are generally not dangerous, provided there is no allergic reaction. Biting insects, however, can spread diseases such as malaria, yellow fever, Lyme disease, and typhus. If the bite appears to worsen rather than improve over time, consult a doctor.

Danger: Bites can sometimes cause an allergic reaction. Call for an ambulance if you notice symptoms of dizziness, nausea, pains in the chest, choking or wheezing, and/or difficulty breathing. A life-threatening situation can develop if the victim goes into shock.

Symptoms

- A raised, red bump on the skin, or several bumps clustered together
- A small hole may be visible in the center of the bump
- The area is itchy and swollen, and may be painful

Treatment Goal

Treatment involves easing symptoms of itchiness, pain, and swelling, and preventing an infection from developing.

Conventional Medicine

Conventional treatment involves alleviating pain, treating or preventing an allergic reaction, and dealing with any side effects of a bite.

Remove the insect: If it is still present, the stinger or in some cases the insect should gently be removed without crushing or squeezing the area of the bite. Use a straight-edged object (such as a credit card) to scrape away the stinger. To treat tick bites, it is essential to remove the tick without compressing the body parts. Apply gentle traction until the tick comes out. If a red rash appears around the tick bite within one to three weeks and begins to spread, consult a doctor, as it could be a sign of Lyme disease.

Topical treatments: Apply an ice pack wrapped in a cloth to the bite. Hydrocortisone cream (0.5%), calamine lotion, or a baking soda paste (made from baking soda and water) can be applied after the ice and thereafter three times a day as needed.

Antihistamines: Diphenhydramine (Benadryl®), which is commonly used to treat symptoms of allergic reactions, may be needed if severe itching is present.

Treating an allergic reaction: Observe the victim for any signs of breathing difficulty, excessive swelling, dizziness, or shock. If any of these symptoms are present, go to hospital immediately. Moderate allergic reactions are also treated with epinephrine, which can be injected with an "epi pen." A doctor will evaluate the patient's airways, breathing, and circulation and treat any complications.

Tip: USE INSECT REPELLENT

Take preventive steps by using an insect repellent on the skin. There are many formulas available that are made from natural ingredients.

Traditional Chinese Medicine

Herbs: Combine 15 g of Jin Yin Hua (honeysuckle flower) and 15 g of Jing Jie (schizonepeta stem and bud). Boil the ingredients in 5 cups of water for five minutes, strain the liquid, and add it to a container that is large enough to bathe the affected area. Soak the bite in this herbal bath once a day for as long as required.

Acupressure: Press the Tai Yang, Hegu, and Feng Chi points gently for about one minute twice a day. The Tai Yang point is at the temple in the depression between the lateral end of the eyebrow and the eyelid. The Hegu point is located on the back of the hand between the thumb and first finger. The Feng Chi points are at the back of the head at the base of the skull, about 2 inches on either side of the center point.

Diet: Eat a balanced diet that includes fresh vegetables, and reduce your coffee intake, since caffeine dehydrates the skin. Fruit such as pears, cranberries, blueberries, and bananas are recommended. Mung beans, red beans, bamboo shoots, and purslane are also good. Avoid food that is rich and fatty, as it has drying and warming properties that can make symptoms worse.

Naturopathy

Supplements: Take 3–5 g of omega-3 essential fatty acids a day as they have anti-inflammatory properties that may help protect against the extreme reaction of anaphylaxis and other allergic responses to insect bites. Quercetin, when taken before being bitten, can lessen the severity of an allergic response. If you have a history of an allergy to bees, wasps, or other insects, consider taking 250 mg of quercetin supplements three times a day. Vitamin C, which can be taken at 500–1,000 mg three times a day, is essential for healing and a strong immune system to avoid infection.

Bioflavonoids work synergistically with vitamin C and have anti-inflammatory properties. Take 250–500 mg two to three times a day.

Topical herbs: There is a variety of herbs that can be used topically to prevent insect bites from occurring, or encourage existing bites to heal. Arnica can be used as a topical herb to treat inflammation from insect bites. Place 3 drops on the bite and massage it into the affected area. Lemon balm, which is another traditional treatment for relief of insect bites or stings, can be applied in the same way.

Tip: USE AN APPLE CIDER VINEGAR SOLUTION

To relieve the discomfort of insect bites, make up a solution of water and apple cider vinegar in a 1:1 ratio and apply it to the bite for a few minutes. Rinse with warm water.

You can also apply aloe vera gel to the affected area for two weeks, or until it is healed, to relieve inflammation. Calendula cream is used as a natural insect repellent, and also soothes skin irritations. Comfrey cream promotes tissue healing, and tea tree oil can be used as an antiseptic to prevent infection. Citronella is a lemon-scented plant that has long been used as an insect repellent. It is also the active ingredient in several commercial insect repellents that you can apply to either your skin or clothing. Pure citronella oil can be irritating to the skin and should never be ingested. If you want to use the oil, dilute it by adding several drops to a vegetable oil base. You can then rub the diluted oil directly on your skin. Citrus essential oil has aromatic qualities that repel insects. Dilute it by adding several drops of essential oil to a vegetable oil base, and experiment by using different combinations of essential oils together to customize your own insect repellent. Lemongrass is a cousin of citronella and has many of the same insect-repelling compounds. If you have access to the fresh herb, simply crush some and rub it directly on your skin. Plantain is also excellent for bug bites and can also be rubbed directly on the skin.

Homeopathy

Any of the following remedies can be used to promote recovery from an insect bite in those who do not have a history of allergic reactions.

Ledum: Use this remedy to treat stings that cause the affected area to feel cool to the touch. Discomfort is relieved by contact with cool air, applying cool compresses, and cool bathing. The skin that has been stung is also likely to look red and slightly swollen.

Apis: This remedy can be used to treat bites that show symptoms of localized inflammation and swelling. The affected area is likely to be raised and look puffy, feel worse for contact with warmth, and feel soothed by exposure to cool applications.

Tip: LAVENDER ESSENTIAL OIL

Diluted lavender essential oil can be immensely soothing and healing when applied to skin affected by an insect bite. Dilute a few drops in a vegetable oil base before applying it directly to the skin.

Urtica urens: If bites trigger strong burning sensations around the edge of the affected area, use Urtica urens. There is also localized itchiness and a stitchlike discomfort that is aggravated by contact with cool air and cool bathing. This remedy can also be effective in easing lingering and itchy sensations that refuse to clear up.

Staphysagria: If insect bites cause severe itching and localized stinging sensations that trigger strong feelings of irritation, use Staphysagria. The least touch to the affected area is uncomfortable, while warmth and scratching give temporary relief. This remedy can also play a useful role as a prophylactic when used by those who know that they tend to attract midge bites.

Herbalism

Stinging nettle: Although it seems counterintuitive to put stinging nettles on an insect sting, this plant may be beneficial. The suggested dosage is to drink a tea made from 1–2 g of the leaf two to three times daily. The infusion may also be applied topically. Many health food stores now sell stinging nettles in standardized extracts as freeze-dried capsules. You may find this a more convenient mode of delivery. Stinging nettles may cause upset stomach and nausea, and there is the potential for an allergic reaction.

Chamomile: This herb can help calm the inflammation and irritation associated with insect bites. Make a poultice from a handful of fresh chamomile flowers and apply it directly to the affected area.

Plantain: The fresh leaves of this plant are best administered by crushing and applying as a poultice. Plantain has an anti-inflammatory, soothing effect, and has antihistamine properties. It helps to soothe any pain and irritation from the insect bite. A combination of plantain, nettle, and chamomile may also be taken as an infusion.

Thyme: This herb may help to relieve the sting of insect bites when used topically. Apply 1 drop of the essential oil in a little base oil, such as apricot kernel oil, that help to nourish and moisturize the skin. Thyme oil has been associated with a few toxic reactions when taken internally, so only use the oil topically to treat insect bites. 🌿

Tip: APPLY A POULTICE

Mash up a clove of garlic and place the poultice on the affected area. This will prevent an infection from developing. You can also use a wet tea bag as a poultice, since the tannic acid in tea helps to reduce the swelling associated with insect bites. Black tea is the most effective.

Cuts

Diagnosis

Cuts can either be minor injuries, involving minimal bleeding, or more severe, incurring significant blood loss. Either way, it is important to control the bleeding and prevent infection. Lacerations are caused by blunt objects that tear or crush the skin, particularly around bony areas of the body such as fingers or knees. These types of injuries also tend to result in swelling and leave jagged edges, so problems with healing may occur. Incised wounds are caused by objects with sharp edges that slice into the skin. These types of cuts tend to be deeper, damaging underlying tissue. Sharp-edged objects can also pierce the skin, resulting in a stab or puncture wound. Minor cuts, where the skin does not gape open, should be washed carefully under cold running water, and gently patted dry. You can also sponge the wound clean.

DANGER: If the bleeding has not stopped after 10 minutes, or the wound is gaping and may need stitches, go to the emergency room of your nearest hospital.

Symptoms

- Bleeding from an open wound
- Stinging or throbbing pain
- There may be swelling around the area

Treatment Goal

To stop the bleeding as soon as possible, to encourage the cut to heal, and to prevent the wound from becoming infected.

Conventional Medicine

Blood loss following a cut can be minimal to severe, depending on the area where the injury has occurred and the vessels cut. A cut artery constitutes a medical emergency, since a pumping artery can release the entire blood supply in a short period of time.

Apply pressure: Remove any clothing around the cut and immediately apply direct pressure to the area from which blood is flowing. This should be done using a cloth folded under the hands. If possible, apply a sterile dressing and bandage it in place by wrapping it with tape or gauze so that some amount of pressure is continually applied to the wound. If the bleeding continues, the injured area should be raised to above the level of the heart. Continue to place dressings over the bandage as they become saturated, rather than removing one and replacing it. Of course, if a heavy amount of bleeding occurs, you should call an ambulance.

Keep the area clean: Wounds should be kept clean and dry. Waterproof bandages are helpful, and an antiseptic such as Neosporin® or Bacitracin® can also be applied.

Tetanus shot: If the wound has occurred in an area that is dirty, get a tetanus booster if it has been more than 10 years since your last one. This will prevent tetanus, a serious disease of the central nervous system caused by the infection of a wound by soil-dwelling bacteria, from developing.

Diet and supplements: The rate at which a wound heals is influenced by a patient's nutritional status, especially their zinc levels. It may be helpful to take 40 mg of zinc daily, and assure that the diet is high in protein and fresh fruit and vegetables. Large amounts of processed foods and sugar should be avoided.

Antibiotics: If redness and heat spread around the immediate area of the cut or if the cut becomes purulent, it should be assessed to determine whether it is infected. If this is the case, antibiotic therapy is required.

Traditional Chinese Medicine

Herbs: Chinese herbs are not used to treat cuts.

Acupressure: This method of treatment is not used to treat cuts.

Diet: There is no specific dietary advice other than maintaining a healthy and well-balanced diet that includes plenty of fresh fruit and vegetables, and grains. Also drink plenty of water every day.

Naturopathy

Diet: Foods such as green, leafy vegetables, apples, and citrus fruits are rich in vitamin C and will help blood capillaries heal quickly. It is best to eat these foods raw, as vitamin C provides enzymes that are destroyed by heat. Other brightly colored foods, such as peppers, berries, and carrots, contain bioflavonoids, which help to heal all kinds of cuts. Avoid sugars, refined carbohydrates, hydrogenated oils, and trans-fatty acids found in fried foods and junk foods, as they interfere with the healing process and promote inflammation.

Supplements: Vitamins A, C, and E, as well as zinc are traditionally used to treat minor wounds and cuts. They can be taken orally or applied topically. Take 15,000 IU of vitamin A a day, 1,000 mg of vitamin C three times a day, 400 IU of vitamin E a day, and/or 15–30 mg of zinc a day. Creams that contain these ingredients are readily available from natural food stores.

Herbs: Gotu kola is thought to have general wound-healing properties, as well working to prevent or treat heavy scars. The recommended dose is 20–60 mg three times a day of an extract standardized to contain 40% asiaticoside, to be taken for two to three weeks. The aloe vera plant has long been used to treat skin conditions. Remove an outer leaf from a plant, slice it lengthways, and then apply the clear, thick gel inside the leaf to the skin two to three times daily. You can also purchase aloe vera gel from good health food stores. Calendula is also helpful for treating minor wounds and rashes, and contains antimicrobial properties. Apply a calendula salve, found in health food stores, to the injured area two to three times daily.

Homeopathy

The following remedies can encourage a minor wound to heal promptly and efficiently.

Arnica: This should be the first remedy you reach for after a minor accident or trauma, and is useful when cuts and bruises have occurred together. Although it can be taken appropriately as an internal remedy, never apply Arnica cream to an open wound; in this case use Calendula cream instead.

Hypericum: This remedy can be used after Arnica if a cut has occurred on an area of the body that is especially rich in nerve supply, such as the fingers or toes. Symptoms include intermittent pains that shoot through the injured area, which tends to be hypersensitive and very tender.

Staphysagria: This remedy is specifically used to heal incised wounds. An episiotomy (cutting tissue to enlarge the vagina) as a result of childbirth is an excellent example of the kind of wound that calls for Staphysagria. It is appropriate for wounds that involve sharp stinging pains, and that are sensitive to touch. It can also be used to ease residual pain once stitched areas have healed.

Herbalism

Tea tree oil: This is perhaps the best and most effective herbal therapy for treating cuts owing to the oil's antibacterial and antifungal properties. Apply a thin layer of tea tree ointment or salve that contains 5–10% tea tree oil to the cut for the first day or two. Tea tree can be strong, especially on open skin, and after one or two days the body is generally able to fight off any lingering bacteria on it own. Dermatitis is the only significant side effect associated with the prolonged and repeated topical use of tea tree oil.

Calendula: This herb is valued for its anti-inflammatory and wound-healing properties, which are due to the flavonoids, carotenes, carotenoid pigments, and volatile oils contained in the plant. Steep the flowers in hot water, let them cool slightly, and then soak a clean cloth or piece of gauze in the liquid and apply it to the affected area as a compress. A poultice can also be made, which involves applying warm or hot (but not hot enough to burn the skin) masses of plant material to the affected area. 90% alcohol tincture can also be obtained from a herbalist. High alcohol content tinctures extract healing resins from calendula much more effectively than water extracts.

Comfrey: This herb contains the constituent allantoin, the same active compound secreted by maggots to dissolve wound secretions and promote healing. Comfrey should not be used on fresh, deeply cut, or broken skin. Once some healing has taken place, and the wound isn't fresh and open, comfrey may be used. To use comfrey, prepare a decoction of the freshly peeled root and leaves and apply it as a compress. Add 2 oz of fresh, peeled root to 4 cups of water and boil for five to seven minutes. Add 2–4 oz of fresh leaves and let them steep for 5–10 minutes. When the decoction has cooled to a warm temperature, strain the decoction and soak a clean cloth or piece of gauze in the liquid. Hold the cloth against the cut for 10–15 minutes. The compress can also be covered in gauze and wrapped with a bandage to hold it in place.

Burns

Diagnosis

When the skin becomes burned, nerve endings are damaged causing intense pain. Burns are classified according to their degree of severity. First degree burns involve damage to the top layer of skin and present as reddening and soreness but no blistering. They are painful, but not serious. Second degree burns damage two layers of skin, and are very red, raw, and blistered. They are considered minor if they involve less than 15% of the body's surface in adults, and less than 10% in children. Third degree burns are extremely serious, and involve damage to all the layers of skin and sometimes blood vessels and nerves as well. These kinds of burns cause the skin to look charred and blackened. Third degree burns should be treated by emergency medical services.

Symptoms

First degree burns
- Painful burning sensation on the skin
- Skin is hot and sensitive to touch
- Skin is red and raw

Second degree burns
- Skin is red, raw, and blistered
- Skin appears moist
- Clothing may be stuck to the skin

Third degree burns
- Skin is blackened
- Difficulty breathing
- Result in severe scarring

Treatment Goal

Treatment involves relieving the pain and soreness caused by the burn and promoting healing with as little scarring as possible. If the burn appears to be anything more than superficial, seek medical help immediately.

Conventional Medicine

First degree burns usually heal within a week or two, and anything more severe should be evaluated by a doctor. Patients who have serious burns should be taken to the hospital where specialized treatment can be administered to resuscitate, block pain, prevent infection, and deliver oxygen when necessary.

Cool the skin immediately: The skin should be cooled to reduce its temperature and thereby stop any further burning of the skin. Run cool water over the area for 20 minutes. Do not put an ice cube directly on the burn, as this may cause further skin damage.

Topical treatment: Bacitracin ointment, a topical antibiotic, is commonly used to treat superficial wounds. Burns are usually covered with petrolatum gauze. Some doctors use collagenase, an enzyme that promotes the production of collagen, to treat second or third degree burns, which take months to heal.

Debridement and skin grafting: A doctor will remove dead tissue to prevent an infection from occurring. Skin grafting may also be necessary to help cover the wound.

Treating chemical and electrical burns: Chemical burns may be treated differently from case to case, depending on the substance that has caused the burn. Consult a doctor for advice. Electrical burns are of particular concern because they can sometimes involve electrocution, affecting cardiac and other essential body functions. After removing the source of the electricity, make sure that the breathing and heart rate of the patient are not compromised. If this is the case, begin cardio-pulmonary resuscitation (CPR) and call for an ambulance.

Tip: MINIMIZE THE RISK OF AN ACCIDENT

Most minor burns and scalds happen inside the home, so take steps to prevent this kind of accident from occurring. Check the temperature of any radiators and bath water, especially if there are young children in the house. Also ensure that kettles, saucepans, and mugs of hot drinks are kept well out of the reach of children.

Traditional Chinese Medicine

Herbs: Mix 5 g of Jin Yin Hua (honeysuckle flower), and 3 g of Bo He (field mint) in a teapot. Add boiling water and let the herbs steep for a few minutes. Sip the tea throughout the day for five to seven days. You can also apply Chinese medicine oil, such as Wan Hua oil, to the area.

Diet: Generally, light, fresh food that dispels dampness and heat is recommended. These foods include mung beans, watermelon, lotus root, purslane, wax gourds, red beans, bananas, and grapefruit. Avoid foods that promote heat and dampness such as pepper, dried garlic, cloves, dried ginger, leeks, green peppers, liver, mustard greens, mutton, and green onions, as these may make the burn worse.

Tip: APPLY GINGER

Crush fresh ginger, squeeze out the juice, and apply it to the burn with a cottonwool ball to reduce pain and help reduce swelling and blistering.

Naturopathy

Diet: Drink plenty of fluids and electrolyte drinks to avoid dehydration. Brightly colored foods, such as berries, citrus fruits, papaya, carrots, and squash contain high amounts of bioflavonoids, which strengthen the immune system and assist in healing. Most of these foods also contain high levels of vitamin C, which contributes to tissue healing. Essential fatty acids found in fresh salmon, walnuts, and flaxseeds are also important for tissue repair.

Supplements: Vitamin E helps tissue to heal and is an excellent antioxidant. Take 400 IU of mixed tocopherol vitamin E a day, or apply a vitamin E oil or cream to the affected area. These substances can be purchased in most health food stores. Take 1,000 mg of vitamin C, to promote skin healing. L-glutamine is helpful in preventing infections from burns and also assists in tissue healing. Take 500 mg three times a day. Zinc is essential for skin healing and increasing immune function. Take 30 mg of zinc a day. Zinc can deplete the body's stores of copper, so 3 mg of copper should be taken with this supplement.

Essential oils: Lavender oil is one of the only essential oils that can be applied directly to the skin without dilution. Lavender oil will take the sting out of the burn, and heal it quickly. Its calming aromatherapy properties will also help to ease the emotional upset of a painful burn. Apply 3–5 drops of oil to the affected area and spread it with a gauze pad.

Tip: TAKE AN APPLE CIDER VINEGAR BATH

Apple cider vinegar baths are effective for large burn areas. Use a brand that has been wood-aged, bought from a health food store, rather than one from the supermarket that may have been chemically aged. It helps to restore the skin's acid/alkaline balance. Add 2 cups of apple cider vinegar to a bathtub of cool or warm water. Soak in the water for 15 minutes. The skin will be calmed and soothed, and much of the pain will be immediately relieved.

Homeopathy

The following remedies can be helpful in stimulating a prompt recovery from a minor domestic burn that covers a surface area of less than 1 inch in diameter. A burn that is more severe than this requires professional medical attention.

Tip: USE HONEY TO EASE PAIN

Uncooked, raw, natural honey (found in health food stores) eases the pain of a mild burn. Its antimicrobial and hydrating properties work to keep the area free of infection and well-moisturized. Gently apply a thick coat of honey to the burn and cover it with gauze to keep the honey from getting on to clothing. Apply honey twice a day until the area is no longer sensitive.

Arnica: This is a useful all-purpose homeopathic remedy for calming the shock of even a minor accident. Patients tend to deny needing any help, and just want to get on with things with a minimum of fuss.

Cantharis: If there is a severe burning sensation around the affected area and blisters form rapidly, use Cantharis. Because of the high degree of inflammation and smarting, being touched causes great distress, while bathing the burn in cool water provides temporary relief.

Urtica urens: To treat minor burns that sting and are accompanied by slight signs of blistering, use Urtica urens. Unlike minor burns that respond well to Cantharis, those that respond well to this remedy feel more sensitive and uncomfortable when bathed in cool water.

Herbalism

Aloe vera: Most people will tell you that nothing soothes a burn better than cooling aloe vera. The clear gel-like substance that oozes from freshly cut leaves of aloe has been used for many years to treat a wide array of skin conditions. To treat a burn, apply the gel from a fresh cut aloe leaf directly to the affected area. If fresh leaves are not available a variety of gels and lotions containing aloe vera can be purchased at a health food store or pharmacy. Some aloe vera gels contain alcohol as a base to contribute to its cooling effect. Be aware that alcohol will sting on any open skin, so avoid any alcohol-based gels if a burn is accompanied by a break in the skin.

Calendula: Also known as marigold, holly gold, and Mary bud, calendula can be applied topically to a burn in the form of an ointment three to four times daily. Use an ointment with a 2–5% concentration of calendula if possible, which should be readily available at your local health food store. Alternatively, a dilute tincture or a decoction may be used. A 90% alcohol tincture is particularly useful for healing as this effectively extracts the resin content from the herb. Calendula has very few contraindications and causes few adverse reactions when used topically. There is a small potential for an allergic reaction on the skin; should this occur, discontinue using calendula immediately.

Slippery elm: The bark of elm produces a slippery, mucus-like substance with medicinal properties. Mix 1 tsp of the powdered root with about ¼ cup of boiling water to make a paste. Allow the paste to cool and spread it directly on the burn. Leave the paste on for 5–10 minutes, and repeat two to three times a day. Adverse reactions to slippery elm when applied topically are rare, but if the burned area worsens, or you notice new symptoms, discontinue use and consult a medical herbalist.

Things to Discuss With Your Practitioner

If you have existing allergies you must discuss these with your practitioner so that they may safely prescribe a treatment. If you have any medical conditions or are taking any type of medicine, it is imperative that you inform your practitioner, who will be able to advise you on safe use of complementary treatments.

Sunstroke

Diagnosis

Sunstroke is a very serious condition and in some cases can even be life-threatening. It often occurs when someone is in a hot climate that has higher temperatures than those they are used to. It can be exacerbated by dehydration and exertion. The first signs are often dizziness, fatigue, a headache, rapid pulse, rapid breathing, and muscle cramps. The condition becomes serious if the skin is flushed and the person is no longer sweating, has a high body temperature, is confused, or loses consciousness. When the body temperature rises even a couple of degrees it can have a significant effect on the way the metabolism works, and an extreme rise can cause many of the body's vital systems, including the heart, lungs, kidney, and brain, to fail.

Symptoms

- Throbbing headache
- Feeling dizzy and sick
- Thinking you are going to pass out
- Feeling very ill and unwell
- Feeling incredibly hot
- Flushed face and red skin
- Falling unconscious
- Sense of fatigue and the need to lie down
- The next day you may feel like you have a bad hangover with a headache and nausea

Treatment Goal

Treatment involves relieving symptoms by cooling the patient down and restoring fluids to the body.

Conventional Medicine

To treat heat exhaustion: Heat exhaustion occurs when a person is overheated, but does not have a fever and remains mentally alert and conscious. Place the patient in a cool, shaded area, and feed them ½ liter of fluid an hour to rehydrate. If possible, add ½ tsp of salt to each liter of water to prevent any complications developing as a result of low sodium in the body.

To treat sunstroke: Sunstroke occurs when a person is overheated and has a fever, and their mental status and possibly their vital signs are compromised. The patient should be transported to a hospital where intravenous resuscitation and support is available. Remove the patient's clothes and place them in a cool, well-ventilated room. Their body temperature should be monitored carefully, with the goal being to lower it to 102°F or less over a 30–60 minute period. Spray the patient with cool mist, and if possible place fans around the body. The use of ice packs is controversial as they may constrict the blood vessels and cause shivering, thus driving the temperature back up. Sometimes treatment for low blood pressure and seizures is required, as these conditions may accompany severe heat stroke. Acidosis, a life-threatening condition that results from a lack of insulin in the system, is another complication, which needs to be addressed in the hospital. Most people recover from sunstroke completely in 48 hours.

Traditional Chinese Medicine

Herbs: Mix 5 g of Jin Yin Hua (honeysuckle flower), and 3 g of Bo He (field mint) in a teapot. Add boiling water and let the herbs steep for a few minutes. Drink throughout the day when in a hot climate as a preventive measure.

Tip: DRESS APPROPRIATELY

Wear light, loose clothing, such as cotton, so sweat can evaporate. Better yet, wear clothing suited to exercise in hot weather, which wicks away moisture from the body to keep temperatures low.

Acupressure: Press the Feng Chi and Hegu points with the tip of your finger or thumb for one minute, and repeat twice a day. The Hegu point is located on the back of the hand between the thumb and first finger. The Feng Chi points are at the back of the head at the base of the skull, about 2 inches on either side of the center point.

Diet: Drink plenty of water every day and eat fresh fruit and vegetables, including bitter melon, watermelon, mung beans, tofu, radishes, and celery. Avoid food that has heat and warming properties, such as hot chili peppers, beef, and lamb. Avoid deep-fried food, and eat less fatty and greasy foods since they also create more heat in the body, which can make symptoms worse.

Naturopathy

The best naturopathic treatment for sunstroke is prevention. There are various methods of keeping cool in the heat, but if you do start to feel overheated by the sun, move to a cool place indoors or into the shade and loosen your clothing.

Diet: Eat a plain, light diet that primarily consists of fruit and vegetables. Celery, cucumber, watermelon, and oranges are particularly useful due to their high water content. Add salt to your food freely to keep electrolytes in check, unless you suffer from kidney disease or hypertension. Electrolytes are any of various ions, such as sodium, potassium or chloride, required by cells to regulate the electric charge and flow of water molecules across the cell membrane. Drink plenty of water and make sure that your body stays hydrated. Drinking lots of fluids in the heat is vital. Replacing any water, salt, and potassium lost by the body due to sun exposure will help prevent sunstroke from occurring. Eliminate caffeine, hot drinks, and alcohol from your diet, as they keep you hot and contribute to dehydration.

Prevention: Wear a hat that provides shade and allows ventilation. Also wear loose, light clothing, such as cotton, that allows sweat to evaporate.

Homeopathy

Severe sunstroke requires prompt medical attention as potentially serious problems can arise. Even the mildest cases will need to be monitored closely. This becomes an even greater priority in cases that affect the very young or the elderly. However, one of the following homeopathic remedies can be used alongside any conventional medical support to help encourage recovery.

Belladonna: Consider using this remedy to treat sunstroke symptoms that develop swiftly and dramatically. Symptoms include bright red, hot, dry skin, and throbbing pains. Headaches are also common, and pulsating pains radiating from the head down the body. Sufferers become irritable when feeling unwell.

Veratrum album: If symptoms of sunstroke include localized burning sensations, as well as an associated feeling of being icy cold, use Veratrum album. Nausea is likely to accompany a headache, and patients generally feel faint and chilled.

Herbalism

Sunstroke is a medical emergency and must be treated by a medical professional in an emergency setting. Do not delay medical treatment by instituting home remedies, although you should try to cool down the patient and administer liquids.

General advice: Once the very first signs of sunstroke appear, go indoors as fast as possible and begin self-help measures. Replacing fluids must be a priority. Also loosen any restrictive clothing around the neck and waist in order to help the body cool down and become more comfortable.

Sunburn

Diagnosis

The painful inflammation, redness, and blistering of the skin caused by overexposure to the sun is known as sunburn. In severe cases, blood vessels as well as skin cells can become damaged. Repeated sunburns increase the risk of developing skin cancer, and can also cause signs of premature aging. Burns result from the ultraviolet (UV) radiation produced by the sun. UVA and UVB are different wavelengths in the light spectrum. UVB is more damaging to the skin and is linked to skin cancer, while both UVA and UVB are responsible for premature aging and sunburn. Tanning beds also produce UVA and UVB rays and improper tanning bed use can cause sunburn. Always use a sunscreen with a high protection factor when you are outside for extensive periods, and be sensible when it comes to how long you expose your skin to the sun.

Symptoms

- Areas of bright red skin
- Skin may radiate heat and feel hot to the touch
- Burning skin that is painful to touch
- Blistering and peeling skin
- In severe cases, faintness, nausea, and vomiting

Treatment Goal

The best treatment is prevention by protecting your skin from the sun and UV exposure. If a sunburn does occur, treatment aims to relieve pain and discomfort, and prevent blistering and peeling as much as possible.

Conventional Medicine

Prevention: Sunburn is best avoided. Apply a waterproof sunscreen with SPF30 and UVA blockage to your skin at least 20 minutes before going out in the sun. A plant called Plypodium leucotomos, found in a product called Heliocare®, has been used for many years to prevent sunburn and associated skin damage. Heliocare® can be taken orally and used in conjunction with sunscreen.

Pain relief: Once a sunburn has occurred, treatment involves relieving pain and inflammation, and caring for the skin. Aspirin or non-steroidal anti-inflammatory drugs (NSAIDs) can be used to manage the pain, and cool topical soaks can also provide relief when applied during the first 24 hours. Lotions that aid skin repair and soothe the burn include Sarna® (which contains menthol and camphor), pramoxine lotion, and Aveeno® anti-itch, which is a combination of pramoxine, calamine, and camphor. If a lotion is refrigerated before being applied it is more soothing.

To treat blisters: If blisters develop, medical treatment should be sought to evaluate the extent of the burn. Blisters should not be popped, as they are a method the body uses to protect itself.

Traditional Chinese Medicine

Herbs:
• Ru Yi Gao: This external herbal medicine is a paste that can be applied gently to the skin twice a day to relieve sunburn.
• Jin Yin Hua tea: Combine 5 g of Jin Yin Hua (honeysuckle flower) with 3 g of Bo He (field mint) in a teapot. Add boiling water and let the herbs steep for a few minutes. This tea can be sipped throughout the day for 10–30 days to assist the healing process. It can also help to prevent infection from occurring. Jin Yin Hua tea can be used in combination with Ru Yi Gao.

Diet: Drink plenty of water and eat fresh fruit and vegetables, such as watermelon, bitter melon, mung beans, tofu, radishes, and celery. Avoid food that has heat and warming properties, such as hot chili peppers, beef, and lamb. Avoid deep-fried food, and eat less fatty and greasy foods, as they also create more heat in the body.

Naturopathy

Diet: Eat a plain, light diet that primarily consists of vegetables and fruits. Celery, cucumber, watermelon, and oranges are particularly beneficial because their high water content will keep you hydrated. Drinking lots of fluids before, during, and after exposure to heat is vital. Sip on water or sports energy drinks every 15 minutes, as hydration will speed up the healing process and keep the body cool while you are in the sun. Do not drink alcohol, hot drinks, or beverages with caffeine while in the sun; they increase the rate of dehydration.

> *Tip:* USE SUNSCREEN
>
> Use sunscreen to prevent sunburn. Natural brands are available in most health food stores.

Supplements: Vitamin A nourishes the skin and destroys free radicals, which can harm cells in the body. Take 50,000 IU thoughout the day, but do not take more than 10,000 IU a day if you are pregnant. Vitamin E aids in tissue repair and helps heal scar tissue. Take 400 IU a day. Also take 4,000 mg of vitamin C throughout the day to help with tissue repair of the skin.

Herbs: Calendula cream has been used for many years to soothe sunburns. Apply a small amount of a cream containing calendula two to three times a day. Using oatmeal can also heal and cool the skin. Use a soap made from oatmeal, available from most health food stores, or wrap oatmeal in one or two cheese cloths, tie them with string, and add them to your bath water.

Homeopathy

Any of the following remedies can be helpful in supporting the body in recovering from mild to moderate sunburn. Severe sunburn may need conventional medical therapy, but you can also seek advice from a homeopathic practitioner.

Belladonna: If symptoms of sunburn, including bright red, throbbing, hot skin, develop rapidly, use Belladonna. Additional symptoms include a pounding headache, and feeling irritable. Being exposed to chilled air, and an inability to perspire make discomfort worse, while resting while slightly propped up under light covers feels soothing.

Carbo veg: If sunburn is combined with a feeling of exhaustion that nears the point of collapse, consider using Carbo veg. The body tends to feel cold, while the head feels hot. There may also be low-grade dehydration, which tends to make symptoms worse. Contact with cool air or being fanned feels soothing.

> **Tip:** USE URTICA URENS CREAM
>
> Applying Urtica urens cream to the affected area can do a great deal to ease the heat, discomfort, and general inflammation of a mild bout of sunburn.

Glonoin: When this remedy is helpful the affected areas of skin look and feel flushed and itchy, and symptoms set in rapidly after overexposure to the sun. Classic symptoms include a throbbing headache that is temporarily soothed by contact with cool, fresh air, and made more uncomfortable by using an ice pack.

Herbalism

Aloe vera: Most people will tell you that nothing soothes a burn better than cool aloe vera gel. The clear gel-like substance that oozes from the fresh-cut leaves of aloe has been used for years to treat a wide array of skin conditions such as burns, bites, stings, and generally dry, scaly skin. To treat burns, simply take the gel from a fresh-cut leaf and apply it directly to the affected area. If fresh leaves are not available, a variety of gels and lotions containing aloe vera can be purchased at a health food store, pharmacy, or stores that specialize in herbal medicines. Some aloe vera gels contain alcohol as a base to contribute to its cooling effect. Be aware that alcohol will sting on any open skin, so avoid any alcohol-based gels if your burn is accompanied by breaks in the skin.

St. John's wort: Ironically, the herb that can potentially cause photosensitivity when taken and exposed to too much sunlight, is wonderful for topical use on sunburnt skin. It is most often used as an infused oil, which is moisturising and nourishing to the skin, but also helps to soothe heat and inflammation in the skin. Lavender essential oil can be added to the St. John's wort-infused oil for an added soothing effect.

Hangover

Diagnosis

A hangover is a condition that develops after a period of heavy drinking, and the symptoms, which include headaches, fatigue, and nausea, are largely due to the by-products that alcohol leaves in your system. It can take the body up to 24 hours to break down the toxins and recover. The most serious consequence of heavy drinking is dehydration, which causes throbbing headaches. Waking up with a thick head and a raging thirst is your body's way of telling you that it lacks sufficient fluids to perform normally. Alcohol causes your blood sugar levels to drop, which can contribute to the general feeling of malaise. Alcohol also acts as an irritant to the lining of the stomach, which is why drinking can cause nausea or even ulcers if you drink heavily on a regular basis.

Symptoms

- Dehydration
- Fatigue
- Headache
- Sensitivity to light and sound
- Trembling
- Red eyes
- Muscle aches
- Vomiting
- Disturbed sleep
- Extreme thirst
- Dizziness
- Depression, anxiety, and irritability

Treatment Goal

The primary goal is to rehydrate the body, which will ease many of the symptoms.

Conventional Medicine

Prevention: Factors such as the type of alcohol drunk, genetics, nutritional status, and hydration seem to affect the intensity of a hangover. Drinking to the extent of feeling drunk, however, usually means a hangover is likely to occur. There are several steps you can take to prevent this, or lessen alcohol's side effects. Avoid drinking on an empty stomach or when overly tired, and avoid intense physical activity while drinking. Taking vitamin B6 prior to drinking also seems to lessen the effects of a hangover. Brown or red alcohol seems to incur worse hangovers than white/clear alcohol, as many dark, fermented alcohols have toxic by-products including methanol, aldehydes, and heavy metals. Drink plenty of water when drinking alcohol, and afterwards, to decrease the intensity of the hangover by hydrating the body.

Diet: If you are experiencing a hangover, avoid eating grapefruits (and drinking their juices) as they have properties that decrease the liver's ability to clear the by-products of alcohol. Fatty meals should also be avoided. Avoid saunas as they can dehydrate you further and cause you to become overheated. Exercise is encouraged as long as you stay adequately hydrated.

Herbs: Some herbal products may help clear the hangover by enhancing the liver's ability to remove toxins. Liver detoxifiers sold in herb shops (Liv 52 is one example) may help if taken on a regular basis. Glutathione and milk thistle may also be helpful.

Medications: A drug called tolfenamic acid may help to relieve the symptoms of a hangover, and is safer to use than acetaminophen and ibuprofen. These pain relievers can usually be taken safely, however, unless extremely large amounts of alcohol have been consumed.

Traditional Chinese Medicine

Herbs: Mix 5 g of Ye Ju Hua (wild chrysanthemum flower) and 3 g of Shen Gan Cao (raw licorice) in a teapot. Add boiling water and let the herbs steep for a few minutes. Drink the tea three to four times a day.

Acupressure: Use the tip of your thumb to press the Hegu, Tai Yang, and Feng Chi points with strong pressure for one to two minutes. The Hegu point is located on the back of the hand in the depression between the thumb and the first finger. The Tai Yang point is found at the temple in the depression between the lateral end of the eyebrow and the eyelid. The Feng Chi points are at the back of the head at the base of the skull, about 2 inches on either side of the center point.

Diet: In general, cranberries, blueberries, pears, and bananas are recommended, along with mung beans, red beans, bamboo shoots, and purslane. Avoid foods that are rich and fatty as these increase heat in the body, worsening symptoms.

Naturopathy

Diet: Always eat a big meal before drinking alcohol. Foods that are high in protein and fat will slow the absorption rate of alcohol into your bloodstream. Alcohol flushes fluids out of the body, leading to dehydration and magnifying other hangover symptoms such as headaches and tiredness. Drink water before, during, and after a night of drinking to counter alcohol's diuretic effects. Drinking Gatorade® is another effective method of replacing lost electrolytes and hydrating the body. Avoid drinking coffee as it is a diuretic and may lead to further dehydration. Bananas are an excellent source of potassium, a mineral that is lost when drinking alcohol. Magnesium, which helps control blood sugar levels, is reduced by alcohol. Bananas can help replace magnesium as well as vitamin C, which will make you feel better. Eat one banana before drinking alcohol and another afterwards. Also eat a slice of bread or some crackers spread with honey, or any other food that is high in fructose, after a heavy drinking session. The fructose (a natural sugar) helps the body burn off alcohol faster. Other good sources of fructose are apples, cherries, and grapes. You can also try eating an

umeboshi plum—these have long been reputed to cure hangovers. They are available at Asian markets and health food stores.

Supplements: B-complex vitamins may be helpful in restoring energy after a night of heavy drinking. Take a high potency B-100 before drinking, before bedtime, and again the next day if you are hungover. Vitamin C helps relieve hangover symptoms and boosts the immune system. Take 1,000 mg before drinking, and 1,000 mg after. N-acetyl-cysteine (NAC) helps your liver detoxify by making glutathione. Take 1,500 mg before drinking and 1,500 mg when you wake up the next day.

Herbs: Ginger can help settle an upset stomach and ease feelings of nausea. In fact, some studies have shown that ginger may be up to three times more effective for treating nausea than common over-the-counter medications. Take 1–4 g daily in pill form or drink ginger tea until the hungover feeling dissipates.

Homeopathy

Appropriate holistic measures can shorten the duration and severity of a hangover. If hangovers are becoming a regular feature of life, attention needs to be paid to lifestyle issues that may benefit from professional advice and support.

Coffea: Symptoms that respond well to this remedy include nervy exhaustion and a crushing headache. Hangover symptoms are made more severe by drinking a strong cup of coffee, while warmth and rest feel helpful and restorative.

Nux vomica: This is a classic cure if symptoms have developed as a result of overindulging in alcohol, food, and cigarettes. Sufferers are irritable and have an emotional short fuse due to lack of sleep, constipation, and a queasy headache that lodges at the back of the head. Vomiting may also be a symptom, but it tends to be unproductive and does not bring relief.

Bryonia: If a hangover is a result of dehydration, use Bryonia. Headaches are likely to be severe and are generally located in the front of the head. The scalp may also feel very sensitive. Symptoms intensify with the slightest movement. Rest and keeping still brings relief, as do long drinks of water.

Tip: REST AND REHYDRATE

These should be the priorities if you are suffering from a hangover. Replacing fluid is a necessity due to the dehydrating effect of alcohol, but do not force yourself to eat if you feel queasy. If you do feel hungry, opt for light items that are easy to digest, such as soups, salads, fruit smoothies, and natural, bio-yogurt. Avoid fatty foods that will put extra strain on the liver, which will already be under considerable stress.

Tip: ADD GRAPEFRUIT ESSENTIAL OIL TO A BATH

Grapefruit has a reputation for encouraging the body to detoxify. If you are hungover, add a few drops of grapefruit essential oil to warm bathwater, or invest in a good-quality commercially produced bath or shower gel that includes this essential oil.

Herbalism

Dehydration is perhaps the salient cause of a hangover. Although there is no specific herbal therapy that has been proven to cure a hangover, there are many theories regarding which herbs are most effective. Fresh, clean water is perhaps the most important aid. A hangover is often associated with nausea and headaches, and these symptoms may be alleviated with the herbal therapies recommended below.

Turmeric: This herb contains compounds called curcuminoids that may be effective in easing a headache associated with a hangover. Try drinking a few drops of turmeric tincture diluted in a glass of water. You can also steep a small amount of fresh turmeric rhizome (1–3 g) in boiling water for 10–20 minutes. Allow to cool and drink two to three times a day.

Mints: Peppermint and spearmint are common herbs used to treat nausea and other gastrointestinal disturbances. Many of the medicinal properties from plants in the mint family come from a class of compounds called essential, or volatile, oils, such as menthol, carvone, and limonene. Steep a handful (1–3 g) of mint leaves in a pot of boiling water, let the liquid cool, and drink two to three times a day while you have symptoms. It should be noted that the volatile oils disappear quickly when heated, so your mint tea may be more effective if you cover it while the herbs are steeping. It is also possible to buy a small bottle of the essential oil of peppermint that is specifically for internal use. One drop of the oil taken under the tongue may be enough to calm your digestive tract and stop the nausea. Do not take any essential oil internally for long periods of time or in high doses because it can have adverse effects on the liver.

Ginger: Commonly used for nausea, an infusion of ginger may be useful for those with digestive upset accompanying a hangover. The most research has been carried out on the gingerols and shagoals, and these act directly on the digestive tract; relieving nausea and having an antiemetic effect. The shogaols are potent and present in higher amounts in the dried form of ginger. Heating can also increase shogaol content. One inch of the fresh root may be chopped and added to a cup of boiling water. If no fresh ginger is available, the powder may be used by adding enough to cover the tip of a teaspoon to 500 ml of water, and sipping as required, shaking before use. Capsules are also available from health food shops, or herb suppliers.

Milk thistle: This herb has a long history of use for liver disorders. Some people take capsules of milk thistle prior to an expected heavy night of drinking, or afterward to prevent the untoward effects of alcohol. Milk thistle seems to work best when taken as an extract standardized to 70% silymarin, at a total dose of 200–420 mg per day.

Chickenpox

Diagnosis

Chickenpox is a highly infectious viral disease, which usually develops in children under the age of 10. It manifests as a rash of small red spots that appear on the scalp and face, or sometimes the torso, and then spread to the rest of the body. The spots develop into itchy blisters, and may scar if scratched. Yellow scabs form after a few days, which eventually drop off.

Chickenpox can only be caught by coming into direct contact with someone who has it. It takes between 10 and 21 days for the illness to incubate, and the patient is most infectious before the rash even appears and until the blisters have all scabbed over. Once you have had the disease you are generally immune for life.

DANGER: If the patient still feels unwell once the scabs have healed, complains of headaches, or feels drowsy, call a doctor immediately. Rarely chickenpox can lead to encephalitis (inflammation of the brain).

Symptoms

- Feeling under the weather or cranky
- Headache, sore throat, and general malaise
- Raised temperature and mild fever
- Loss of appetite
- Swollen lymph glands
- Rash of small red spots on the scalp and face, which spreads to the rest of the body

Treatment Goal

To relieve symptoms of itchiness, and prevent scratching and scarring.

Conventional Medicine

Treatment for chicken pox is generally to relieve symptoms until the virus has run its course. One important exception is that any newborn whose mother develops chickenpox up to five days before delivery to two days after delivery should receive an anti-chickenpox immunoglobulin.

Reduce fever: Acetaminophen (Tylenol®) can be administered to bring down a fever. Aspirin should not be used by those under 16, as it has been linked to the development of Reye's syndrome, a lethal disease that affects the liver and other body organs.

Relieve itchiness: Benadryl®, Periactin®, or hydroxyzine can be used to relieve itchiness Taking soothing baths to which baking soda or an emollient such as Aveeno® have been added is also helpful. Topical calamine, chamomile, or calendula lotion is also soothing.

Antivirals: The antiviral acyclovir may be used to lesson symptoms in adolescents and adults. It is also recommended for all immuno-compromised people (those whose immune systems are not working well), and for those who have been on steroids, who have serious lung infections, or who suffer from chronic skin disorders. Valacyclovir or famyciclovir are also used for this purpose.

Antibiotics: If a secondary skin infection occurs, antibiotics are prescribed. Usually antibiotics that target the bacteria streptococcus are appropriate.

Traditional Chinese Medicine

Herbs: Mix 5 g of Jin Yin Hua (honeysuckle flower), 5 g of Fang Fen (ledebouriella root), and 3 g of Bo He (field mint) in a teapot. Add boiling water and let the herbs steep for a few minutes. Sip the tea throughout the day for 10–30 days.

Acupressure: Press the Tai Yang, Hegu, and Feng Chi points with gentle pressure for about one minute every day. The Tai Yang point is located at the temple, in the depression between the lateral end of the eyebrow and the eyelid. The Hegu point is located on the back of the hand, between the thumb and first finger. Press this point on both hands. The Feng Chi points are at the back of the head at the base of the skull, about 2 inches on either side of the center point.

Diet: Eat light, fresh food, such as turnips, celery, spinach, eggplant, purslane, wax gourds, and mung beans. Gentle foods, such as organic green vegetables, radishes, bitter melon, and pears can strengthen the immune system. Green tea is also beneficial since it has a gentle cleansing effect. Avoid ginger, chilies, mustard greens, and mutton, as they are pungent and irritating and increase heat in the body, which may make the condition worse. Also avoid seafood, and fatty and spicy food.

Naturopathy

The following therapeutic suggestions apply to both adults and children unless otherwise specified.

Diet: Drink raw fruit and vegetable juices. These cool the system and hydrate the skin. Lemon juice is considered to be especially beneficial. Drink lots of water (about two 8 oz glasses of water every hour throughout the day) to prevent dehydration. Avoid all dairy products until the skin lesions have resolved, as dairy is a major allergen and may worsen symptoms. A soup prepared from carrots and coriander has been found to be beneficial in the treatment of chickenpox. Use about 100 g of carrots and 60 g of fresh coriander cut into small pieces and boiled. Eat this soup once a day.

Supplements: The dosages provided in this section are for adults only. The supplements are also available from health food stores for children and the instructions on the label should be followed. Take 400 IU of vitamin E

Tip: USE BAKING SODA

Baking soda is a popular remedy to control the itchiness caused by chickenpox. Add some baking soda to a glass of water and sponge the affected area with the liquid. The soda will dry on the skin to keep the patient from scratching the lesions.

Tip: NEEM LEAF BATH

Soak 2 cups of neem leaves in a tub of warm water for 30 minutes. Add cool water and some ginger and soak in the tub for 30 minutes to relieve itchiness.

a day to promote healing and provide the body with powerful antioxidants. Applying vitamin E oil to the skin is also beneficial in treating chickenpox as it makes the marks left by the virus fade more quickly. Take 25,000 IU of vitamin A twice a day to boost the immune system and also help with skin healing. Pregnant women should not take more than 10,000 IU of vitamin A a day. Vitamin C, which can be taken at 1,000 mg three times a day, also helps to stimulate the immune system and it is important for tissue healing. Bioflavonoids work similarly and synergistically with vitamin C. Take 500–1,000 mg two to three times a day. Also take 15,000 IU of beta-carotene a day to heal tissue and stimulate the immune system.

Herbs: Apply sandalwood oil to the rash until the scabs start to fall off to help reduce scarring. You can also sip on a tea made from mildly sedative herbs, such as chamomile, marigold, and lemon balm, several times a day. This can help to relieve the distress caused by itchiness.

Homeopathy

Any of the following remedies can be helpful in easing itchiness and in shortening the duration of an acute episode.

Aconite: This remedy can be useful during the first, feverish stage of chickenpox. Restlessness and fear may develop quickly at night, and a fever may be accompanied by thirst and dry skin. Use Aconite before the chickenpox rash has actually appeared. Once a rash develops, you will need to change remedy.

Belladonna: This remedy can also be used to ease a fever associated with the early stage of chickenpox that develops rapidly. Symptoms include a high fever with bright red skin that radiates heat and irritability. Once a rash develops, choose another remedy.

Ant tart: If a rash is slow to emerge, and if chickenpox is associated with a persistent cough, use Ant tart. When the rash does develop, spots tend to be large, have a bluish tinge, and leave a red mark behind as they

Tip: USE CALENDULA TINCTURE

The extreme itchiness and irritation caused by chickenpox can be eased by applying a diluted tincture of Calendula to a saturated cottonwool pad and placing it on the affected areas. Dilute one part of tincture to 10 parts of boiled, cooled water. For a prolonged soothing effect, apply Calendula cream following the tincture.

Tip: TAKE SPONGE BATHS

Avoid bathing your child during the feverish stage of this illness, since hot baths make a rash more irritated and itchy. Instead, sponge your child down in a comfortably warm room, making sure they do not get chilled in the process. Once the spots have become crusty and dry, be careful not to knock them off when towel drying.

heal. There is also a thick, unpleasant coating on the tongue. Becoming overheated or bathing worsens symptoms, while contact with cool air and coughing brings a sense of relief.

Rhus tox: To treat spots that are itchy at night, causing restlessness, use Rhus tox. Spots may be moist and blistery at first, then become crusty. Resting and undressing make the rash more irritating, while rubbing and changing position provide temporary relief.

Pulsatilla: To treat the later stage of chickenpox, where the spots are slow to appear, or linger longer than is expected, use Pulsatilla. Symptoms include feeling chilly but disliking hot conditions, and having a dry mouth and white-coated tongue but not feeling thirsty. Children who are normally cheerful may become weepy and clingy when suffering from chickenpox.

Herbalism

The common complaint with chickenpox is, of course, itchiness. Herbal therapies can be very beneficial in relieving this symptom.

Oatmeal: This herb is the first choice for treating itchiness due to chickenpox: it is inexpensive, widely available, and there are virtually no known side effects. Chickenpox commonly affects large areas of the body, so an oatmeal bath is most effective. Add approximately 1 cup of finely ground oatmeal (grind oatmeal in a food processor or coffee grinder) to a warm bath. Soaking will allow the oatmeal to lightly coat the skin and relieve the itchiness and irritation. This method is particularly effective because chickenpox lesions can be extensive and sometimes hard to reach, so topical treatments can be difficult to administer. A few drops of lavender essential oil may be added to bath, to offer a more soothing effect.

Chickweed: This herb has a great antipruritic effect. Often available in herb or health stores in a cream or ointment, this herb may be applied topically when required. Herbalists often use infused oils of this herb. It can also be added to the bath, so that it may be easier to apply to the whole body. Agitate the water before stepping into the bath, to disperse the oil a little, so it may come into contact with more affected areas.

Elderberry: Naturally rich in Vitamin C and flavonoids, elderberry juice can support the immune system in fighting the virus, and specific formulations of juice can be bought at your local health food store. The formulated juice can be taken orally at the onset of symptoms for three to five days. Diarrhea and vomiting have been reported in some following the use of elderberry juice.

Index